'We love the inspirational and hopeful stories that Sabine Vermeire shares in this book! She opens the door to her therapy room to offer illustrations of a variety of creative ways to accompany children and their carers in facing extremely challenging circumstances. It is clear that Sabine draws these stories from years of hard-won experience. She never pathologizes or loses hope, and oftentimes she finds ways to bring humor and play to heartbreaking situations. The ways of working she offers are never simplistic, and they take the wider context of marginalized lives into account. For us, the heart of the book is the attitude she conveys toward the children, parents, and carers she works with. If all therapy could be practiced with her attitude, we are sure that both the lives we touch and our own would be better for it'.

Jill Freedman (MSW) and Gene Combs (MD), *authors of Narrative Therapy: The Social Construction of Preferred Realities*

'This is a beautiful book by an exceptional family therapist who works with children who lived their lives within stories of trauma, violence and neglect. Sabine's therapeutic focus is on ways to find connection and on setting out on journeys of discovery and healing. There always is a group of friends, family and other supporters who root for the child on their long expedition. Sabine wonders with them whether princesses ever go to the bathroom, she wants to learn everything there is to know about dinosaurs, she is concerned about poisonous question marks, and she has no doubt that white rabbits can write beautiful letters. Playfulness definitely can help a family therapist to do a better job!'

Professor Peter Rober, *PhD, clinical psychologist, family therapist and family therapy trainer at Context-Center for marital and family therapy (UPC KU Leuven)*

'This elegant book brings rich ideas from family therapy, narrative practice and playful approaches of working with children. Sabine has brilliantly weaved in her skillful and highly nuanced work with children with such clarity and sparkle. She has brought in multiverses of complexities that children's lives can get sucked into in the face of trauma and adversity. And yet, at the same time, thrown light on how we can position ourselves through playful curiosity to "do hope" and steps we can take to respect children's voices and lived experiences, invite agency and practice solidarity. This delightful book will be my companion for life, and I would highly recommend it to all practitioners who work with children, families and their networks'.

Shelja Sen, *Narrative Therapist, Writer, Co-founder Children First, India*

Unravelling Trauma and Weaving Resilience with Systemic and Narrative Therapy

Unravelling Trauma and Weaving Resilience with Systemic and Narrative Therapy is an innovative book that details how clinicians can engage children, families and their networks in creative and collaborative relationships to elicit change within the context of trauma and violence.

Combining systemic, narrative and dialogical theoretical frameworks with clinical examples, this volume focuses on therapeutic conversations that can help children, and those involved with them, deconstruct their experienced difficulties, and create more hopeful stories and alternative ways of relating to one another through a sense of play. Vermeire advocates for serious playfulness as a way of directly addressing trauma and its effects, as well as along 'trauma-sensitive' side paths. Puppetry, artwork, interviews and theatre play are used to weave networks of resilience in ever-widening circles and this approach is informed by the awareness that individual problems are always to be seen as relational, social and political.

This book is an important read for therapists and social workers who work with traumatised children and their multi-stressed families.

Sabine Vermeire is a systemic and narrative psychotherapist, supervisor and trainer. She works at Interactie-Academie, Antwerp, Belgium.

The Systemic Thinking and Practice Series
Series Editors: Charlotte Burck and Gwyn Daniel

This influential series was co-founded in 1989 by series editors David Campbell and Ros Draper to promote innovative applications of systemic theory to psychotherapy, teaching, supervision and organisational consultation. In 2011, Charlotte Burck and Gwyn Daniel became series editors and aim to present new theoretical developments and pioneering practice, to make links with other theoretical approaches, and to promote the relevance of systemic theory to contemporary social and psychological questions.

Recent titles in the series include:

Emotions and the Therapist: A Systemic-Dialogical Approach
By Paolo Bertrando

Creative Positions in Adult Mental Health: Outside In-Inside Out
Edited by Sue McNab and Karen Partridge

Ethical and Aesthetic Explorations of Systemic Practice: New Critical Reflections
Pietro Barbetta, Maria Esther Cavagnis, Inga-Britt Krause and Umberta Telfener

Working Systemically with Refugee Couples and Families: Exploring Trauma, Resilience and Culture
Shadi Shahnavaz

Psychotherapeutic Competencies: Techniques, Relationships, and Epistemology in Systemic Practice
Laura Fruggeri, Francesca Balestra, and Elena Venturelli

Systemic Perspectives in Mental Health, Social Work and Youth Care
Anke Savenije, Justine van Lawick, and Ellen Reijmers

Unravelling Trauma and Weaving Resilience with Systemic and Narrative Therapy

Playful Collaborations with Children, Families and Networks

Sabine Vermeire

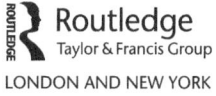
Routledge
Taylor & Francis Group

LONDON AND NEW YORK

Designed cover image: Detail of 'Solution', 2022, mixed media on canvas, 200 X 220 cm, Tatjana Gerhard

First published 2023
by Routledge
4 Park Square, Milton Park, Abingdon, Oxon OX14 4RN

and by Routledge
605 Third Avenue, New York, NY 10158

Routledge is an imprint of the Taylor & Francis Group, an informa business

© 2023 Sabine Vermeire

The right of Sabine Vermeire to be identified as author of this work has been asserted in accordance with sections 77 and 78 of the Copyright, Designs and Patents Act 1988.

Trademark notice: Product or corporate names may be trademarks or registered trademarks, and are used only for identification and explanation without intent to infringe.

British Library Cataloguing-in-Publication Data
A catalogue record for this book is available from the British Library

ISBN: 978-0-367-76639-9 (hbk)
ISBN: 978-0-367-76638-2 (pbk)
ISBN: 978-1-003-16786-0 (ebk)

DOI: 10.4324/9781003167860

Typeset in Times New Roman
by Deanta Global Publishing Services, Chennai, India

Contents

Series editors' foreword

Many of us struggle with how best to work with children who have undergone trauma and experienced violence. Professionals and the organisations within which we work often rely on theories of child development and models of intervention which try to provide certainty. They are often named as evidence-based, but they so easily carry unintended consequences for children and their families who remain captured by notions of 'damaged identities' especially when help is provided without exploring children's and families' own creative resources.

We are therefore thrilled to have this inspiring book in our series. Sabine Vermeire throws open windows, unsettles rigidities and invites us to consider fresh and invigorating ideas. She takes us on her journeys with young people and their families and caretakers through circumstances that can make the heart sink. She is determined not to repeat what others have done before when it has such limited and sometimes even harmful effects. Her ability to spark the interest of silent children who do not wish to be in the room with her or their family members and have little hope that anything could be different, to invite them into a space of curiosity while respecting their world view is as engaging of them as it is of us, the reader. What will be unfolded next? How are these stories going to develop and which important questions will Sabine and these young people and their family members research together? What is love? How have others managed when one of their loved ones 'stepped out of life' (Sabine's poignant and poetic phrase for suicide)? And what playful resources can bring forth hopes, strategies for survival and resilience?

Sabine Vermeire is an experienced, highly respected and talented systemic and narrative therapist from Belgium who draws on her creative therapeutic work of over 20 years with children and families who have experienced trauma. Her clinical work is continually interwoven with clear and accessible theoretical explanations which bring together systemic, narrative and dialogical theoretical frameworks to attend to the micro-processes in therapy as well as the ways that wider contexts inform therapeutic talk and relationships.

She has developed a therapeutic stance from which she is able to skilfully engage reluctant children and families in collaborative relationships, and challenge those professional and societal beliefs which contribute to constraining the possibilities for these children. Instead, she accompanies them in an effective and enriching process of change. Sabine includes many extracts from her videotaped clinical work which bring the children and their relationships and the therapy to life, and from which professionals of any orientation will gain enormously and be able to relate to their own work contexts. Importantly Sabine invites us to develop our own stances and creativity, as she does the families and networks she works with, rather than offering a rule book which has proved so constraining in other approaches.

We predict that this book will become a touchstone for your work with multi-stressed children, their families and their networks. It will perturb your ideas and open up new ways to think and develop your practice. Sabine Vermeire illustrates in vivid and practical detail how we, together with young people and their families, can weave resilience into their relationships and contexts to enable them to go on with their lives following trauma and violence. This book makes a powerful and significant contribution to the systemic, narrative and dialogic field and to all those working with the aftermath of violence and trauma.

We are so proud to be able to include this book in our series.

Charlotte Burck and Gwyn Daniel

Foreword to *Unravelling trauma and weaving resilience with systemic and narrative therapy*

Glenda Fredman

An amuse bouche

This book invites us to walk alongside a talented practitioner, Sabine Vermeire, 'meandering, zigzagging, back and forth' with her as she guides us along the ups and downs, twists and turns of her practice. Along the path, she gives us the opportunity to witness, listen and learn from her art of unravelling frozen, fragmented or chaotic stories that encapsulate trauma and then weaving alternative stories of resilience that restore a sense of coherence, agency and belonging with children, young people,[1] their families, carers and the professionals who serve them.

From the start we meet Sabine as she sets the scene with three stories of her practice. And throughout the book we come to know her through rich stories of her personal and professional life. She draws on her vast experience as a trainer, supervisor and therapist working with children, young people and families in a wide array of contexts including prisons, foster care, residential care and psychiatric units and we get warming glimpses into her family life around her kitchen table.

Sabine does not promise to solve all problems for us, but to help us bring into view 'new more liveable pathways'. She offers us a 'multitude of possible entrances and walking routes, useful "footholds" and guidelines and creative ideas for practitioners to find ways through the "complexity, dilemmas and paradoxes"'.

Underpinning her practice is a rigorous systemic and narrative approach that she uses lightly, as a compass, to guide her in navigating her way through conversations, carrying these in her 'backpack' as tools. She weaves in scholarly works from systemic and narrative theories as well as from attachment, developmental and social theories and offers us refreshing access to new writings outside of the English speaking literature.

As Sabine takes us by the hand, pointing out multiple possible pathways that intersect and intertwine and showing us how we might unravel complex knots of suffering, she draws our attention to some familiar and some overlooked pitfalls. She shares honest accounts of going 'wrong' that we all have met and can relate to, like asking questions that are too intrusive or inviting young people to tell, confess or relive unwanted experiences that can bring forth hesitation and suspicion. She points out the common urge in many of us to act too quickly in our well-intended efforts to make it better, fix problems, explain, clarify or remove shame or blame that risk losing sight of the child's experience and wishes and ignoring what many people involved have to offer. As she shines a light on stories that include little moves like gently saying to a child, 'You don't have to explain what is happening at home … I just want to give it a name …', or asking 'What were your escape routes' (from a named problem)', we gather practices that help us stand back, stay present and invite the young person to unravel how they came to a life-diminishing conclusion, explore if this is a preferred place they want to be and if this feeling or state is helpful to them.

Our attention is drawn to the dangers of repeating known and familiar attitudes and practices blindly. For example, we are alerted to taking care with the words we use as 'our words are not innocent'. A simple word like 'trauma' might seem a quick, easy shortcut for us, but if it does not fit could cause harm or strengthen a sense of failure for the young person or carers. It could even entangle us all in 'highly compelling discourses about victimhood' that risk 'reproducing subtle practices of violence or abuse'. We see how Sabine uses different words to describe adverse experiences, choosing to name in ways the child and those involved prefer, so that together they might 'unravel their multiple meanings'.

Sabine shines a light on the 'web of complexities' we get called into as soon as we start out to work with young people in these situations. She helps us see how 'the polyphony of voices gathers' representing not only individual people but also institutions, society and political and professional discourses. She encourages us to go slow, considering our own position in relation to these voices that come from 'different worlds' (judicial, medical, educational, psychiatric, social care), each representing different interests. I appreciate how her work shows us ways to respect the differences by tuning in to listen and learn how each world constructs and frames and hence find ways to connect with colleagues who 'inhabit' these worlds.

At the heart of Sabine's approach is *centring the child*. From the outset she moves away from positioning the young person as 'in need' to approaching children and young people as 'full agents' who actively take part in shaping their own lives. Therefore, she works creatively, playfully and sensitively to bring the voices of the young people to the foreground so she (and we) can learn from them. She shares a rich assortment of novel ways that she has learned from the children she works with to invite the young person to become an active participant at the centre, for example inviting children into positions of co-researcher, and giving the child a pretend microphone to interview practitioners about issues of importance to them.

These practices offer us antidotes to getting caught in webs of expert problem definitions like diagnoses and labels that might lure us into blindly perpetuating dominant views of 'normal' childhood as white, middle-class and Eurocentric and reifying these descriptions as attributes of the individual child thus overlooking children's actions to resist, or losing sight of important relationships that sustain them. By enabling us to stay connected to the young person's perspective we are also helped to avoid the 'temptation of the unhelpful dances' like veering from deficit to strength and optimism.

As well as enabling children to develop a sense of coherence and agency, Sabine is committed to enhancing a sense of belonging in the young people she works with. As we move through the book we join her as she 'widens circles of important others' who get to know about the worries of the children and thus enhances the relational agency of all involved. She offers us creative ways to link lives beyond the therapy room through showing how she builds support teams of significant people who can contribute to create a 'riverbank' position from which children and all involved can reflect on painful experiences. Always centring the child, she invites them to choose whose voices and knowledges to invite into the room, positioning the child, for example, as reporter, scientific investigator, interviewer or videographer thereby offering a safe place in which to stand and ask questions that occupy their mind.

I love the expansive nature of Sabine's work. Just as we are grasping and looking forward to creating networks of support and solidarity with and for the child and their parents, she goes further, inviting children as directors to include peers, networks and wider communities not only for the child but also for the carers and practitioners since, as she tells us, 'it also takes children to raise a village'. Then she goes even further collecting, collating and curating these new knowledges, initiatives and skills into works of art, plays, books, raps and songs to share with others in similar situations so that the young people begin to experience themselves as able to make valuable contributions to the lives of future generations.

Sabine invites us to her kitchen table to share and witness stories. I felt she was there with me as I joined her on the journey – following in her footsteps, meandering, tripping, stumbling – her catching me before falling, occasionally pausing to take my own diversion to another path, connect with aspects of my own work, stories in my own life and marvelling as new ideas emerged. One practice that captured my attention, is '*suggesting different conversational settings*'. I have selected this practice since, in this book that offers a plethora of creative and elaborate methods and techniques, it might slip past because of its apparent simplicity. I also want to illustrate how these apparently small offerings of Sabine can flourish and bring about huge effects.

Sabine reminds us that 'each conversational setting will create possibilities and limitations to collaborate, speak, explore, transform'. From the stories she shares, I notice that '*conversational setting*' refers not only to the environment (where we meet) but also to the relationships (who joins the conversation) and the atmosphere (how we meet). I have spent the majority of my professional life working within public services where it has been taken for granted that we meet people in 'clinics'. Depending on the service, the rooms may be small or large, with or without windows, furnished for medical procedures or even be used mostly as a storeroom. It has usually been clear that we should be grateful for a room – and often told not to move anything. Depending on the service we are also expected, and often prescribed, to see either individuals, families, couples, together or separately, and rarely are children or parents offered a choice. Therefore, I was drawn to Sabine's reminder that 'each choice (of conversational setting) creates a context in which certain meanings can emerge and others fade into the background' and the 'conversational setting influences the process of meaning making and so the therapeutic process'. These phrases highlight why, as public service practitioners, we respond with sadness and frustration, and sometimes even tears, when we are required to meet people in unsatisfactory spaces or to have prescribed who joins the conversation and who does not.

What Sabine's stories sparked for me was the possibility to have important conversations with young people and their carers about conversational settings. For example, even when there is no choice, that the only room we can meet in is a disused ward now used to store empty water cylinders, we can still talk together about this room to open space for building the best possible conversational setting together by starting with exploring: 'What is like sitting here together?' 'Is it comfortable for our being together?' 'How does this space enable/constrain the sorts of talking, listening, learning we can do?' 'What might we do to make it feel more welcoming?'

I have also taken away a repertoire of ideas and practices for conversations with young people, parents, carers and professionals about who joins our conversational setting. Honouring all involved and taking care to respect their position in relation to the child 'as valued partners and co-researchers' is a useful first step and the phrase 'caring for carers from the start is a means of caring for the child' is a mantra I take with me.

Throughout this book, Sabine illustrates how she respects each practitioner's world and worldview as adding something valuable in these complex situations in the interest of building a sense of relational agency for all involved where everyone experiences themselves as relational agents. The opportunity to witness how she appreciates the possibilities of these different worlds, as well as their limitations, without compromising her values or colluding with injustice, opened space for me to have a useful conversation with a colleague in supervision.

My colleague, who works in a hospital with children facing cancer treatment, was concerned that the paediatricians were insisting that children are present at all meetings to discuss their treatment. My colleague had witnessed these meetings causing distress and confusion to children when doctors had 'used language way above their heads', parents had asked questions that brought forth distressing hypothetical information and children had been terrified by misunderstandings. For example, recently, a seven-year-old boy and his parents were meeting with the paediatric oncologist and the nurse. The nurse and doctor had taken care to prepare the room with toys and art and craft materials and a small table and chair for the child to choose to sit if he preferred. However, very soon into the meeting, after brief introductions, the doctor started to explain the procedure for the forthcoming biopsy and the nurse explained that the little boy would come to hospital the night before and 'we will starve him so he is prepared for anaesthetic the next day'. Parents were grateful for the clear explanations and opportunity to ask any questions. Only my colleague noticed that the boy was sitting frozen with eyes glazed. When she asked if he had any questions, he shook his head and began to cry. That night, at home, still very tearful, he asked his mother 'when will they starve me' – and 'will they put me in a cage like Hansel and Gretel until my arms are chicken bones?' This episode led my colleague to propose to her medical colleagues that, in the future, they initially invite parents separately to explain the medical procedures. The doctors, however, were adamant that it was 'good paediatric practice' to always include the child.

I introduced my colleague to Sabine's concept and practice of 'conversational settings'. Naming 'medicine' and 'cancer services' as 'different worlds', I asked if she had any idea how come the world of paediatric medicine and childhood cancer would view 'always including the child' as good practice? My colleague was aware that there were clear professional guidelines for paediatricians to 'ensure that children and young people are fully informed about their health', 'empowered to take an active role in their health care' and 'have a choice and a voice' and complained that these guidelines are often 'rigidly' enacted by 'always including the child without thinking or careful preparation since consultations are so rushed'. Inviting my colleague to reconnect with 'the very good intention' informing this directive opened space for her to have a conversation with her paediatric oncology team about the opportunities and constraints for children, parents and practitioners of including children in all meetings. This conversation has since generated a request from the team for my colleague to facilitate some 'reflective practice sessions' where they might reflect on and practise what kinds of conversations they might have with whom, how to talk in different conservational settings including the words to use, making medical information accessible to the children at different ages and so on.

In this book Sabine shows us 'how to do with' rather than 'what to do'. She gently leads us from the 'well-trodden pathways of therapy' with a guideline, 'do not repeat what has already been done' (so as not to reproduce practices of injustice), which I have been holding as another sort of mantra since reading the book. I have found it very hard to select from such a rich abundance of creative practices and so have offered tasters of what stood out for me; I encourage you to read the book slowly, savouring, digesting and reflecting, going back and forth between chapters, allowing yourself time to pause and think about the people you work with, the webs you get caught in, the voices calling you.

Note

1 I go on to use the term 'child' or 'young person' interchangeably to refer to both children and young people.

Introduction

Three stories to set the scene

In The Little Prince *by Antoine de Saint-Exupéry (1995, p. 22), the main character, the little prince, with some indignation but also full of wisdom, exclaims: 'When you say "The proof that the little prince really existed was that he was enchanting, that he laughed, and that he wanted a sheep", people will shrug their shoulders and treat you as if you were a child. But if you say to them: "The planet he came from was Asteroid B-612", then they will be convinced and leave you in peace from all their questions'.*

More than 25 years ago

I worked as a systemic psychotherapist-in-training in a home for children placed there by the family court. David, eight years old, was brought in by the police together with his two little sisters. There was a history of domestic violence in the family and his father had tried to attack his mother with a knife while David was watching, hidden under the kitchen table. His father was sent to prison and his mother was admitted to a psychiatric hospital. David didn't speak to anyone. He nodded sometimes when we had a request. When someone got physically closer than one metre, he started to growl and yell. In school he wet his pants several times a day and in the classroom he kept silent. Soon he was bullied and when children got too close he wildly thrashed about. The atmosphere in the children's home grew grimmer and a sense of helplessness overtook everyone.

The team of carers were very worried about David. Nothing seemed to work or make any difference. How could we make contact with him without being too intrusive? How could we invite him into even only a small conversation? How could we respond to his silence, his outbursts, his pants-wetting, etc. in a supportive, helpful way? How could we understand what was going on in order to find ideas and openings for connection and change?

Certainly, there were many more questions than answers that occupied our minds. There was also much more uncertainty than guidance. The team searched very hard for solutions. We were wondering whether sending him to child

DOI: 10.4324/9781003167860-1

psychiatry could be helpful. It was also a time that PTSS (post-traumatic stress syndrome) and all the extensions of this diagnosis like 'complex trauma', 'developmental trauma' or 'early childhood trauma' weren't that common in our vocabulary. Although at that time the notion 'insecurely attached' and the diagnosis 'Reactive Attachment Disorder' were already quite popular to grasp what was happening in front of our eyes, they didn't seem to offer us enough guidelines or support in our struggles with David.

As I often did, I came in the living room of the children's home after schooltime.

David sat in a corner far away from the other kids next to a large box filled with little toy soldiers. One by one he picked them out of the box, brought them before his head and let them fall on the ground while each time making the noise of an explosion 'Kaboom'. In front of him on the ground were already lying more than 50 little toy soldiers. The moment I came near, he stopped and looked up from the corner of his eye. I noticed out loud that it seemed hard working that he was doing. He nodded and went on until all soldiers were out of the box laying on the floor.

The next day around the same time I entered the living room. He was sitting in his corner dropping the toy soldiers one by one, making the sound of exploding bombs. Again I approached him, staying at a reasonable distance and asking if he had still a lot of work to do. He shrugged and when I asked if he could use some help, he shrugged again and went on bombing.

One day later, almost the same scenario but this time I sat next to him and made sure that I carefully respected the distance of one metre. I took a toy soldier out of the box and asked if it was okay to help him. He nodded. While I dropped a soldier and tried to make the noise of an explosion, he silently watched me. I asked if I was doing it right. He nodded and restarted his own bombing. When all the soldiers were dropped on the floor, he put them back in the box and left the room.

This repeated itself for a few days until, at a certain moment, I came into the room and he immediately divided the heap of soldiers in half and pushed a pile towards me. For the first time I got a sense of collaboration and moving into new directions. More and more he gave me instructions how to become a better bomber and when I asked why he had to do this daily work he answered: 'Making sure nobody can be hurt!'

This 'bombing together', engaging in his actions and trying to make sense out of it became a stepping stone for a discovery journey together about 'violence, being hurt, feeling safe ..., family, taking care, etc.' but also for re-connection with what was important and valuable to him and who mattered. We invited the other carers into our investigations as well as his sisters, grandparents and over time also his parents in all kinds of ways. It didn't 'solve' all the problems but new, more liveable, pathways to walk on became visible.

Ten years ago

At that time, as a therapist and supervisor I was involved in a project 'Narrative ways to re-(dis)covery'. We were searching for ways to re-connect with youngsters placed in youth prison, a secured psychiatric unit or living in a youngster's home where their stay was under pressure. As a child, they often experienced trauma, violence or abuse and became violent themselves, they were often struggling with addiction problems, self-harming or sometimes ended up in contexts of sexual exploitation or delinquency, etc. We started to invite these youngsters for a biographical interview in the presence of professionals, family members and important people of their network (as witnesses). During these interviews we hoped to find stepping stones and new entry points for the youngster, the professionals and the network to go on. At the same time we hoped it would open doors so their experiences, responses and stories could be acknowledged and some alternative storylines, new perspectives and meanings would emerge. While travelling through problem stories and alternative stories of their lives we tried to weave threads so that a sense of coherence and connection could emerge and new ideas about the future came to the fore.

Yana lived the first year of her life mainly in squats and on the street with her mother, a Moroccan teenage mum who was struggling with a drug addiction. After that year she was placed by children's court in foster care. Unfortunately there was a lot of tension and partner violence in this family. Over time, the relationship between her and her foster mother also became violent. As the problems and the abuse were escalating at the age of 11 she was placed in an institution. At the time I met her, she was 15. She refused to go to school. She didn't get out of her bed in the morning and wanted to be dead. We organised a biographical interview in the hope of finding some ways to go on. Reluctantly she agreed.

Visibly hesitating she entered the room accompanied by her mentor, her social worker and a school friend. Although asked, she clearly didn't want a family member as witness. After thanking everyone in the room for coming, we shared our hopes and wishes for this gathering. I put the witnesses a little bit aside and asked Yana's permission to record this interview so she could take the stories told with her afterwards. The first ten minutes of the interview she didn't look up, hiding herself behind her long hair and only answering with a quiet little voice 'yes' or 'no' or shrugs shoulders '… Don't know …'.

The interview seemed to be going nowhere. My questions about what brought her here and what occupied her mind did not lead to a conversation, nor did they invite curiosity into the room. On the contrary, they rather seemed to invite 'resistance'. Maybe they felt it too intrusive just evoking more hesitations and suspicion? Before I knew it, we were trapped in an unhelpful dance. Yana appeared more and more as a vulnerable, depressed victim who was almost unable to respond. At that moment I realised that we were getting stuck. I noticed that I asked questions that had been asked probably a hundred times, so there was nothing new to tell. The exclamation my systemic psychotherapeutic trainer used when we, her trainees, became stuck in our conversations was 'Don't repeat what has already been done!' So, out of the blue, I offered Yana a completely different question, hoping to find some safe ground and some support for our conversation.

S: *When you were three or four years old, did you have a cuddly bear?*
  For the first time she raises her head and a smile appears on her face.
S: *Can I ask you a question? How did this cuddly bear look like? ... Or is this a too*
  big confession??? ... Shall I ask the witnesses to close their ears? ...
Y: *No. ... I still have him.*
  And again a smile pops up.
S: *Really?*
Y: *Yes, ... Very embarrassing ...*
S: *Even though ... I'm going to ask 'What kind of cuddly bear do you have?'*
Y: *It's a big bear. His name is Little Orange.*
Y: *Very embarrassing, isn't it?*
S: *I don't know... Because ... If you still have this bear ... Maybe this says some-*
  thing about the importance of this bear.
Y: *Yes, that's true.*
  ...

Yana told how Little Orange sits next to her watching television, he joins her when she is staying with friends. He even went on holidays with her. Throughout her life he became a big support to her.

S: *Do you reach for him when times are difficult?*
Y: *Yes ... Without him I can't sleep.*
S: *It seems that it is also thanks to you that he still walks around in this world?*
Y: *We take good care of each other!*
S: *Apparently you know something about caring? Is he also sometimes your*
  advisor?
Y: *He can't talk isn't it? ... Secretly? On the sly?*
S: *On my opinion, cuddle bears give sometimes good advice ...*
Y: *I don't know ... I never really listened.*
S: *We're going to do a bit crazy ... If he could give you some advice ... How would*
  it sound?
Y: *(thinking deeply) Don't know ... Maybe ... 'Just go on ... Even when it's dif-*
  ficult ...'

Once when we offered a chair to Little Orange to join our conversation, a little bit of lightness came in. We had some safe ground to stand on and Little Orange became an appreciated member of our team of support. We could ask him for forgotten stories, advice, inspiration, etc. when we got stuck in the conversation or locked up in unhelpful dances.

A bit later Yana explained she loved going to elementary school as it was a distraction from home. So I immediately became curious about what was happening at home that she needed to be distracted from. Her head went down again, she shrimped and refused to answer my question.

A dead end again. So, I negotiated about how we could name the things that happened at home without her having to tell, confess or relive some experiences.

Could we put it in a kind of container and find some words to express and to put these experiences in?

S: *You don't have to explain what was happening at home... I just want to give it a name. The troubles at home? The shit at home? Or the hassle ...?*
Y: *It was a whole hassle at home.*
S: *So can I write 'the Whole Hassle' on a piece of paper?*
Y: *Yes.*
   While I put the piece of paper with these words on it between us, I asked how old she was when 'the Whole Hassle' came along for the first time.
Y: *I remember a few things when I was in preschool. At the age of six it disappeared for a while but when a new dad came, 'the Whole Hassle' started all over again.*
S: *When 'the Whole Hassle' was at home, what were your escape routes?*
Y: *Going to my room.*
S: *What did you do in your room? I suppose that Little Orange was there?*
Y: *Yes. ... Crying.*
S: *Is this a period that you cried a lot?*
Y: *Yes, until the age of 15.*
   ...
S: *What did 'the Whole Hassle' ruin?*
Y: *My youth!*
S: *Completely?*
Y: *About 60–70 per cent.*
S: *What is in this 30–40 per cent that you tried to protect?*
   I tried to keep in mind that children and youngsters always take steps in endeavouring to prevent the trauma they are subject to, and, when preventing this trauma is impossible, they take steps to try to modify it in some way or to modify its effects on their lives (White, 2006c, p. 28). People always take steps to protect or keep up what and who is important or valuable to them. I ask Yana how she tried to respond to '*the Whole Hassle*'. First she answered she had done nothing. So I asked how much she had worried in her head and if there were some survival techniques she developed.
   ...
S: *Yana, you said: 'I went sitting in my room, I cried, ... I found support and consolation by Little Orange ...' What exactly were you thinking?*
Y: *Running away and never come back ...*
S: *What were you running away from and maybe protesting against?*
Y: *'The Whole Hassle', once I made my suitcase. I wanted to go to the neighbours.*
   I just wanted a normal life. *It was always a relief when I could go out with the dogs.*
S: *Where the dogs sometimes your consolation?*
   ...

Suddenly Yana said that it was her fault that things went wrong. '*It's my fault because I didn't communicate.*' At that point the urge to make Yana clear that it wasn't her fault became huge. Often this isn't helpful because it doesn't bring a new perspective on what happened. Through experience I have learned to invite them to unravel how they came to such a final conclusion and explore if these feelings or convictions of guilt were helpful in their life.

S: *Are these thoughts of being guilty taking a lot of time on your mind?*

Y: *Yes, mostly in the evening. When I'm lying in my bed.*

S: *Are these helpful thoughts?*

Y: *No, not really.*

S: *When you start to think 'It's my fault', does it become difficult to follow the advice of Little Orange 'Just go on'?*

Y: *Yes, I start to cry and at the same time I try not to cry. I don't want this.*

S: *What is important to you that you don't want this?*

Y: *I don't want to be pitiful. I still want to make something out of my life.*

As the conversation further develops, step by step we discover aspects that show she still cares, that things and persons still matter and that she still wants to be meaningful.

After the interview her mentor, the family worker and her friend were asked what resonated with them and what they wanted to take with them from these stories that had been told. The family worker was touched by the story of Little Orange. Although she was 48 years old she still had her own cuddly bear from the time she was a child. She was also surprised by the many efforts of Yana to keep going on. A few days after the interview she took her cuddly bear to the children's home and both bears got introduced to each other. It became a friendship for years but the most important thing: it opened many long conversations between Yana, the family worker and the two bears about how to go on after times of hardship and how to relate to the people who played a part in these hard times. As Yana received a letter as well as the recorded interview on a DVD, a few months later she watched the DVD together with her foster mum.

A few weeks ago

At Interactie-Academie, a training institute and group practice for systemic psychotherapy and family counselling, we are engaged in a foster care programme to prevent breakdown placement. Esma, nine years old, and her grandparents come to see me for a conversation because the situation is becoming untenable and her grandparents are very worried. Esma lived until the age of seven with her parents who both are mentally challenged. After several incidents of domestic violence and the disclosure of sexual abuse by her uncle the juvenile court decided to place her in foster care with her maternal grandparents. Her mother stays in a psychiatric unit, her father returned to Turkey, his homeland, and her uncle was imprisoned. A few months ago emotional outbursts appeared: one moment Esma cries and is inconsolable; another moment she screams and kicks around. At the school playground she already had several panic attacks and she developed several ticks. When her grandparents, the schoolteacher or others ask her about these emotional moments she freezes. Her grandparents are worried, as they don't know what to think or how to respond to these difficulties. When I meet them in the waiting room, Esma disappears behind her grandma's skirt and mumbles something in a toddler's voice. She carries a small backpack in her hand. I ask if this is her school bag. She shakes her head 'no'. The bag contains her favourite books and the photo album of her childhood and family. Her 'Top' favourite book turns out to be *Peter Pan*.

Quickly I find out that Wendy is her favourite character. In the evening she has long conversations with Wendy. She hopes to become someone like Wendy who takes good care of the lost boys and brings warmth to their hearts. Once in the therapy room her grandparents start to explain what goes wrong and Esma makes herself very small on her chair. The more grandfather tells that she is really all right for them although things are sometimes very difficult the more tears start to run down her cheek. Grandma exclaims rather desperately: *'She has to learn to believe in herself!'*

As I fear these ways and directions of exploring will only silence Esma's voice, I gently interrupt her grandparents and I address myself to Esma. I ask her if we can invite Wendy into the conversation, and while asking, I offer Wendy a chair. In the meantime a 'KAA Ghent' football club supporters scarf drops out of her bag. It seems Esma's dad is a great supporter as well as her grandfather. She keeps all the scores of this team in a small notebook to report to her dad when he hopefully returns from Turkey. I ask her if we also have to offer a chair to her dad, the football team and maybe Turkey in our meeting. She nods enthusiastically, takes the scarf and lays it on another chair. I quickly consult doctor Google to find out with her where Turkey is situated and how many miles it is away from here. Together with grandma she draws a flag of Turkey and they place it on the chair of her father. I suggest to draw a line from her chair to the one of her father and we write '2709 kilometres in bird's eye view'. Esma insists to add 'feels like 100.000.000.000 kilometres'. We explore step by step who else is part of her team of support and solidarity.

The grandparents agree firmly when I notice that Esma is surrounded by a solid team. I ask them if they know what these different people appreciate the most about Esma. Grandma immediately says 'her caring for everyone'. So I check with Esma if this means she works hard for all the people she loves. She nods with a little smile on her face. This makes me wonder why she is living with her grandparents. Tears pop up and she freezes. I ask her if she could make a drawing at the flip chart of all the people in her heart and how big her worries for all these people are.

She tells her heart becomes smaller and smaller each time she thinks of her family. She is afraid that her heart will shrink and disappear because of all these tears, while her hands are enlarging because of the worries she carries with her.

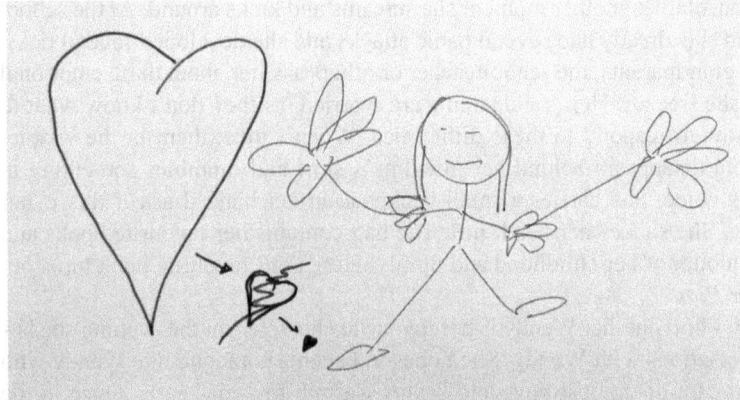

Figure 0.1 Drawing of a girl and a heart. Photograph by the author.

Can I do some guesses about the tears and can all the people present (live and imaginary) lend us a hand? I focus my attention to the large audience and drop some questions. Silently, from the corner of her eye, she listens to the questions.

Could it be that Esma works very hard to keep the tears inside? What kind of sadness is occupying her heart that she tries to hide from everyone? Is there anyone who has some expertise about this sadness?

With a soft voice Esma says that when Wendy is nearby *The Sadness* (about all the things that happened) passes much quicker. I look surprised and become very curious what kind of magic is happening between the both of them that makes a difference.

Could it be that it is very frustrating that keeping the tears and *The Sadness* inside sometimes doesn't work? Could it be that sometimes *The Sadness* becomes extremely large and takes over control?

Esma draws how *The Sadness* makes her head crazy.

A bit mysteriously I step towards Esma and 'whisper' in her ear 'Do you think grandma and granddad also have some sadness in their heart? Or would it be a different sadness?'. Esma responds that she has no idea but she assumes they also have some sadness in their heart. I ask her if she could interview them about their heart and pretend to put a microphone in her hand. Enthusiastically she steps towards them and starts to interview them.

We decide to put all the worries and different kinds of sadness in a small box in the form of coloured beads and try to find out who can be helpful in bearing all this grief. Esma hides the little box with sadness in a safe place in the puppet house.

There is one bead she doesn't want to be put in this beautifully decorated box. The bead that represents 'The bad things that happened with her uncle', we have to put that in a separate box. Together with her grandparents we think of a suitable place for this box. While talking, sharing and exploring, Esma sits more and

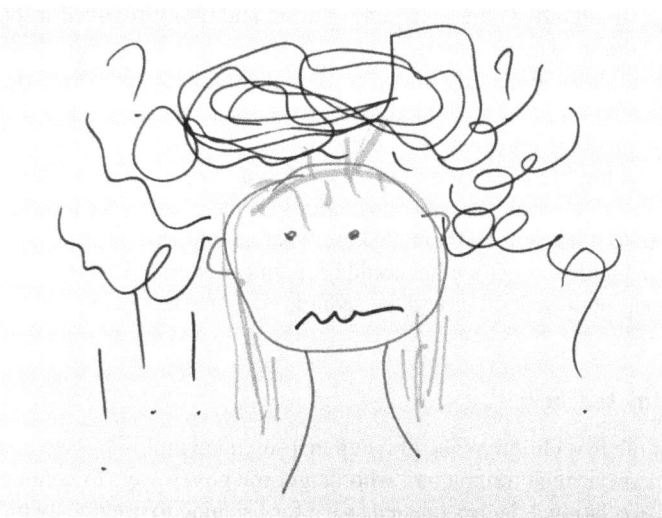

Figure 0.2 Drawing of a girl with exploding thoughts. Photograph by the author.

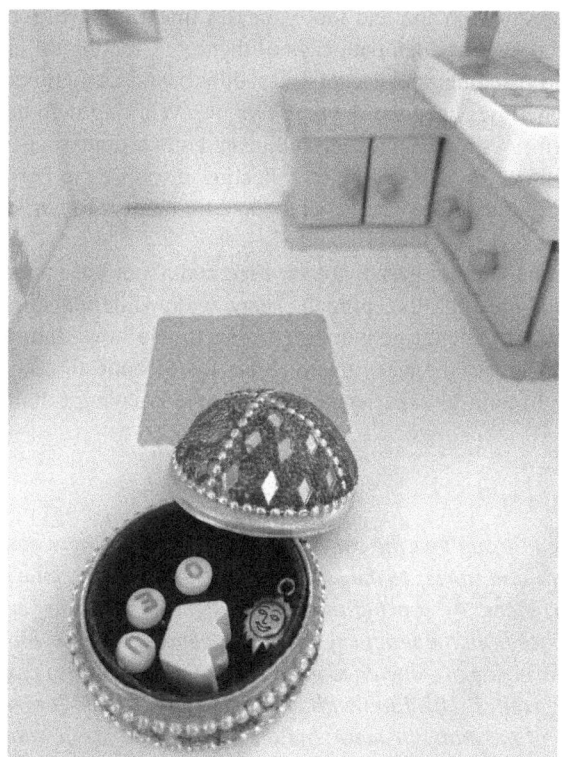

Figure 0.3 Box in puppet house. Photograph by the author.

more upright. Her grandparents are also getting more and more involved in our research. New 'relational dances' emerge.

Later on we do a partly imaginary interview with the different significant persons from Esma's network talking about their worries, their viewpoints and their reflections on our meeting together. We search for small actions of Esma that make a difference in the life of her grandparents and everyone imaginary present in the room. We list all their skills and contributions on the board, take a picture of it so they can take it home with them. Asking what an important purpose and hope of our working and talking together could be, Esma answers: 'That everyone somehow gets along with each other and the sadness becomes less heavy'.

Three of my many teachers

David was one of the first children who grew up in a so-called multi-stressed context in which he experienced trauma and who taught me novel ways to connect. Stepping in playful relational dances opened space for listening to previously hidden actions, sharing unknown experiences in a safe way and developing new, alternative stories and meaning.

The biographical interview with Yana and the witnesses made me aware of the importance of leaving the well-trodden pathways of therapy. Creating different contexts of speaking and listening, and accepting 'cuddly bears' as members of teams of support, can sometimes open the doors to therapy. Working with her helped me realise it is often possible to uncover subjugated stories, alternative perspectives and new meanings, by, for example, collecting responses to hardship, or by being curious about actions towards what and who matters to her, or is valuable to her.

In conversations with Esma and her grandparents, I learned about the importance of safe grounds to stand on, and of keeping the scope wide while reflecting and co-acting with children's relational networks. I began to see how sharing experiences, creating shared local languages opens doors to re-connection and to the collective processing of painful experiences as collective weaving trauma through the fabric of life.

Dear reader,

From the very beginning and throughout the entire book, I aspire to bring voices of children, their experiences and stories to the foreground, especially in contexts of adverse childhood experiences. By sharing these three stories, from the very beginning I want to emphasise both the uniqueness and the commonality of each therapeutic journey. Therefore, you are invited to get a taste of a multitude of possible entrances and walking routes. This links with my hope for this book. It aims not only to echo the voices of the many insiders, but also to provide useful footholds, guidelines and inspiring ideas for the many professionals who, together with these children and people involved, must find a way through the complexity, the dilemmas and the paradoxes so that it can, in turn, help these children and their families to move on in life.

Along the way we can encounter many obstructions and pitfalls, so we must be well equipped and leave well prepared. A rich systemic and narrative tradition of thinking and practices serves as a compass to navigate throughout our conversations and common therapeutic journey. My backpack is filled with their principles, concepts and ways of doing as possible helpful tools.

I will use different words and descriptions for the adversities and traumatic experiences which the children went through because I do not want to get into the discussion of what can or cannot be called trauma. This counts as well for the impact and effects of the adversities. As much as possible, I will choose to name it in ways in which the child and those involved refer to it and try to unravel together their multiple meanings. During our therapeutic journey these children and all involved often continue to face challenges in everyday life, wounds can easily be reopened and relational injuries and pain are not 'over', so we have to take into account this will constantly cross our path, just as the many voices involved interfere constantly in a web of reciprocal influences.

Reflection is required on which life areas and relationships we need to visit and explore first in order to create safe and solid grounds. As no child is an island, we require a team of mutual support and solidarity. We are faced with a multitude of possible starting points and valuable routes for our journey, each with their own possibilities, pitfalls and limitations. Is it best to talk to the child, carers, family or network separately first or do we bring them all together at once? Is our main focus on the present, the past or the future? Do we have to talk about problematic actions, painful emotions, ruminating thoughts, intangible body reactions or do we need to focus on the relational injuries? In my opinion, these are not decisions that the therapist should take alone, but that result from a collaborative engagement in ongoing dialogues about how to shape our therapeutic journey with the child and the many others involved. This also means that, with the exception of the chapter on first meetings, the order in the book does not reflect what I would see as an ideal sequence of steps in the therapeutic process. Just like I do not want to give the illusion, through the many stories about what proved to be helpful and actually made a difference, that our journey is a smooth and straightforward process towards a 'happy end'. These journeys follow a more meandering, zigzagging, back and forth path. Sometimes we even get lost on side paths and end up in a swampy bog. Transformation rather happens over time than overnight.

The reader will encounter a multicoloured mosaic of travel routes to undertake with children, carers and their networks. The aim is always to foster a sense of agency, a sense of belonging and a sense of coherence by collaboratively weaving networks of resilience. It is important for the reader to bear in mind there is no predetermined end point other than the hope that the adversities will become woven into the fabric of their lives and people have found more satisfying ways to go on.

It is also important to point out that the paths I take therapeutically in this book should be taken as inspiration, and not as an instruction of how the work has to be done. It will always remain the responsibility of the therapist or counsellor themselves to make choices on the spot, while immersed in the here and now of embodied dialogues with those present as well as the many physically absent third parties involved. I hope this book will inspire the reader to find the courage to step into invigorating participatory transformative processes of their own making.

Before I briefly address the various chapters, a final word on how I refer to myself. I will alternate between 'I' and 'we', because of course I am the author of this book, and I take full responsibility for its content, but on the other hand I want to honour the many people I 'carry' with me, some of whom have become indistinguishable from myself in my ways of looking at the children and families we meet in therapy.

In Chapter 1, I will present the web of complexities in which we can get entangled with children, their families and networks in the case of adverse childhood experiences. By making some of the complexities and the many voices visible, I hope to create an awareness of these influencing relations and contexts and of the necessity to find a position to relate to them.

In Chapter 2, I will show the importance of collaborative and inviting practices to connect to the insiders' perspective of the child, family and many involved. Our systemic and narrative perspectives on trauma, adversity and the possibilities of fostering resilience processes are discussed. Based on ideas of what creates well-being we make explicit the importance of facilitating and enhancing a sense of agency, a sense of belonging and a sense of coherence. Doing hope, just as serious playfulness and playful seriousness, will appear to be indispensable aspects in weaving networks of resilience.

Chapter 3, on first meetings, will offer the reader a lot of ingredients to begin therapeutic journeys well equipped, and to create safe grounds. Issues of speaking versus keeping silent as well as many other sources of hesitation are discussed. Opportunities to move within them are explored. Taking the idea of 'walking our talk' as a guideline, I will present an alternative approach to starting therapeutical journeys and discuss possibilities and limitations of different conversational settings.

Chapter 4 focuses on what I like to refer to as the tentacles of trauma and adversity. We will zoom in and at the same time zoom out on the presented difficulties. We will introduce all kinds of playful ways of unravelling trauma and its many effects.

Chapter 5, in turn, offers reflections on the often intricate relational complexity in the here and now, and will introduce, in Chapter 6, some paths for dealing further with 'wounded relationships' and family members who were offending. In Chapter 7 we explore some helpful ways in engaging more directly with the parents and carers getting lost in all of these entanglements. We will address issues of (parenting) support and acts of solidarity that help to strengthen the bonds with their child.

Finally, in Chapter 8, using methods such as timelines or life review interviews, the collected pieces of the puzzle are brought together, enhancing a sense of coherence. In that final chapter we further explore 'compassionate witnessing', creating 'a sense of belonging' and the possibility of weaving experienced adversities into the fabric of life.

My special thanks goes to all these children, youngsters, families and carers for the confidence they gave me, the many stories they shared and the courage and willingness to embark on such journeys. Their original, often surprising, but above all relentless attempts to create for themselves and their loved ones a life and a place in this world worth living continue to amaze. Their gathered and shared wisdom forms a lasting source of inspiration that accompanies me all the time. Also the many conversations, collaborations and projects with my former colleagues at the children's home as well as with my current colleagues, associated trainers and students at the Interactie-Academie and other training institutes each time again offered fruitful perspectives and ideas.

Over many years, our sturdy wooden kitchen table became a place where friends and colleagues from all over the world gathered, in person and online, to continue the relentless search for what works for these children, young people, families and their networks. Many seeds were planted here for projects that give children a voice or that open up opportunities to re-experience that they still matter and belong. I also want to mention that all the stories presented are altered, disguised and are used with the consent of the children, youngsters and families involved. Many of them are really proud to share their stories and hope that we as practitioners can learn from their experiences.

The piles of books and articles by systemic and narrative thinkers and practitioners on our kitchen table also contributed significantly to this book and to the development of my thinking and acting. Writing is a lonely job where authors often have no clue about the significance of their writings. So I want to thank them all.

Nevertheless without the invitation of Charlotte Burck and Gwyn Daniel to write this book for the systemic thinking and practice series, believing in the value of my work and the support of this book, this would never have been written. So many thanks!

Last but not least, I want to thank my mum who taught her children from very early on what kind of care and support can truly make a difference in life. At the age of three, her own mother disappeared from her life and she was raised by her grandparents. She showed me how, despite adversity, it is still possible together with others to find ways to live a life worth living. Just as my father taught me the importance of doing justice, raised in a family at the margins of our society. They both inspired my sister, brother and me to build teams of support and solidarity as valuable companions through all kinds of waters of life.

Finally I would like to mention explicitly my pillars of strength, my partner Luc and son Jonas. Their contribution is invisibly present in every sentence of this book. Without them, it would never have come about. As the book was mainly written at our kitchen table, they brought a cup of coffee or tea or the perfect piece of chocolate, a joke or a smile at the right moment but were also always available for discussion or to hear my frustrations, struggles and sometimes even hopelessness ☺. For their constant encouragement and, above all, their never wavering belief in the value of this book, I am deeply grateful.

Warm wishes,
Sabine

Chapter I

Dis-covering a web of complexities

Introduction

Our starting point is the idea that when children get caught in multi-stressed contexts or traumatic life histories, we enter a web of complexities. When children are hurt, a whole lot of different 'agents' become involved. To use an analogy, whenever we start working with a child and their family or network it's as if a polyphony of voices gathers (Gergen, 1999). Some voices sound very loud, others are rather quiet, and tend to become overlooked. Often they are contradictory, sometimes they are overwhelming, sometimes they invite reflection, sometimes they impose action. The voices represent very different kinds of actors, some being persons, others being institutions, or society itself or some can even be non-human actors. They are all affected and triggered. Many of them become committed to the same cause: helping the child and their family to thrive.

After an escalation of violence between his mother and his stepfather, Xander (11) is placed by the youth court at a crisis unit for children. His mother was brought to a secured psychiatric unit so he couldn't stay at the caravan park where they all three lived together. His mother is diagnosed with borderline personality disorder and his stepfather struggles with an alcohol addiction. There were regularly incidents of violence and Xander was several times heavily beaten by his stepfather. Social services call the situation of Xander 'a serious case of neglect and physical and emotional abuse'. At the age of two, his father disappeared after a quarrel with his mum and throwing Xander on the floor. There are three adult half brothers and sisters but there is no contact with them.

At the crisis unit, Xander keeps on crying, refuses to go to school and sometimes he smashes his fists against the wall until they bleed. It takes hours to get him calmed down. At night, he has nightmares in which he repeats desperately 'I want my mum! Bring me to my mum'. The judge decided he can't visit his mum until she is 'stabilised'. The carers no longer know how to respond, a child psychiatrist prescribed a mild anti-depressant and trauma therapy is hoped to be a possible solution. In attempts to understand what is going on, the terms 'insecure attachment' and 'complex, developmental trauma' have been used several times.

DOI: 10.4324/9781003167860-2

The urge to act

Van der Kolk (2014) warns against intervening immediately to fix the problems. When children are physically, emotionally or mentally hurt the taken-for-granted foundations of society have been damaged and the 'agreed' world order has been shaken up. Although Xander is presented as a child with complex trauma who urgently needs help, there are many more people around him affected and in distress. The urge to act is voiced by many parties involved. The exclamation 'this must stop immediately' can be heard as an intention, a hope or wish for the child. Unfortunately this urge doesn't answer the question of what are appropriate ways to stop 'this' and what exactly has to be stopped or has to be stopped first. *The violence? The drinking? The emotional abuse? Living in bad conditions? The crying of Xander? The head banging? The relationship with his mother?* Such a cry of distress can sound as if a simple solution for an interwoven multiplicity of problems, obstacles, worries in specific multi-stressed contexts is to be identified and to be found.

The call for immediate action in fact conceals the complexity. We risk drifting away from what Xander thinks, feels, wants or what his worries, relational involvements and understandings of the problems are and what this means in relation to the important people in his life. Likewise we risk ignoring the commitment of many more actors, and experiencing them as annoying or even disturbing.

Being aware of this collective 'pressure' to help out offers the possibility to take a more reflective stance towards both the complexities entering the room, as well as what it is that occupies Xander and the people concerned. Before entering into the quest of unravelling this polyphony of engaged voices, let us first take a closer look at what is often a starting situation, and the challenges it entails.

Actions, emotions and the body hijacking the therapy room

As soon as Xander, his mentor and the crisis unit psychologist are seated, the psychologist explains to me why they bring Xander to therapy. Immediately Xander starts to cry. It almost sounds as the howling of a wolf. He scratches his arm with his finger nails and his mentor tries to stop him.

It is worth remembering that children and young people with a background of violence, abuse or neglect are often 'brought' to a therapist. Coming to see the therapist in order to work on the problems or process traumatic experiences is often not a response they invented themselves. Once entering the room, the impact of the experiences and the child's responses can accompany them. Expressions of sadness or anger, for instance, in the form of temper tantrums or crying or scratching, refusal to speak, etc., can become excessively present. Bodily (re)actions and stress can be all over the place. Tics, shaking, black-outs, panic attacks can make talking impossible.

Because the acute problems are sometimes so intrusive, we cannot ignore them and we have to be careful not to get caught up in this crying, the anger, the feelings of helplessness ourselves. We are challenged to find ways to respond in supportive ways that allow us to acknowledge these expressions of pain or suffering and at the same time open the possibility to get relationally involved.

Taking some handkerchiefs from my desk, I ask Xander since when these tears accompany him and if it is always the same kind of tears that overwhelm him. He looks up as if taken by surprise. I go further, asking 'Are they such a kind of tears that can be comforted by handkerchiefs or are these too small to catch all the sadness that the tears carry with them?' Tears keep on rolling over his cheeks and sobbing he answers: 'You would need a whole swimming pool'. A little smile appears on his face when I wonder out loud how for heaven's sake I can be helpful to him if I don't have a swimming pool in this therapy room. I don't think my boss will allow us to dig a swimming pool in the garden.

There are at least two possible ways of conceiving of the child's behaviour and overwhelming emotions or bodily responses. We can look at them as utterances expressing internal representations that were caused by traumatic life experiences. Taken as such, these behaviours, and the underlying representations, are problematic, and one needs to find ways to change or fix them. But we can also understand their behaviour as communicative actions and interactive in nature. Inspired by Pearce and Cronen (1980), we believe that if we want to make sense of children's acts we need to be curious about the meaning given to contexts that are not directly observable. The challenge then becomes to engage in meaningful interactions where all the participants are able to make sense of both their own and the other's actions. Children's behavioural, bodily or emotional utterances can be understood as contributions to the unfolding therapeutic relationship (Fredman, 2004; Lang in Kristensen, 2007; Vermeire & Sermijn, 2017).

The temptation of unhelpful dances

Through the years parents or carers, even adults and people in general, haven't been experienced as reliable, caring or helpful to children like Xander. Children who suffered from such painful relational experiences sometimes start to claim, but also to reject, the care that their 'carers' and other adults are trying to give to them. Although they seem to require adults' total attention at the same time they reject it (Golding & Hughes, 2012). They develop an overly sensitive sense for unsafety. Any unfamiliar situation, as for instance an unknown therapist or therapy context, can evoke feelings of suspicion. Neither do their bodies take a risk: they often immediately go into a state of hyper-security. The child's habitual ways of responding to contexts of insecurity can lure the therapist into unhelpful dances.

Explaining this is a safe place, trying to convince the child we are reliable or trustworthy or trying to reassure with words, often result in the opposite of what we intend. Feelings of anxiety and suspicion easily get fuelled. Connecting with the child is complicated because there always remains a hierarchy between adults and children however hard we as adults try to minimise it. The height of our bodies, the amount of words we know and the way we overlook the world, amongst others, constitute big differences. As we can't escape our 'adulthood', we can easily engage in a one-directional 'caring' relationship in which the adult is self-evidently positioned as the helper giving advice, and the child is positioned as needing help and as having to accept and follow the advice given (Vermeire, 2017).

When I check with Xander if this is a strange situation to him, as he is sitting here with three adults in a therapy session, he immediately answers that we don't have to assume this will be helpful because none of us can bring his mum back to him. He wants all these stupid adults to stop explaining that he has to understand that it is for his best. 'No one can understand what it means living my life, like no one can understand what it means to miss my mum'.

In this response, Xander in fact (to the careful listener) offers helpful instructions for our collaborative relationship: 'Sabine, don't explain all kinds of things to me' and 'Sabine, don't think you understand what it is I am trying to deal with'. Xander warns me not to take, at this moment, an expert position towards his experiences and the things happening in his life.

So from the very beginning we face the challenge Alan Jenkins (2009) named the importance of intervening without reproducing subtle practices of abuse or violence. This is particularly important when we consider that many children who experienced trauma lost touch with a valued sense of who they hope to be or believe they are. They reached negative conclusions about their lives, their relationships and their identities (Sheinberg & Fraenkel, 2001). Their 'sense of self' is sometimes diminished to such a degree that it becomes very difficult for them to give any account of what they value in life (White, 2006c). We have to tumble in interactions that do not reinforce their sense of failure nor strengthen their experiences of trauma. So the question 'How not to repeat what has already been done?' will be an important guideline throughout the rest of this book.

Embracing complexity

As children are considered important in our societies, it should not come as a surprise that many voices are taking part in dialogues on the best interests of the child. We believe it to be helpful to give an overview of what kinds of voices are engaged. Some of these voices are informing our own, others are very distant from ours.

In what follows, we will briefly discuss various voices that participate in our therapeutic conversations, and especially when unnoticed may deeply influence the course and outcome of the therapeutic process. We discuss 'scientific theories', 'expert knowledge' and 'social institutions'.

Scientific theories

Theories of child development, moral development, attachment, trauma and resilience inform how people think about children, how they talk with them, what they ask them, and how they make sense of issues they are dealing with (Vetere & Dowling, 2005). The ideas, viewpoints, beliefs and social representations that go along with these theories and discourses circulating in our communities will also co-construct the lens through which these children look at and think of themselves, their family and relationships, their life and the painful things that happened.

Xander was sent to special education at the age of six because the school team was convinced that he was mentally challenged. Nobody took into account that his mum was Romanian. At home he spoke a mix of Dutch and Romanian. He didn't attend kindergarten and mainly interacted with adults at the caravan park. During his first years at primary school, there was no one who spent time in following up on homework or who valued his efforts in school. For a long time, he was seen through the lens of a mentally challenged child, not only by school but also by his parents and even by himself. His timid, withdrawn attitude and the fact that he barely spoke were understood within this context. Luckily there was the owner of the park shop who noticed Xander was interested in books. She gave him imaginative, exciting books that he used to read in the storage room of the shop. Later on she also started to challenge him with extra homework. At secondary school he discovered the possibilities of street dance and writing rap songs. This allowed him to become part of a new community of peers.

According to Semin and Gergen (1990), social sciences as psychology and educational sciences contribute to broader society conversations concerning, for instance, development or attachment. Regarding the voice of **developmental psychology** it is good to keep in mind that the predominant view still is a *retrospective* developmental perspective, which is to be distinguished from the less familiar *prospective* or open perspective on development. Retrospective theories construe development as a unilinear and unidirectional process with limited interindividual and intercultural variations (Breeuwsma, 2001). The final stage, adulthood, as well as the different intermediary stages to reach this final stage are clearly described. This can be helpful in assessing what a child or youngster can understand of what we are saying or trying to explain. This account offers ideas about how to adjust our way and level of speaking so that it connects with how the child conceives of their world and expresses themselves in their world at that particular developmental stage. This developmental framework shows also the expectations of our society on behalf of the child. This can help us to notice that a child in these contexts is mainly behaving as an adult or just acting as a toddler instead of an eight-year-old boy.

We should be aware that developmental theories that see children as active participants in their own development by changing their environment are less influential. Valsiner (2000) inspired by Vygotsky (1986), for instance, proposes to understand development as a never-ending negotiation process between parents, child and environment. Such less predominant developmental voices depict an open, dynamic, more prospective stance towards development.

When children experience adversity, developmental metaphors are often used that align with the idea that personality is firmly rooted in early life and that psychological development is inhibited or even halted when an important phase has been missed (McNamee & Gergen, 1992). Disturbances, mainly in the first five years of childhood can, according to this view, disadvantage later developmental stages (Verhofstadt-Denève et al., 2003). We need to be aware that this tape recorder model voices a rather deterministic and perhaps pessimistic linear viewpoint regarding the developmental possibilities of the child.

We should also be aware that attachment and attachment theories have become default in thinking about these children. For many parents, educators, and therapists the language of attachment has become part and parcel of the language in which they describe and understand their children, themselves and their relationship. So it's not surprising that, also in the context of developmental trauma or complex trauma, professionals as well as laypersons rely on **attachment theories** to make sense of the difficulties that arise. This voice typically tends to stress the importance of early attachment in children's lives, and to minimise current bonds and the importance of relationships other than parent–child.

Xander can easily be seen as an insecurely attached child in relation with his parents and carers. The bond with his mum can be labelled as unhealthy and too close, and even symbiotic. His relationship with Mary, the owner of the camping shop, their secretly gossiping and making little jokes risks not to be noticed as a meaningful attachment relation.

From a therapeutic stance, as well as in daily life, it is a pity that many of his actions, e.g. making himself invisible during quarrels, being quiet in the morning, or withdrawing himself or constructing a shelter in a small grove at the end of the caravan park, and so on, are hardly to be detected as helpful, and adaptive actions in unsafe contexts.

Crittenden and Claussen (2003) shifted the focus of their research from individual characteristics of children, towards characteristics of contexts. They investigated how children in threatening contexts reduced danger, how their strategies evolved during their development and how they influenced the way they conceived of relationships. They concluded that all attachment patterns can be considered as adaptive depending on the contexts in which they emerge. These behaviours make sense if the actual relational and cultural contexts are taken into account. In systemic therapy, attachment behaviour can thus be conceived as an often unnoticed or misunderstood relational response as well as a relational invitation, within a particular context, that can evoke emotional connectedness. Attachment then is not seen as a reified attribute of an individual child, caused by unsafe context, but rather as an emergent context-dependent quality of dynamic relational processes in which the therapist can actively take part (Vermeire, 2020).

Next to the voice of developmental theory, and the voice of attachment theory, **theories of socialisation** also can sound very loud. In the latter field of research, the less common idea that children are full agents, who actively take a part in the shaping of their own lives, and those of important others, is gaining momentum (Kuzcynski & De Mol, 2015). Whereas the taken-for-granted stance in these theories was, and perhaps still is, that parents, and other adults, influence the development of the child unidirectionally, more and more research is available that shows how these processes are in fact better conceived of as bidirectional. In clinical settings it has been argued that children can also regain a sense of relational agency, in the sense that they, for instance, can notice, sense and perhaps become reassured, that they contribute to the relationship with their parent, and more importantly, also that what they do, and what they refrain from doing, adds to the quality of the lives of their parents in many senses (De Mol et al., 2018). The voice that claims that these children are 'full agents' is understandably often hard to notice in these contexts.

Xander's actions towards his mum such as preparing dinner, throwing bottles of vodka in the kitchen sink when she is sleeping, ... aren't easily appreciated as valuable actions of relational involvement. On the contrary they are more often seen as tasks that are not in accordance with his age. Still, noticing and acknowledging such actions often does contribute to a sense of relational agency.

The great merit of trauma theories is that they have raised awareness of the fact that children can suffer severely from adversity, which can also have serious effects on them later in life. This also makes it possible for their sufferings to be recognised. At the same time, many **trauma theories and approaches** add to the idea that these children are victims, and as such no (sense of) agency is attributed to them. This downplaying of children's agency is strengthened more as discourses on trauma are interwoven with highly compelling discourses about victimhood. Also in folk psychology children in contexts of complex trauma or developmental trauma easily get represented as victims for life. Such reductions threaten to make the many other aspects of identity disappear from sight and urge us to describe the children and adolescents mainly in a language of negative effects and deficits. 'They cannot build a relationship', 'They are damaged', 'They are lost' are just a few examples of this reduction (Wade, 1997). Bystanders are moved and often try to help with actions that can be perceived by the child as pity and that provoke negative conclusions about themselves and their self-worth.

A few months later in our therapeutic journey Xander takes a seat and, heavily agitated, he says: 'I hate it when they look at me with their Harry Potter eyes! They all should leave me alone'. First I don't get what he wants to say. He continues that at a friend's birthday party, the mum of this friend gave him a whole package of clothes adding the sentence 'Please, I am sure you can use these'. This action made him angry but at the same time he felt he had to say politely 'Thank you'. He doesn't want to be looked at with 'pity'.

As therapists we are also attracted to these theories and social discourses, and are inclined to follow them blindly. If, in our urge to support, we address or frame children mainly as victims, in agreement with these social discourses, we might not be noticing what these relational difficulties or life events mean to them and we may overlook their actions to resist or to keep on going (Vermeire, 2011). Wade (1997) points out how these children's acts of resistance often aren't recognised for what they are. Some therapeutic approaches try to respond to these reductions by highlighting the force and strength of these children, carers or families. Seeing them as victims, as well as 'strong' both risk to ignore the pain and to cast them in single identity stories as 'survivors' or 'heroes' negating the dynamic, multifaceted, relational and contextual character of identity stories.

Sometimes, compelling ideas about processing trauma inform people's thoughts and actions in their conversations with and about children and youngsters. 'Trauma therapy takes a long time, it is something drastic and you really have to go through it to get rid of the consequences of the trauma', 'you have to learn to talk about it', 'as long you can't talk about it, it isn't processed', ' untreated victims become perpetrators', etc. It is probably better to realise that these viewpoints are simply there so we can reflect on them and take a critical stance towards them as a lot of children and families in these contexts, as well as therapists, fall into their grip and feel the pressure of the social instructions or social prescriptions contained in them.

Expert problem definitions

Another 'voice' that, often unmarked, contributes to addressing child adversity is what we might call 'expert problem definitions', together with its counter voice of critique of diagnosis.

In Xander's story, 'Post Traumatic Stress Disorder', 'Complex Trauma' and 'Attachment Disorder' were some of the naming in order to get a grip on the problems in the here and now and find a way to deal with them by the carers.

Diagnoses can provide recognition that the suffering is real, and not imaginary or exaggerated. Sometimes the diagnosis takes on the meaning that something harmful was actually done to them. They offer words and language to share and talk about the difficulties and are often considered a necessary condition to provide therapy. It needs to be stressed that, for instance, DSM diagnoses are deemed very important in our society. Although often a gap remains between *knowing what* is wrong and *knowing how* to go on in helpful ways.

It is worthwhile to address some of the expected controversy surrounding diagnoses. If we take language to be constitutive of our social worlds (Carr, 2012) naming difficulties for instance as attachment problems, PTSS or developmental trauma can on the one hand help to get a grip on the complex realities, but at the same time it can have a reducing effect on the child's 'self' and the range of their possible actions (Gergen et al., 1996; Vermeire, 2020). Indeed, any such diagnosis can evoke and reinforce a whole range of images, ideas and perspectives of the child as well as of parents and significant others. Sometimes diagnoses enhance blaming and shaming discourses about the parents and the child. Some diagnoses seem to inform the possibilities and impossibilities of their relationships with each other and with the outside world (Weingarten, 2003; Dallos, 2006).

Van der Kolk (2014) points out that diagnoses have a profound influence on how children define themselves. It can enhance their feelings of falling short or being worthless. These diagnoses for sure can offer recognition and acknowledgement of the suffering, but as meaning-making processes are dynamic, relational and contextual, at a later life stage they can feel oppressive and isolating. At the same time such a diagnosis can feel a relief for the carers while for the parents a curse, or vice versa. Unfortunately, a diagnosis doesn't tell us how this unique child themselves understands the problems and what experiences and meanings given to these experiences occupy their mind. Neither is the child invited to become an active participant in this research of what is going on, or the naming of the problem what White (2007) called experience-near ways.

Voices critical of diagnoses point out that they tend to obscure the social, cultural and economic contexts as well as these contexts' interconnectedness with the presented problem. Minuchin et al. (1967) emphasised the impact of poverty in his book 'Families of the slums'. Children from lower socio-economic backgrounds appear to be more often 'disorganised' with carers who are often heavily burdened by economic and family instability (Van der Kolk, 2014). Poverty, it is remarked, is not a risk in itself, but it makes it more difficult to raise children well (Rutter, 1999). White (2011) noted that it is much harder to conceal abuse in lower class social living contexts than, for example, in middle-class households.

More recently, the voice of neurosciences became very popular in explaining what is going on which is consistent with a biological perspective on behaviour. It seems obvious that situations of abuse also affect the body and the brain. They can be, as it were, 'registering' and 'inhabiting' themselves in the body. In different but related contexts and relationships, these influences of the past can become activated. Much research has been done on the impact of stress on the development of the brain and the imprints in the neural networks, the memory and stress hormone systems. I think it is important to take this viewpoint into account but also keep in mind that it is one of multiple ways of understanding what is happening in the here and now. Perry (2006, 2017) makes a plea not to disconnect the brain from how it evolved to respond to a complex social world. Genetic predispositions were shaped by evolution to be exquisitely sensitive to the people who surrounded it. As such, trauma and responses cannot be understood outside the context of human relationships. Recent research also indicates the neuroplasticity of the brain, which refers to the capacity of neurons and their networks to be altered by experience so that the impact on the brain can adjust based on treatment and a strong social network that surrounds and supports them (Perry, 2017).

According to a family and systemic therapy approach it is important not just to focus on the aetiology of problems and get stuck in a never-ending search for explanations. This means we have to pay special attention to the interpersonal and social processes and dynamics that maintain, increase or decrease these difficulties (Fruggeri, 1992).

On a social constructionist account, diagnoses, problem definitions, viewpoints on the problems are preliminary conclusions of many interpersonal, societal dialogues and negotiations. They inform our own viewpoint on the problems and influence, in their turn, my view on the child, on their family, etc., and on the conversation. They can offer guidelines for me as a therapist but at the same time the questions I ask and the directions I take in the conversation will be coloured by these. As the main focus is on what is wrong, many of these children's creative, often unusual responses to the traumatic experiences aren't recognised as such and their relational efforts can get ignored. Just like it can be important not to explain each action or problem of the child through the painful experiences but stay open-minded for the many influencing relations in the here and now.

Carr (2012) reminds us that the assumption underlying this approach is that the therapeutic value of diagnoses and narratives doesn't lie in their being 'true', but in their ability to provide guidance, supply rich meanings and to contribute to change and well-being.

A multiverse of worlds

When Xander starts to cry, I can imagine that at that very moment his mum is implicitly joining us in this meeting. His stepfather is looking with suspicion upon our conversation and the whole team of carers of the crisis unit is present by putting all their expectations on my shoulders. But also the children's judge and the child psychiatrist are whispering instructions in our ears while we are trying to start a conversation.

The above mentioned parliament of voices (Beckers, 2016) often includes, next to parents, family members and their networks, representatives of a 'judicial world', a 'medical-psychiatric world' and an 'educational world' that are involved each with their taken-for-granted assumptions, their logics and languages, their ideas of what has to be done and how it should be done. Each anonymous institutional sphere has its personal representatives. They often have different interests, purposes and goals and thus different things to do. These differences will colour the conversations with children and networks. The policeman, the social worker, the headmaster or the children's judge will all address Xander differently, will ask different questions, in a different way, while inquiring for instance about his relation with his stepfather, or his experiences in the caravan park. What he tells them, or doesn't tell them, will be heard and responded to very differently.

After an interrogation of Xander, before he was brought to the crisis unit, a police officer writes in a report that Xander declared being left alone several days a week. He had to collect food and cook for himself. He witnessed how his parents got drunk and got into fights. He sometimes tried to interfere and there is proof of several physical incidents where Xander is beaten by partners of his mum.

A judicial world is focused on facts and truth-finding. They need to compose a complete and clear picture of what factually happened. They represent society's interest. They listen to the stories told as witness statements. Their search for proof and thinking in terms of 'who is guilty', 'wrong and right', 'true or lies' and so on not only influences the conversation with the child or youngster but can bring them in difficult positions and relational struggles with their family members afterwards.

When Xander starts to think that his mum is brought to a secure unit because of the things he told, feelings of guilt aren't far away. Maybe he even has to punish himself for the things he revealed. Maybe he just told half of what happened the previous years, does this make him a liar? What does this interrogation mean for further conversations with adults he doesn't know and who say 'You can tell everything, what you tell is in confidence'.

It also means that I have to be aware that these experiences can influence my conversations with Xander. I'll have to find a clear position that differentiates the therapeutical from the judicial sphere. My first focus is the interest of Xander, the important people in his life and his network and I am interested in the stories he tells and the meanings that emerge. I am not trying to find the truth but the well-being of Xander and the people involved are my concern.

This is not to downplay the role or importance of the judicial sphere in any way. Convictions of the people who used violence or abused children by court can mean a firm recognition and acknowledging of children's suffering. Decisions taken by juvenile courts can free the child from the pressure of being able to make a 'right' choice.

Each of these institutional worlds can add something valuable in these complex situations so it is important to be aware of the possibilities of each world as well as their limitations and pitfalls. We have to reflect carefully on how we can help the child and people involved to notice and make these distinctions.

A few years ago, I had conversations with Farida, an 18-year-old girl who had been raped by her uncle for many years. After all these years of silence, she went to the police and her uncle was brought immediately to prison. An extended investigation started and she was questioned several times by the court psychiatrist. At one of these investigation moments he asked her how it was possible to still have a boyfriend and a sexual relationship. She was perplexed by these questions, mumbled something, rose and stepped out of the room. For hours she wandered around town no longer knowing where she was or who she was. A few days later we had an appointment. Immediately she dropped a barrage of questions: 'Do they think I invented everything? Won't they believe me? Am I getting crazy? Is still having a boyfriend abnormal in my situation?'

It was clear that I hadn't prepared her well enough for these meetings with the court psychiatrist whose job it is on behalf of the judge to investigate what the impact and effects are on her. His job isn't enhancing 'well-being' at that moment. If she had had a clear frame of what to expect and what the purposes and goals were of these interrogations, this could have given her the necessary support in that moment.

Next to the discussed institutional worlds, informal social networks as for instance the family, the football club, the parents of school friends or neighbourhood have an important influence on how the therapeutic process can unfold. Not only are these children part of all kinds of networks of relationships, as a therapist I am linked to all kinds of commitments. So sometimes my colleagues interfere with their thoughts and reflections on the situation or my partner and friends look over my shoulder giving some remarks on what I am doing in the therapy room.

Wider social and political contexts

Next to these 'agents', or voices that unexpectedly and in a taken-for-granted manner can and will enter our therapy, it is important to also take the voices of the broader, societal and political context into account.

Xander is 11 years old, wears trousers immediately showing that they are second-hand and his shoes are too small. The school he attends has a heavy reputation and he lives at a caravan park outside town. His mum immigrated years ago from a small ethnic community in Romania so I can hear he speaks with a different accent than mine.

According to White (2011), it is never a question of whether or not we bring politics into the therapy room, but whether or not we are willing to acknowledge its existence, and to what extent we are willing to be complicit in its exercise. He asks: 'How could the therapy setting be free of gender, race and class politics?' and 'How can therapy be exempt from the politics associated with hierarchies of knowledge and the politics of marginalisation in this culture?' When people enter the therapy room, they bring with them the politics of their relationships. And when people enter a therapy room, they enter a context that is structured by politics (Freedman & Combs, 2002). But how can the 'voice of politics' be noticed and heard?

Burnham (2012) developed the helpful acronym 'Social GRACES' to represent aspects of difference in beliefs, power resources and lifestyle that are visible or invisible, voiced or unvoiced. The term 'GRACES' refers to gender, gender identity, geography, generation, race, religion, age, ability, appearance, culture, class, caste, education, ethnicity, economic scan, spirituality, sexuality, sexual orientation. Burnham's acronym can help to keep us alert to our own biases and acknowledge the sometimes evoked micro-aggression moments. Social GRACES enhance therapeutic reflexivity: 'How am I attending to these differences in this moment, in this interaction, with this person?'

When Xander enters the room, notions about being privileged and disadvantaged are present. How can I be accountable as a white adult middle-class woman who is a mum herself? I am situated in a different position than Xander and his mum so how can we still become allies in our therapeutic journey without ignoring the differences or hiding practices of marginalisation?

Just like Xander noticed in a conversation: 'For you and the carers it is easy, in the evening you all are going home and sleep in your own bed with your own family. You don't know what it means to have to live with nine other crazy kids in the same house quarrelling and making all the time crazy noises day in day out. The carers in the children's home even get paid to annoy me'.

This brings us to the voice of institutionalised discrimination. Through this often unseen perspective, the way society organises care, the structures that are available and attainable, also influence and put limits to what is and is not possible in and outside the therapy room, what can be negotiated or not. Despite acknowledging the diversity of children and conceptions of childhood (nationally and globally), the care system may still continue to perpetuate the dominant developmental view of a 'normal' child(hood) as middle class, white and Eurocentric that romanticises the image of the innocent child(hood).

The solutions our societies provide can disadvantage the children, youngsters, their parents and even can be experienced as traumatic. Sometimes taking a child away from their home seems the least bad of all the bad solutions at the time. Our help can create a growing sense of alienation from their families and communities.

At a later point in the first conversation, Xander yells he is perfectly capable to take care of himself. Why doesn't anyone believe him? He knows how to fry an egg and he can even bake pancakes. Why can't he go back to the caravan park? Maybe the situation at home wasn't ideal but he was at least with his mum. This was home and felt familiar and known. Now he has to live with other children who make him crazy and carers who don't understand him. This is much worse than the life he had.

As a therapist I choose to try to be aware of these power dynamics. I don't believe I can, or should be, non-political. I want to take into account the impact and effects of our care systems and my ways of thinking and practising care. So the question becomes 'how can I be accountable and "response"-able in my work with Xander as my actions and responses also contribute to, and endorse, the social worlds created?'

Later in the therapeutic process, after another cry of frustration from Xander, we send a letter to the juvenile court. Xander's aim and hope was to give the judge a notion about what his mum meant and still means to him and how 'the missing' is devastating to him. Luckily, the judge was charmed by this letter and invited him for a conversation at his office. This didn't exactly bring the desired change in the situation as Xander did not obtain the permission to visit his mum (something he silently was hoping for) but it nevertheless gave him a sense of agency as his worries as well as his relational efforts were taken seriously by the judge.

Vikki Reynolds (2020) points out that we have the choice to situate the personal suffering in its socio-political context and resist the individualisation of suffering when there is structural oppression. In considering this choice I can ask myself 'What does "justice-doing" actually mean in these contexts?' in order not to reproduce practices of injustice (Reynolds, 2020; Afuape, 2011). In Reynolds's view, justice-doing goes beyond the scope of anti-oppressive practice, which aims not to replicate oppression, but entails actually being just and ethical with people, which requires engaging the activist project to transform the social contexts in which suffering and oppression occur, and to do this in ways led by persons with accountability to their communities.

After a few years enduring a lot of obstacles and problems, Xander still lives in a youngsters' home. Promises to live at home each time again were quashed by the juvenile judge because there was a relapse of his mum, new violence incidents in their partner relation, struggles in the institution etc. At the age of 15 he says, 'No one can understand what it means to live the life I have to live', and 'I can't stop the craving for living with my mum'. So I ask if it would make a difference for his life and himself if there were some people who would have a notion. As he thought it would make a huge difference, we decided to collect all the letters I wrote to him after each conversation, cut and pasted fragments, brought them together in a small book and chose a new name for himself in the book. We edited this book and added an envelope at the last page so people could respond to him after reading and resonating with the landscapes of his life. Our hope was that many people, especially carers got a different notion in relation to children and families in these contexts and maybe got inspired to relate in different ways. Xander never thought someone would buy this book, let alone that anyone would read it. In the meantime 900 books were sold and he received more than 50 letters. It encouraged him in writing rap songs and to edit his rap songs.

In a systemic view we shouldn't isolate or cut off our therapy room and our conversations with the child (and the carers) from the social world they are living in. The child has to live their life in their communities outside of the therapy room. So we have to be aware that everything spoken and thought of has to be linked with the people involved and their community. It has to be meaningful and appropriate in their daily life. So instead of feeling disconnected and maybe marginalised, we have to find ways to enhance a sense of belonging and this from a stance of 'justice-doing'.

Conclusions

The multitude of voices and agents that in one way or another are involved in the therapeutic processes, can urge us to act quickly, before we appreciate the complexity of the situation. Acting immediately is not to be confused with having a 'sense of agency', but rather the opposite. We tried to list some of the most important 'influences' we can meet when working with children and families in contexts of severe distress and painful life experiences. We hope to convince the reader to embrace this complexity. Acknowledging this complexity can help us to hold on to the belief that children are full agents, although their sense of agency is often lost to themselves. It can also prevent us falling into one of two extremes, for instance on the one hand focusing on deficits, and what is wrong versus on the other hand engaging optimistically, with the strengths of the child, or of other members of the network. The aim is to stay connected with the first-person perspective of the child and to remain aware that children, and the people who are involved or care for them, are always engaged in relationships of interdependence.

Although a child is not just a passive receiver of what is happening in their world and their relationships, their actions and responses are often no longer seen as valuable, communicational and relational involvements. Before we know it, we no longer approach them as active participants in the whole meaning-making process. What is more, an outsider's perspective is taken that removes us from the first person's perspective of the child and the people involved.

Getting lost in the complexity and the multiple interwoven obstacles and problems, our attempts to regain a sense of grip can force us to simplify the world and to get caught up in single stories. We are moved away from the versality, multiplicity and diversity of their world and the dynamic layering of meaning-making processes in a multitude of contexts.

Chapter 2

A collaborative therapeutic journey

Children and the many people involved are interwoven in a network of continuous, mutual influences and exchanges. In order to notice and take disadvantages and relational commitments seriously, we take a collaborative stance. Our compass consists of a systemic and narrative approach, but also draws on research on resilience and resilience processes. As we strive for experiences and discoveries that regain and enhance a sense of agency, of belonging and of coherence, we stress that this journey should not be a *dyadic* quest of a therapist and a child insulated from their lifeworld. On the contrary, we need to keep in mind all involved. The importance of a working alliance and therapy with all the significant people as a collective journey cannot be underestimated. Subsequently, we introduce serious playfulness and playful seriousness as a strong force throughout our therapeutic journeys that provides a powerful antidote to the tentacles of adverse childhood experiences. This playfulness can also open new ways in sharing stories and conversational settings. Finally, but perhaps most importantly, we show the importance of weaving networks of mutual support and solidarity through the whole journey as networking resilience.

An insider's perspective

Among the multitude of voices, those of the children in the first place and others directly involved are in danger of not being heard or listened to. Because we do not want to repeat what has already happened, namely that their experiences, perception and view were not noticed, or were rejected, we try to bring their story to the foreground. We are inspired by Mullender et al. (2002) who argued that in the context of domestic violence, we should do research *with* children rather than conducting research *about* children. This means taking children, their families and carers seriously, seeking to understand children as people in their own right, acknowledging children as actors in the social contexts of their own lives, acknowledging children as playing a role in society as a whole and conceptualising children as having their own life arenas, their own concepts and their own use of time.

After the first conversation with Xander and his carers, I wrote him a letter, documenting his worries, relational involvements, the disadvantages in his life, etc.

DOI: 10.4324/9781003167860-3

I put it in an envelope, put a stamp on it and sent it to Xander at the children's home. (Children in care seldom receive post, except letters from youth court often announcing that their placement is extended.)

Ghent, 2nd of May,

Hello Xander,

As promised, I write you a letter. You liked to have our conversation on paper so you can keep up what we discuss. Maybe you will show this letter to the juvenile judge so he knows what is important to you.

Monday evening you came with David, your mentor and Stacey, the psychologist. You told me what in the previous months happened to you. Many things felt 'heavy'. You still find them awful. They make you sad and angry at the same time. It even makes you cry the whole day and bang your head.

Being placed in a children's home by the judge is the worst thing they could ever do. You know exactly how many days and nights you are already there (2 months and 28 days). This means you can't see your mum and you miss her enormously. The children in the group are quarrelling all the time. This makes it very busy in your head.

You can't sleep well because your mum is also all the time in your head. Sometimes you have a 'lucky day' but at night the nightmares can come and spoil this lucky day. In some of the horrible nightmares you can't find your mum! She is surrounded by doubles and you can't track down who your real mum is. You also get crazy by promises that aren't kept.

Xander, these dreams seemed to tell how important your mum is to you. You explained how important you are to her. You are a son that helped already a lot. You can comfort her by sitting next to her but also by ensuring she doesn't drink too much.

I was really impressed how you keep an eye on everything. You clearly see the difference between water and vodka, even if your stepfather tries to reassure you it's water. Emptying bottles while they are sleeping is just one of your attempts to make your mum drink less. Maybe this also shows much courage. Knowing that your mum has an implant, reassures you. When she got Antabuse in the form of a pill she sometimes kept drinking.

You told me your mum hadn't had an easy life. She comes from Romania and has no family over here. Only by the phone you sometimes hear your grandparents. You visited them long ago. When your mum was 17 she ran away from home to Amsterdam. Later she came to Brussels and met your father. Your mum told that there happened bad things at that time. She always tried to protect you. Your second stepfather was not good either. Dirk, your current stepfather, you find the best of them all, also to your mum.

Your mum has a lot of depressions and borderline. You don't trust the doctors who told this because they gave her medication that isn't helpful. It makes you sad that Dirk and your mum had such a big fight that your mum ended up in the hospital. You really hope that everything will be fine. Despite the difficulties you still love your mum. You had already many good moments. You want to go home as quickly as possible but don't know what exactly you have to do. First they said: 'Listen to the judge', than they said: 'Stay calm', but none of this makes a difference. This makes you worry a lot. Everyone is in charge of you and even when you try hard to do your best, nothing changes.

Many people say you are too mature for your age. You noticed that this can be true. You can take care of yourself like cooking an egg or do shopping. Despite these skills and knowledge people also say you are too small and immature to deal with all the difficulties. You have to learn to make friends and play with peers. Most of them you find just stupid.

When I asked what your mum would wish for you when you are grown up, a whole list appeared. She says regularly:

- *Don't do the same as us.*
- *Choose a good partner.*
- *Don't do stupidities and don't become depressed.*
- *Try to have fun in life and be happy.*

Writing this down I was wondering if you know what to do now to become happy later? Is this something we have to talk about later?

The sadness and the tears, you can't just stop them. Each time you have to think of your mum they pop up. These tears accompany you already for ages. Luckily there are sometimes the lucky days. When people say 'Stay strong!', it goes in one ear and out the other ear but it keeps a little bit hanging in your head. It is one of the small things that sometimes helps. Mary, the lady of the shop at the caravan park, knows best how to deal with this sadness. We decided to talk at a later moment a bit more about this ongoing sadness because each time we started to talk about it the tears took it over.

At the end of our conversation we asked David and Stacey what touched them in your story. They both were impressed by your thoughtful acts of caring towards your mum. It gave them a better understanding of how important she is to you and how much you miss her.

Xander, we agreed to meet again within two weeks. Just let me know if I have forgotten important things in this letter or didn't accurately reflect what you told. In the meanwhile I hope there are some 'lucky' days and that things go better with your mum.

Warmly,
Sabine Vermeire (2015)

Children and families in contexts of adversity need to be listened to carefully and meticulously. The impact and effects of the painful experiences cannot be simply known nor named from the outside and from the outset. What exactly is traumatic and what will be considered traumatic is embedded in a multitude of dialogues and dynamic reciprocal contextual influences (Decraemer, 2010). The painful events and their meanings at the time become intertwined with many exchanges and experiences later and now in a continuous process of meaning-making. Traumatic events can colour subsequent events and vice versa. Likewise the 'zeitgeist' and larger socio-cultural attitudes continually influence our modes of understanding. This means each time we have to step in dialogues in which we become co-researchers unravelling trauma and its effects.

A systemic and narrative approach

According to World Health Organisation 'Adverse Childhood Experiences' (ACEs) are defined operationally as childhood events, varying in severity and often chronic, occurring in a child's family or social environment that cause harm or distress, thereby disrupting the child's physical or psychological health and development. Physical, emotional and sexual abuse, neglect, household challenges like substance misuse, mental illness, domestic violence, etc., and other adversities like bullying, community violence, natural disasters are all types of adverse childhood experiences. Research shows that experiencing a higher number of ACEs can increase the risk for disease, early death and poor social outcomes. In general, in the Western world around 10 per cent of the population comes into contact with four or more ACEs and 3 per cent of the children have to deal with serious forms of child abuse. We can say that this is a global social health problem and that everyone is affected by it, directly or indirectly.

From a systemic point of view, we try to understand traumatic experiences, profound life events and their effects in the interconnectedness between a child and their relational and social worlds. In these complex mutual exchanges all kinds of experiences originate, persist or disappear. What people do, say, think, feel and refrain from doing, or saying, constantly influences others and vice versa and is always embedded in a multiplicity of contexts. Bateson's famous dictum is still worth referring to: '*Without context, words and actions have no meaning at all*' (Bateson, 1979, p. 15). Bateson and his co-researchers, very early in the history of systemic therapy, substituted information for energy (Ruesch and Bateson, 1951; Watzlawick et al., 1967). This was an important step, that allowed practitioners to take a less mechanistic and intrapsychic view of psychological suffering. Moreover, they emphasised the importance of the body and body language in communication. Afterwards other systemic practitioners substituted interpretation and ways of understanding for information (Mattheeuws, 1977; White & Epston, 1990; McNamee & Gergen, 1992). In this 'interpretative' account, A's behaviour doesn't cause a reaction in B, neither is it a message that contains information, but B interprets whatever A does or refrains from doing, whenever they are together. This interpretative stance means that verbal as well as non-verbal communication is consequential, context-related, multilayered and multiple-interpretable (Wasserman & Fisher-Yoshida, 2017). Pearce and Cronen (1980) stressed that interpretation, or meaning, stands in a reflexive relation to action and that its participants recursively create relational or interactional patterns, constructive as well as unhelpful, that can become very hard to defy, or to change for the better. I will sometimes refer to such patterns as relational dances. White and Epston (1990) took the narrative or story as the most important frame for people to understand their lives (Bruner, 1986). Their account stories, however, not only contribute to understanding what happened and happens or to predicting what is going to happen but are also constitutive of lives (White & Epston, 1990; McNamee & Gergen, 1992).

In more recent years, systemic therapy has paid more attention to people as embodied beings and to emotions as relational and contextual (Fredman, 2004). Influenced by enactivism, the focus shifted also to the interplay between bodies and objects, emotions and meanings. For example, during play, this point of view can lead to an openness on the side of therapist and clients alike for the emergence of new meanings and actions (Rucinska & Reijmers, 2014).

Last but not least, in systemic therapy, there was an early interest and involvement in the real social conditions of people (e.g., Minuchin, 1967). In addition to the influence of the many ongoing interpersonal influences, larger influencing systems and structures were also taken into account. Some were inspired by the French philosopher Foucault (1980, 2007), others by the social psychologist Moscovici (1984). It soon became clear that the many complex circuits of influence are neither neutral nor equivalent and power dynamics are always present (Foucault, 1980; Dell, 1989). The plea for practices that pay attention to both influence and power also resonates with the increasing demand to do justice to people's dignity and experiences (Afuape, 2011; Reynolds, 2012; McCarthy & Simon, 2016; Audet & Paré, 2018).

Although all these meaning-giving contexts are interwoven and influencing, in our therapeutic journey and conversation we always have to start somewhere without being ensured of a good outcome. From a systemic perspective it is considered impossible for a therapist to have an overview and 'knowledge from outside'. It requires repeatedly looking, reflecting and negotiating together in therapy which contexts and relationships we should highlight and take as our starting point. It is impossible to know in advance what meanings/actions will be subscribed to or undertaken, will shift or be newly developed. This means it is necessary to continuously assess throughout our journey whether things change in more hopeful directions, or whether the sessions unintentionally sustain unhelpful relational dances and narratives.

As systemic practitioners we resist the tendency of individualising traumatic experiences by disconnecting a person from the people and communities they belong to. Instead, as systemic therapists, we embrace the multiplicity of contexts and social worlds children and families inhabit. This applies both to how we look at problems and to ways of dealing with them. We treat children, youngsters and their families not as passive receivers of what happens in their lives while we do recognise and acknowledge that their sense of agency has often decreased. We widen the scope to include more than what is wrong and what supposedly causes the problems.

We can consider adverse childhood and traumatic experiences as wounds in what children hold precious in their relationships, communities and life (Sheinberg & Fraenkel, 2001; Weingarten, 2003; Reynolds, 2020). The body, the mind, the spirit and relationships with others can be hurt (Walsh, 2007). These experiences can affect the child's physical, emotional, psychological and relational well-being and their sense of continuity and coherence, but also of the people involved and even their communities. The connectedness with what matters, who matters and the community gets disrupted. In other words, these experiences and their impact affect a sense of agency, a sense of belonging and a sense of coherence.

The adverse effects interact with each other in a complex way and mutually influence each other and undermine the child's sense of self-worth. These children, birth families and carers are often stuck in single stories and solidified meanings about their experiences, relationships and lives. They tried to interpret and make sense of what happened. The construction of these stories and narratives is always embedded in many ongoing interpersonal dialogues and broader social, cultural narratives. Many ideas about the adverse childhood experiences, the child and their family circulate, some endorse the single stories, others contradict them or do not take them seriously and reject them. It is important to keep in mind that these ideas are informed by social discourses about trauma, victimhood, family relations and so on.

When the multiplicity and fluidity of meaning in different contexts becomes obscured the child or youngster can become isolated and alienated from their families, significant people, peer groups and their communities.

What creates well-being?

From a systemic and narrative stance, we can look at well-being and enhancing well-being as an ongoing dialogue in which children, their families and carers can be understood and understand themselves in a multiplicity of contexts and are able to situate their experiences and themselves in a frame of interconnectedness. In doing so they no longer understand their experiences, their relationships and themselves in one single, solidified story but in a multiplicity of stories. In this account it also makes a difference if children and families still have a sense of agency, mattering and belonging and at the same time having the experience of being able and allowed to differ from others. The experience of being able to make choices, or having the opportunity to relate to what is important to themselves and their loved ones, is considered helpful.

Well-being also depends on whether people can position themselves in relation to the multiplicity of voices, social representations and discourses or rather experience being in the grip of, or even imprisoned by, these discourses. Experiencing themselves as having ways to bear the complexity of life with its paradoxes, ambivalences, constraints and dilemmas makes it possible to carry on with their lives (https://interactie-academie.be/over-ons).

A systemic therapeutic practice is always situated in the social, cultural, political and economic fabric and zeitgeist. Ideas and beliefs of what creates well-being are constantly (re-)negotiated in society and differ from one period of time to another and from one place to another. Regarding trauma, for a long time the focus has been on stories of victimhood, on pathologising effects of trauma and on how an individual person succeeds (or not) to process traumatising experiences.

During the past decades the focus changed to incorporating the child as an active participant and a full agent and to resilience and resilience processes. In this book I will develop the idea that helping the child to 'process trauma', necessitates the traumatic experiences to be woven into the fabric of life. In collaboration with everyone involved, the focus is on the unravelling of these experiences and addressing their effects, situating them in a multiplicity of life events, and a multiplicity of storylines. The aim is to discover, or rather co-create, new and more liveable perspectives, and to help the child to position themselves differently, or relate in new ways to what has happened so new action can become visible.

In doing so, I follow the saying that many roads lead to Rome. I want to add that the road is not a straight highway. There are many points of departure, but also many places in or outside Rome that are worthwhile as temporary destinations. On this journey I hope to keep in mind the polyphony of significant voices. I will try to draw maximally on the potential healing power of relationships and communities, and thus work on creating networks of support and solidarity.

Resilience and resilience processes

Instead of getting trapped in a never-ending research of what causes pathology within the child and family we can also assume that the probability is high that children caught up in trauma and multi-stress life circumstances will present difficulties and get stuck in their relationships and life. This is consistent with the default position and research of Antonovsky (1987). He considered stress and illness as natural aspects of life and concentrated his research on the question 'What creates health?' instead of 'What creates pathology?' His research showed that besides general resources like intelligence, coping, social support and connection, cultural stability, material facilities, etc., an important resource turned out to be '*a sense of coherence*'. He conducted research with women who survived the Holocaust. One-third of these women succeeded in leading a normal, good life. The question that intrigued him: 'What makes that a part of them succeed to live a good life according to themselves instead of being in a bad condition?' Antonovsky conceived of '*a sense of coherence*' as a global orientation where someone has a strong faith in what happens in their life is comprehensible, manageable and meaningful. It is a way of looking at life and to successfully deal with the multiple life-stressors. (Re-)gaining a sense of coherence makes a significant contribution to health, mental well-being and quality of life and is said to have a greater impact than individual characteristics (Antonovsky, 1987; Eriksson & Lindstrom, 2007; Walsh, 2006).

Also, the Kauai longitudinal study of Werner (2005) is often cited to come to an understanding of resilience and resilience processes.

> In the Kauai study, a team of mental health workers, paediatricians, public health nurses, and social workers monitored the development of all children born on the island at ages 1, 2, 10, 18, 32, and 40 years. (...) Some 30% of the survivors (n =210) in our study population were born and raised in poverty, had experienced pre- or perinatal complications; lived in families troubled by chronic discord, divorce, or parental psychopathology; and were reared by mothers with less than 8 grades of education. Two-thirds of the children who had experienced four or more of such risk factors by age two developed learning or behaviour problems by age ten or had delinquency records and/or mental health problems by age 18. However, one out of three of these children grew into competent, confident and caring adults. They did not develop any behaviour or learning problems during childhood or adolescence. (...) Their educational and vocational accomplishment were equal to or even exceeded those of children who had grown up in more economically secure and stable home environments. Their very existence challenges the myth that a child who is a member of a so called 'high-risk' group is fated to become one of life's losers.
>
> (Werner, 2005, p.11)

Through this research three clusters of protective factors were identified: within the individual, in the family and in the community. Most of their findings have since been replicated in a number of longitudinal studies around the world—on the mainland in the U.S.A., and in Australia, New Zealand, Denmark, Sweden, Great Britain, and Germany (Werner, 2005). In all of these studies, one can discern a common core of individual dispositions and sources of social support that contribute to resilience. These protective buffers appear to make a more significant impact on the life course of individuals who thrive despite adversity than do specific risk factors and stressful life events, and they transcend ethnic and social class boundaries.

Resilience has become an important concept in mental health theory and research. Early studies focused on personal traits for resilience or hardiness, reflecting the dominant cultural ethos of the rugged individual. Later on, resilience came to be viewed in terms of an interplay of multiple risk and protective processes over time, involving individual, family and social cultural influences. Walsh (2003) defines resilience as the ability to withstand and rebound from disruptive life challenges. She makes an appeal to view resilience as relationally based instead of individually based. Her family resilience perspective, grounded in a systemic orientation, looks beyond the parent-child dyad to consider broader influences. Significant relationships with kin, intimate partners and mentors, such as coaches and teachers, who supported their efforts, believed in their potential and encouraged them to make the most of their lives proved to be crucial in the development of resilience.

Contextualising the distress and strong connections make a difference. This involves dynamic processes fostering positive adaptation (Luthar et al., 2000) and over time fostering the ability to 'struggle' well to surmount obstacles and go on with life. Ungar (2005) suggests a 'thick description' of resilience that reveals a seamless set of negotiations between individuals who take the initiative, and an environment with crisscrossing resources that impact one on the other in endless and unpredictable combinations.

According to Rutter (1999, p. 119) there is abundant evidence of the enormous variation in children's responses to such painful experiences always in an inter-play of multiple risk and protective processes over time, involving individual, family and larger socio-cultural influences. He offers interesting stepping stones for family therapists to enhance resilience processes as resilience may be strongly influenced by people's patterns of interpersonal relationships. He emphasises that the reduction of 'negative chain reactions' and an increase of 'positive chain reactions' influences the extent to which the effects of adversity persist over time. New experiences which open up opportunities can provide beneficial 'turning point' effects and although positive experiences in themselves do not exert much of a protective effect, they can be helpful if they serve to neutralise some risk factors. There are no universally effective coping strategies although there are certainly responses that tend to be maladaptive in their consequences. He also shows that the chain of resilient outcome is enhanced if there is a cognitive and affective processing of experiences. Finally, our attitudes to ourselves and our confidence in our ability to deal effectively with life challenges is likely to be influenced by how we coped with stress and challenges in the past.

Ungar (2005) emphasises that it is better to use 'looking for resilience' as a roadmap than a destiny. This means in the role as a therapist, the onus is on us to be continuously open to hearing about stories that create and sustain resilience without ignoring their suffering. We see resilience processes as a collective search for the co-creation and weaving of networks of resilience and hope, in contexts of adversity.

An invitation to collaborative practices

Children in contexts of domestic violence want to be seen as active participants Mullender et al. (2002) discovered. Their research shows that children want to be listened to and taken seriously. Noticing their efforts and coping strategies and valuing their involvement adds to the building of a working alliance. They also want to be actively involved in the process of finding solutions and taking decisions, without the burden of having to 'take decisions themselves'.

These children's and often their families' trust has been shaken or dam-aged. This means we have to allow for the child each time again to find out whether the relationship provides the necessary conditions for talking, acting or playing. We need to take their suspicions into account, acknowledge their hesitations or notice their dilemmas in stepping into this therapeutic journey. A humble stance towards their stories, their responses, skills and knowledge is recommended. Searching for resilience and creativity in relation to surviving in difficult emotional stressful situations seems to connect with what children themselves want (Moore & Bruna Sue, 2011). This also means approaching them as experts of their lives while being curious about their subjective experi-ences and understandings which is in alignment with Wilson's children focused practice (Wilson,1998) or Epston and White's (1992) externalising approach. Many researchers and practitioners in the field endorse the importance of build-ing strong relationships with these children and their parents or carers (Barratt & Lobatto, 2016; Vetere & Dowling, 2005). Only when parents, carers and children are confident that the therapist holds each of them in mind, a sense of 'being part of a team' will be established (Wilson, 2021).

This brings us to an important issue about the conversational setting in creating working alliances. Each conversational setting will create possibilities and limita-tions to collaborate, speak, explore and transform but will also be understood in a certain way by the child and other people involved. There can be some discomfort for children as well as for the parents or carers when everyone involved is present. Children are constantly monitoring the alliances in the room, and attempting to maintain a comfortable position of inclusion and working alliance with all parties (Lobatto, 2002; Rober, 2014). There can be children's concerns about the reac-tions of other members to what they are telling, worries about marginalisation of parents' needs, remaining stuck in being 'the problem-carrier', etc.

Based on children's experiences, the idea of the family therapy encounter as a kind of therapeutic circle in which different participants manoeuvre in and out of the circle, can be very helpful (Lobatto, 2002). If children feel ignored or judged as inadequate in front of their family their working alliance with the therapist is faltering. If their position is validated by the therapist and family then their alliances with all parties are strengthened. This counts as well for the parents or carers. The negotiation of each person's position in this circle is an ongoing dynamic process that can even be seen as an important part of the thera-peutic process itself in which each participant is invited to be actively involved. This ongoing negotiation also concerns the choice of our conversational set-tings. Building a strong working alliance requires that we negotiate carefully when, why, how and for what reason we speak with the child or parents or car-ers alone, or with several people involved together. Through our journey, also reflecting on playfully changing settings that can bring movement in meaning can be important. Issues about safety and what happens with the spoken words or stories told will have to be taken into account and discussed in all these dif-ferent settings.

As the child is embedded in a web of relationships, we also have to include all the other important people and institutional representatives. This means making room for each one's main worries, expectations and hopes. In doing so we facilitate their collaboration and invite them to reflect on their possible contribution. We have to weave networks of collaborative relationships not only with the child and its network but also between them. Lang and McAdam (2001) insist on weaving networks of care and Fredman (2014) calls them networks of hope. By weaving textured networks of relationships that connect clients, as threads, with people in their resource-full community, energy and creativity between people can be generated and antidotes to demoralisation offered (Fredman, 2014). From the very first moment we create a context that enhances, for the child and family, a sense of putting our shoulders to the wheel all together in solidarity.

Van Hennik (2021) makes a plea to conceive of the therapist as practitioner who at the same time acts as researcher together with the clients as co-researchers. The output of research is input for therapy in the 'collaborative learning community' constituted together, something that is also emphasised by Lang and McAdam (2001). Research on what works in therapy (Duncan & Miller, 2010) indicates that the extent to which clients are actively involved in the therapeutic process is a significant determinant of the outcome. This makes the quality of our collaboration an important factor and stresses the need to introduce a culture of feedback from the very beginning of the therapy (Rober et al., 2021).

Safe grounds

Children and families in these multi-stress contexts are desperately trying to keep their heads above water in a swirling river of emotional turmoil. They kick around, lose all sense of agency and sometimes have no idea where they are or who they are. Their responses to the traumatic experiences or perceived unsafe contexts sometimes take over. Wetting their pants, encopresis, nightmares, panic attacks, tics, endless black thoughts, etc., can become shameful, unpredictable actions of the body and leave the child with an even greater sense of being out of control.

In order to deal with these effects and responses differently, we will need to find ways to help them, onto the river bank and onto safe, solid ground. A position on the riverbank can help to ease the constant state of alertness, but also makes it easier to look at the river with its obstacles, constraints and difficulties (Kaseke, 2010). Looking at, and trying to make sense of, painful events in relationships is easier when one is not constantly struggling to keep one's head above water. So, an important goal will be to gather small islands or safe ground to stand on together. From the very beginning, therefore, we look for constructive relationships, safe territories and territories of resilience (Rober, 1999; Wilson, 2007; White, 2006a), which include stories of life domains and relational contexts in which the children are not defined by their painful life histories, but in which they appear as active participants in their own lives and relationships (Vermeire, 2020).

Once established, safe grounds also provide places to return to when things start to feel unsafe and unpredictable again. Every step we take can activate a sense of insecurity. We do not so much need an attitude that tries to prevent each enactment of 'unsafety' but rather one that is reassuring that I can handle uncertainty or won't be blown away by feelings of insecurity and that we will find ways to go on. These safe grounds also allow some 'courage' in which we commit ourselves to ask the questions that need to be asked even though they may sometimes be difficult or challenging (Arao & Clemens, 2013).

Re(dis)covering a sense of personal agency

Apart from creating safe grounds, another important condition to fulfil is that our therapeutic efforts always (try to) enhance a sense of agency, which children (and people involved) in the contexts of complex trauma and violence, often have lost.

> A sense of personal agency is the sense of self that is associated with the perception that one is able to intervene in one's own life as an agent of what gives value to and as an agent of one's own intentions, and a sense that the world is at least minimally responsive to the fact of one's existence.
>
> (White, 2006a, p. 150)

White stresses the critical importance of restoration and/or developing this sense of personal agency in work with children who have been subject to trauma as it offers an antidote to the ideas and representations that one is no more than a passive recipient of life's contingencies. Focusing on reconnecting children as agents to their intentions, dreams, values and so on, in an ongoing dialogue with the people and community around them can offer stepping stones to generate new meanings that can lead to more fulfilling actions. Also Van der Kolk (2014) notices that acquiring a sense of agency means discovering what makes them (and others) feel bad and that their actions can change how they feel and how others respond. They learn that they can play an active role when faced with difficult situations.

Social sharing of experiences, emotions and stories

The author David Grossman expressed how important it was to him to find language and words after the death of his son in the Israeli-Lebanese War: 'It is a relief and refreshing not being a product of one's fears and revengefulness'. He calls to not solidify in time and always find new words. It made it possible for him to return to life (Van Riet, 2020).

In our Western culture, children are often instructed to regulate their emotions as it is thought of as an individual process, although since Bowlby (1982) we know that emotion regulation requires interaction with attachment figures. So, it is better to think of it as a social process. The social sharing of emotions, research shows, is a necessary part of emotion regulation, not only in the case of children, but also in the case of adults for that matter (De Mol & Rimé, 2017; Rimé, 2009).

Our therapeutic environment should help children find language (verbal or non-verbal) that helps them to make sense of what happened, and to share these experiences with others. Often this kind of language, or the context to develop it, is lacking. This not only complicates the social sharing of emotions, but also children's inner dialogues, through which they try to make sense of what is happening around them, get stuck (Dallos, 2006). Children, as soon as they are able to, get involved in conversations about emotions with their parents. Depending on the support carers offer, they can learn to give meaning to their own feelings and those of others, and generate stories out of this. Research suggests that children's narrative skills develop differently in safe versus unsafe contexts (Dallos, 2005). In unsafe contexts it can be dangerous to talk about emotions or even express emotions, or it has been made clear to them that certain emotions are wrong.

Emma (17 years old) ended up in situations of sexual exploitation after a long history of violence and abuse in her family. I ask her what she is hoping for in our conversations. She explains she stopped feeling and thinking a long time ago and has no longer any idea of what to feel or think. Often she doesn't understand herself and her actions. People asked already so many times 'Why?', but she has no idea. For a long time 'revenge' seemed to be a good engine. After living in contexts of neglect and being bullied in school, she became a bully herself. She kicked against others and the world. Using drugs helped her to make it to the next day and abusing boys who crossed her path gave her, temporarily, a sense of power.

The co-creation of emotional language will be a necessary component of the therapeutic process, as it makes social sharing of emotions, experiences and stories possible, and helps to develop or discover new and alternative meanings. It will also be important not to limit ourselves to working with the child alone, but to also engage parents and carers, even siblings, peers, etc., in this co-creation process as they can likewise experience a lack of shared vocabulary or language. It can even open opportunities to inspire or help one another.

New relational dances

The effects of the traumatic experiences on children, their utterances of suffering, feelings of insecurity and not finding helpful responses of people involved put their relationships under high pressure. They often end up in painful dances with their parents and carers and this can easily infect many other relationships. As a sense of mattering consists of feeling valued and adding value (Prilleltensky, 2021; Beckers et al., 2021), children and carers become convinced that they can no longer make a difference in the relationship, that they don't matter to each other. They get caught in devilish spirals. They operate more and more from mutual negative internalisations about each other and get caught up by mutual 'misunderstandings'. Carers can become emotionally distanced from the child and the needs of the child are no longer noticed. The 'dialogue of care' is under pressure, and sometimes breaks down (Jakob, 2011). Hughes and Baylin (2012) even refer to 'blocked care' in some of these situations, which is seen as an emotional difficulty rooted in the parent's own attachment history and triggered by child behaviour (Beckers et al., 2021).

In the process of co-creation of language and sharing experiences and emotions, offering different ways of gathering, speaking and listening, we aim to create alternative relational dances between the child and people involved, so they can become supportive to each other. While doing so we develop alternative shared meaningful experiences in which the child, parents and carers get re-connected in more helpful ways. As each one involved has different experiences and understandings of what is going on, Priya Parker (2019) suggests creating new shared meaningful experiences across what she calls lines of difference. This process can be helpful in the reduction of negative chain reactions and even increase positive chain reactions.

Re(dis)covering a sense of relational agency

As painful experiences often happen in relation to the people who were supposed to take care of children, their trust in relationships is fundamentally hurt. Their parents or primary carers often struggle themselves with mental health problems, have themselves experienced trauma through life or live in socio-economic or cultural circumstances that do not leave much room for the child and their needs. The relationships between children and parents or carers can become characterised by uncertainty and unpredictability.

Although these relationships get injured, these children often stay very loyal to their parents or carers. In many of these contexts they don't just have negative experiences with their primary carers or family members. Sometimes the parent or carer who does harmful things is also a wonderful playmate, someone who stands up for them or takes care of them in particular situations. These different aspects of the same person can evoke feelings of ambivalence and confusion. They sometimes notice the struggles and efforts of their parents, try to help them out, and themselves feel powerless.

De Mol et al. (2018) emphasise that in close relationships *a sense of relational agency* is a necessary condition in order to experience intimacy and connection. From their viewpoint, a person's sense of relational agency is constantly constructed through experiences of having relational influence on others and being relationally influenced by them. What we do (and refrain from doing) is meaningful to others and what others do (and refrain from doing) is meaningful to us (see also Anderson & Gehart, 2007). A *sense of relational agency* arises when people realise that they still have relational influence on others and others on them; this influence can be intentional as well as non-intentional. When children no longer experience that they make a difference in the relationship and can be meaningful to the other, themselves and the relationship, this has an impact on their sense of well-being and self-image. The experience and especially the acknowledgement of the experience that a person can please another person or have an influence that is constructive for that other person is of vital importance for the development of a positive identity, self-confidence and a satisfying relationship. In order to experience themselves as relational agents, we have to (re-)embed children, family members and carers in their relational contexts.

Their mutual actions of relational involvement and the relational invitations of the children in relation to their parents or carers often don't get noticed or aren't interpreted as efforts in the relationship. As they no longer have a sense of being meaningful or make a valuable contribution in the relationship, their sense of relational agency decreases.

When children or youngsters are referred for therapy, it often means that parents, carers as well as the child have lost their sense of relational agency and feel alienated from the child. They no longer notice that they make a valuable contribution in the life of the child. This means we have to engage them in the whole process and making room for their worries, concerns, disadvantages, etc. Fostering good relations and caring for 'the parents and carers' is an important aspect in enhancing their sense of relational agency (Richardson et al., 2016).

And, in fact, the same goes for the professional networks, including social institutions such as the youth court, as they can also experience a loss of a sense of relational agency. That's why I strongly believe that investing in the re(dis) covering of a sense of relational agency will be paramount to realise the therapeutic goals.

Re(dis)covering a sense of coherence

Xander tries to explain that his mum is ill because his dad was a kind of monster. His dad almost killed them both. He tried to help his mum but not enough. Sometimes he was playing at the caravan park and didn't take care enough of his mum. He made her worry about him. Maybe he was too much of a troublemaker. Without him she might not be in the hospital. While listening to his explanations and his ways of making meaning out of what happened, I hear between the lines that also feelings and convictions of guilt and shame are nestled in his mind and heart.

Before they came to therapy, the people concerned (as well as the child themselves) tried to make sense of what happened and tried to find out how to understand the problematic behaviour, the overwhelming emotions or the unpredictable ways of relating to others. Thin, often single descriptions about their life, the harmful events, their relationships, their identities and simple linear causal explanations about the problems are presented. Many non-traumatic experiences, constructive relationships and the complexity, ambivalence and contradictions of what happened shift to the background. These children and family members themselves often have solidified stories lacking nuance. In contexts of trauma, simplified explanations can affect their sense of self-worth, induce self-destructive actions like self-harming or increase their negative feelings towards the people around them and the world.

It is because I didn't eat my food properly. It is because we are Muslim and don't fit in this community. It is because my dad hates me.

Carter and McGoldrick (2004) point out that children, youngsters and family members during critical moments or after critical periods can be frozen in time. Some just live in the moment itself, without any connection with the past or future. Others get so preoccupied by the past or focused on future goals that they aren't able to live in the here and now. They try to escape from the past by disconnecting from painful relationships or certain aspects of their history.

Research shows that insecurely attached children often have incoherent (shredded, reduced or unfinished) stories about their history, their family, themselves and their relationships (Byng-Hall, 1995; Walsh, 2006). They lack cohesion and overview. Past experiences seem detached and disconnected. Richardson et al. (2016) emphasise the vital importance of a developmental story of one's life for young people in care, but the immediate network of family to provide a reservoir of memories is often lacking.

The experiences of abuse, neglect or trauma affect their relationships. It is difficult to make sense of the contradictions of love and harm received from the person who perpetrated violence or was neglecting their needs. Questions often keep buzzing around, sometimes for years 'Why?', 'Why me?', 'What does this say about me?' and each time again they have to try to make sense of what happened and of the intimate injured relationships. How the outside world, carers and the care system view their parents or family members also affects how they understand and relate to their family. Children early on get a notion about what a good family should be. Realising that they are different influences how they think about themselves.

The experiences of maltreatment were often different for different family members. Byng-Hall (1995) underlines the importance of developing more coherent narratives about attachment in the family. This helps family members to empathise more accurately with each other's distress and so enable them to respond appropriately and more sensitively to each other's cues, including attachment cues, thus achieving an increase in what he calls interactional awareness. The idea is that the child and family members develop new understandings of what happened and no longer feel powerless or helpless. As such, enhancing a sense of coherence is an important aspect of building resilience (Walsh, 2006). Helping these children and their natural and professional networks requires finding ways to co-construct a sense of coherence.

Re(dis)covering a sense of belonging

Xander sometimes felt terribly ashamed when his mum and stepdad, in a state of intoxication, were singing and yelling at people on the bus. There was also a moment that naked pictures of his mum circulated on social media and one of his class mates had noticed this. These experiences made him speechless. He would have liked to disappear from this world.

As their world is narrowed and they no longer look around them they risk seeing themselves as the only persons on this planet struggling with these problems or being caught up in such painful relationships or life histories. They miss allies in their ongoing struggle. The many networks they are living in aren't felt as supportive. On the contrary, the people around them, agencies or institutes decide what has to be done and how it has to be done. They have no sense of control of what happens to them nor do they feel they themselves play an active role in the directions of their lives.

Their ways of trying to connect with the people around them (often from a suspicious stance) and their hard working to (re)gain a sense of mattering to, or belonging not only with their carers but also other people and peers aren't always considered appropriate or acceptable in the different life areas like the foster home or children's home, school, leisure clubs or neighbourhood. They often get into trouble. Previous experiences, communications and stories become history and context for next gatherings. Several doors are closed to them. They get insulated, disconnected from many people, family and peers and the world they inhabit. A sense of belonging gets lost.

Also, dominant discourses about what a family should be, can have a grip on them and can make them look upon themselves and their family as failing. Shame can inform their actions in school, leisure clubs and neighbourhood as they become anxious about what classmates might think. They often have no appropriate response to the questions they read in the eyes of classmates, peers. They sometimes make themselves invisible, become the clown in the classroom or start to protest.

Children and their families experience neglect, dismissal, humiliation or abuse as 'social wounds'. Care, attention, love and respect (positive social responses) assist people of all ages in filling their being with a sense of worth. Unfortunately, phenomena such as child abuse bring about social wounds in the networks and communities of the child that often leads to people distancing themselves from the child (Richardson & Wade, 2008). In order for the networks to be able to reconnect with the child and develop solidarity, care has to be taken of these 'social wounds'. This means we need to create conditions that allow for the development of solidarity. Involving networks can enhance their sense of belonging.

Hope as a door to possible futures

David Grossman said that hope is always a movement forwards: from a depressing, suffocating reality you throw an anchor to an imaginary future and when it's clamped down, you pull yourself, as a person or as society, towards that anchor. More important than this action is the awareness that you still can imagine yourself a future. That there still exists an enclave, free and not affected through the situation (Van Riet, 2020).

A final prerequisite for our therapies to be helpful, is that they 'do' hope. Walsh (2003) states that resilience has to be seen and understood as a process that can grow when hope and pain can be linked with each other within meaningful relationships. Both children and their carers move from hope to despair, and vice versa. It is important that we as therapists are aware of this, and that we can respond in ways that avoid the polarity between hope and despair. Particularly helpful is the idea of 'reasonable hope' as developed by Weingarten (2010, p. 7): 'Reasonable hope softens the polarity between hope and despair, hope and hopelessness and allows people to place themselves in the category of the hopeful'. Orienting ourselves towards the balance of hope in constellations of hope and hopelessness provides one compass point of therapeutic practice (Flaskas, 2007). Hope is to the spirit what oxygen is to the lungs (Walsh, 2003). It is a future-oriented belief: no matter how bleak the present, a better future can be envisioned. Hedtke (2014) states that hope is an active verb that refers to a process. It is an expression of agency in the face of significant challenges. By weaving stories that feature hope through their experiences and actions, a glimpse of a possible future arises.

Xander tells he had a secret place in a small grove at the end of the caravan park. He built a camp with sticks and sheets to take shelter when things got out of hand between his mum and stepfather. The idea that he could go and live there when things went all wrong, was a very reassuring thought and helped him to keep going on. He set up his shelter with pictures of exotic destinations and took care there were always cookies to survive for three days.

Serious playfulness and playful seriousness

Children have their own ways of expressing and sharing experiences. We can get 'stuck', literally and metaphorically, in the therapy room with children, youngsters and their family when we hold on to our traditional ideas of having conversations. Our predominant Western middle-class idea of how to conduct conversations entails a face-to-face contact, looking each other in the eye, talking (i.e., using verbal means), and so on. This puts high demands on the child when they want to talk about painful issues. In these contexts, children's stories are particularly vulnerable to colonisation and silencing (Smith & Nylund, 1997; Weingarten, 1998). Our meetings can get reduced to poor question-answer dialogues where nothing new is told or nothing new happens (Vermeire, 2017). Although research showed that special attention needs to be paid to the way these children are invited to therapy, noting their preference for a practitioner style that is creative, playful and enjoyable (Herring, 2021).

Geertz (1973) emphasises the necessity of making sense of other people's behaviour in terms of practices of their own culture rather than our own beliefs. Play and playfulness can be considered as an attitude for connecting the world of the adults, which is rich in abstract thoughts and words with the world of children, full of non-verbal expressions, actions and concrete images. It can bridge the differences in positions, roles, even power resources which are inevitably present. *While joining in children's activities and local practices such as cooking in the toy kitchen, fighting as mediaeval knights, doing sports and exercises, making music and writing rap songs or playing chess*, we can engage in dialogues in which we can explore their world in verbal as well as non-verbal communications together. We can comment and negotiate their reality, taking different stances, rejecting or confirming them and feeling connected in interaction. In doing so, we exchange perspectives while emotions, influences and identity descriptions are confirmed, ignored or denied (Rucinska & Reijmers, 2014). Joining in their language and world we meet their worries, problems, obstacles and challenges.

We need to take into account that children often have no words available to give voice to the unspeakable. Their bodies speak for them and react even quicker. Van der Kolk (2014) found that children in these contexts sometimes lose their curiosity about the world. Given the weight and severity that often characterise the stories about these children and the persistency that seems to be a mark of their problems, therapists need an approach that brings with it a certain lightness that can re-open the possibility for curiosity and reflection. This means a platform needs to be created from which child and therapist can discover and create new meanings instead of being imprisoned by problems and obstacles. This also means that we, ourselves, need an openness to, and curiosity for, what children (and people involved) bring to the therapy and conversations, just as we need an openness to whatever is present in the room and in the life of the child that can be helpful in creating possibilities for actions and ongoing dialogues.

Playfulness as an attitude

We conceive of playfulness as an attitude and atmosphere that allows us, together with children, youngsters and their families, to tinker, or to 'cook' with ingredients that are available, in order to create something new that makes a difference in their lives (Vermeire & Van den Berge, 2021). As Koestler points out, the results of creativity can be quite surprising:

> The creative act (…) does not create something out of nothing; it uncovers, selects, re-shuffles, combines, synthesizes already existing facts, ideas, faculties, skills. The more familiar the parts, the more striking the new whole.
>
> (1964, p. 120)

At each stage in the meeting and throughout the whole therapeutic process we can look for stepping stones to creativity or 'disciplined improvisation' (Madsen & Gillespie, 2014). We try to collaborate with their local words, local language and meanings or we try to co-create ways of expressing that fit with their local practices (Vermeire & Van den Berge, 2021). This means we sometimes postpone, put aside or even become irreverent towards more traditional ideas and pathways of doing therapy with children, families and their networks (Cecchin, 1987; Cecchin et al., 1992; Wilson, 2007).

Taking such a playful approach can be quite a challenge. As a psychotherapy trainer, I sometimes invite trainees to look at a taped conversation with a five-year-old boy playing with animal toys and in conversation with the camerawoman. I ask them to look closely and be attentive to what comes into their minds.

The boy is sitting on the floor surrounded by animal toys. He holds two adult hippos in his hand and puts each at one side of a line he has drawn on the floor. Next to each hippo he adds a little 'child' hippo. While setting this scenery he explains to me, the camerawoman, that one child hippo lives with his mum and the other with his dad. The line is important because mums nor dads are not allowed to cross this line. Only the children's hippos have sometimes permission. When I ask 'why?', he responds immediately: 'This is the rule! Otherwise mums and dads start to fight and dads are much stronger than mums'. With a lot of noise and growling he demonstrates what such a fight looks like. The hippos start to bite, beat and kick each other. He also emphasises that sometimes little hippos can get hurt during such a fight and throws a little hippo through the air. He reassures me that the little hippo isn't crying when such a thing happens because he loves his dad.

After watching this small piece of play, I list all the reflections of the trainees on a whiteboard. Mostly words and ideas such as a divorce with high conflict, abuse, violence in the family appear on the board. Thoughts about the boy are often that he is quite aggressive, rather rigid or autistic in playing and maybe traumatised by the events in the family.

Afterwards I apologise for exploiting their taken-for-granted knowledge and ideas. Although this boy, who is actually my son, is in the meantime already 14 years old, I have no knowledge of violence in my family and my partner and I aren't divorced. After everyone has recovered from this little shock, I explain that my son from an early age on has been fascinated by documentaries about animals and in this recorded fragment we are engaged in a dialogue in which he, full of pride, demonstrates his knowledge about hippos and how hippos live. I even presume he tries to impress his mum and make her proud of him.

What fascinates me and what trainees take from this is how our attention is quickly focused on the child, the family and on what is problematic or 'wrong' with them. At the same time this focus makes us blind to many other contexts that can be relevant and expand our view. When I ask afterwards if someone noticed that the boy is wearing his pyjamas, that the house cat is passing by on the screen and that my son twice calls me mum, everyone is surprised.

Staying in playfulness and play in therapy can be quite a challenge. Rucinska and Reijmers (2014) point out that it can easily become an attempt to reveal or uncover 'hidden meanings', to find the right interpretation, or to explain certain behaviours as a discharging of emotions. They propose an understanding of play and playfulness as a dialogue that creates an embodied experience. They endorse a process-oriented interaction (not directed at a specific goal or result) with the hope of changing some of the child's perspectives and creating new meaning together. Play is a communication tool rather than an expression of thoughts and feelings.

Madsen (2007) pointed out that 'An attitude is an intervention'. This means that playfulness not only brings us together in new relational dances and new language games but it can also invite an atmosphere of movement and creativity that allows for new pathways to be discovered and new meanings to be co-created.

A letter from Victor addressed to his family and classmates (Vermeire et al., 2018).

Hello,

I am Victor and I am ten years old. I'd like to introduce you to Monsieur Anger. He is from Paris.

My Dad died a little while ago. He chose to stop living. A few days later I chose to stop crying. I tried my best to help my Mum and my little brothers.

And then ... Monsieur Anger appeared. And then more often! And then bigger and bigger!

I made Monsieur Anger in blue clay. He has short legs, however, he can charge in really quickly. When he is around, he won't leave. He doesn't have a good brain either because he makes me do stupid things like running away, hurting someone ... sometimes really badly ... And that gets me into fights with other people. The worst is fighting with Mum. It is so bad that sometimes he makes me cry. Luckily, he doesn't come to school. I don't want Monsieur Anger anymore!

I sent Monsieur Anger to Antarctica and put up lots of false signposts so he would get lost! But he came back ...

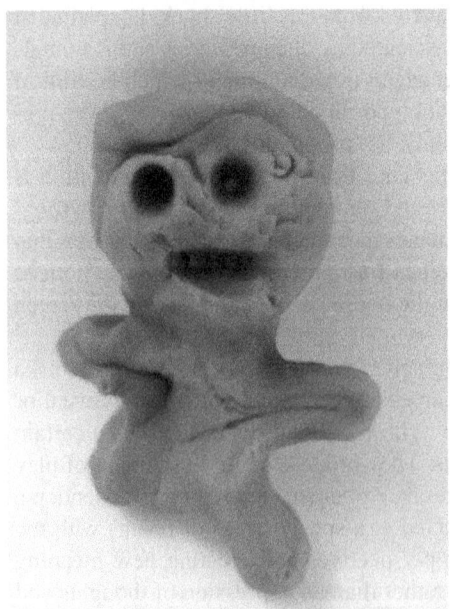

Figure 2.1 Purple clay figure. Photograph by the author.

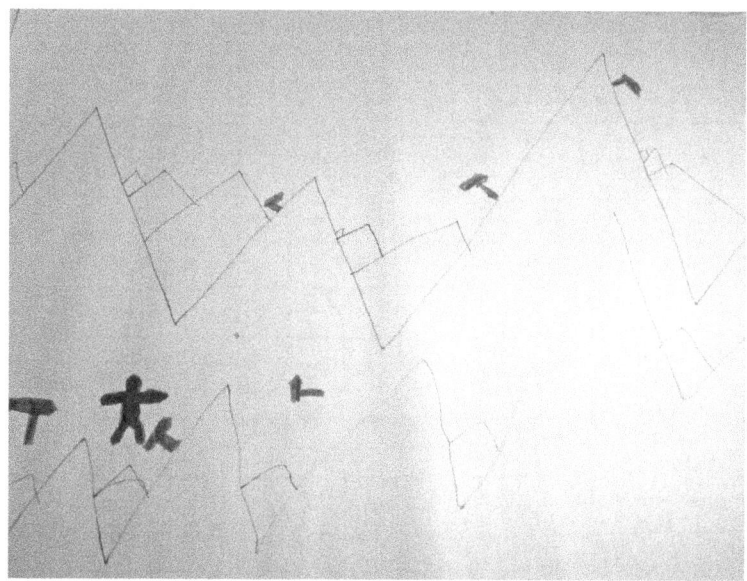

Figure 2.2 Drawing of mountains with signpost. Photograph by the author.

We looked at Monsieur Anger's family and we discovered that his Mum is Mrs Disillusionment and his Dad is Mr Disappointment ... and he has a little sister, Miss Sadness. They all live together under the Eiffel Tower.

In the meantime, my Mum and I have decided to work together to make sure that Monsieur Anger doesn't get a chance to grow that big again. We are taking good care of his little sister, Miss Sadness!

By inviting playfulness in conversations and conversational settings we open up a space for different ways of talking and relating, which is in line with Hughes's PACE (Playfulness, Acceptance, Curiosity, Empathy) (2007). Through playfulness we can find some light points in the darkness, the dark thoughts and feelings (Marsten et al., 2017). That means not just looking in places and directions we are used to, but taking other, alternative entrances together to go on a more adventurous journey with all kinds of side paths and surprising companions, and with an open ending.

Over the years we invited fairy tale characters such as Mowgli and Simba to our meetings but also Messi, Beyoncé, Spiderman and cuddly bears to enhance polyphony. They became interesting inspirators and advisors but also persons through which we can ask questions, through which the child can tell stories in a manageable and new way and vice versa. We offered a chair to a beloved deceased nanny to ask reflections about what she appreciates about the child. We literally went on a quest for the lost prince and climbed a 'mountain' to have a new viewpoint on the situation and restoke hope. Even actually hammering

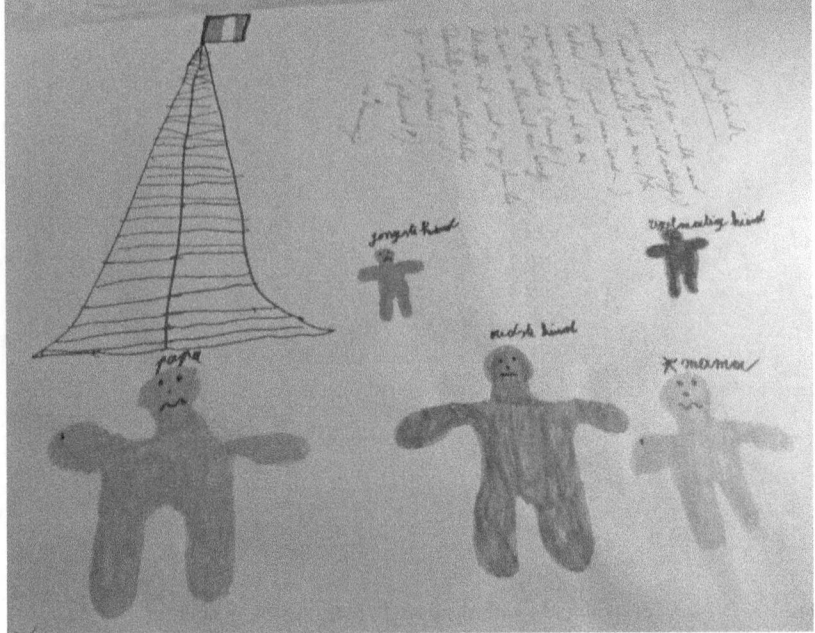

Figure 2.3 Drawing of five figures under the Eiffel Tower. Photograph by the author.

together a boat to travel to safer places and reflect upon what has to be taken in our suitcase opened new directions for conversations and connection. We wrote in moments of despair letters to Santa Claus with special request and send a questionnaire to the queen of Belgium, the judge and children-experts-by-experience.

We propose a rather kaleidoscopic take on playfulness. We allow for, and stimulate, a freedom of movement, that is not only a movement of our bodies but also of our thoughts and feelings. We let go of the reins of language rules and the expectations that are associated with these rules. We aim for a 'language in action' that can open a theatre of possibilities (Wilson, 2005).

Doorways to imagination

Sometimes life events are too horrific, too painful to be simply told and shared in an ordinary conversation. Denborough (2008) noticed for instance that people who experienced hardship often speak of themselves in the third person to create a distance between them and the events. *Playing puppet plays, creating drama performances or theatre plays, songs, films, graphic novels, ... can also offer a pathway to tell the stories they want to tell in an indirect, manageable way.* It also opens the possibility to share experiences and stories and bring insider knowledge into the world in ways that it can be listened to. While creating such a project they can also envision and imagine possible futures. Certainly, when daily life experiences become too hard, too painful it can offer shelter, support and hope.

An invitation to change roles and positions can open surprising perspectives on the world, their relations, themselves or the problems. *One moment I can become a philosopher and the next a king while the child can jump from the table as a super hero and land as a dancing queen.* From these different positions, questions may be asked and answers given that otherwise feel too unsafe or are too vulnerable to express. In a jointly created context and dialogue, we can play, explore and practice what is not yet shared or what actions might mean. It can also create wonder, away from the 'right' answer or the 'truth', so that perhaps new answers to questions can be found, not necessarily according to Western rational logic.

While playing with the frames of what is called 'reality', 'play', 'fantasy', we can create shared words, shared language that open doors to our imagination and vice versa. In an ongoing interplay imagination, mind and actions get stretched and enlarged. Something unthinkable can become thinkable again. Although we aren't exactly magicians in a playful world, magic ideas, imagination and actions can truly be gateways to real life. We can as an example look sceptically at rain dancing (Breeuwsma, 2001). From a Western rational point of view, we can argue that these dances won't make it more probable that rain will fall but for the insiders it is probably more about symbolising an important event that expresses a value, a relational and community commitment.

- *'The Huge Dark-Dark-Black Fear of Death' started to come sneaky at night in Jim's bedroom after his mum stepped out of life. After being reassured that the love of his mum was still around, he decided no longer to allow himself to be overwhelmed by the scaredness. Together with his dad, he burned the painting of this monstrous fear in the garden. The collective burning ritual seemed to be very effective. It didn't resolve all pain nor problems but enhanced sharing emotions through shared new experiences.*
- *Aisha learned from her mother a Somalian incantation that brings peace and helped her going on through hardship. At a certain point in her life she ended up in a situation of sexual exploitation. After a long journey of troubles we invited, together with her sister, a Somalian priest to help us to fulfil the incantation ritual in her new little flat.*
- *Robin and his father made on the top floor of his school an eagle's nest to observe the playground and find answers to the bullies in the classroom. He had been beaten up by two boys and had refused to go to school any longer.*

Playfulness becomes an invitation to engage in new images, new words and new ways of responding and of sharing experiences. Like Sen (2018) invites us to see depression not as 'dementors', the soul-sucking dark creatures from the Harry Potter books, but to cast a 'Riddikulus spell' on them and turn them into shape-shifting and funnily exaggerated Boggarts. By unravelling concepts and ideas in unexpected ways we can discover and collect new, alternative perspectives, re-position ourselves or obtain wisdom. Being on a joint quest enhances our collaboration with children, also youngsters in cooperation with the people involved. They appear more and more as skilled, creative thinkers, inventors and constructors. We can have a performance of new, alternative stories and identities.

Negotiating playfulness

Children themselves often invite us into playfulness. *A school bag, a KAA Ghent supporters scarf, an image on a T-shirt, music on a smartphone, … all can offer openings.* Just noticing what is present in the room or lays metaphorically in words can offer stepping stones. In contexts of hardship there is often hesitation to step into new ways of collaboration, so young children can be invited to playfulness by asking if they are into a game, something new or like to try something 'a little bit crazy'. Youngsters often get easily engaged by some teasing, challenging them a bit or just explaining it doesn't seem to be very helpful to do over and over again what they already tried so maybe they are up for something different. When conversations become too intensive and painful, offering an escape route by jumping into something more playful can be helpful to re-find safe ground. *Every time Toby reaches for the knight's sword, it is a signal that we have talked or 'worked' long enough. The unspoken deal is that we immediately start a fight with the swords.* Van Parys et al. (2014) found in interviews of children with parents struggling with mental health issues that an important aspect to keep going on is 'not dwelling on their own experiences', the problems and difficulties the whole time. Also in our meetings, moments and actions outside these difficulties have to be taken care of.

Leaving the well-trodden pathways, stepping into alternative, playful side paths as co-researchers is an ongoing process of negotiation of how we will collaborate together and try to do the work that has to be done. These negotiations don't just apply to the child or youngster but also to their carers and people involved. Sometimes we have to ask carers' permission to leave the traditional, well-known pathways in the conversation but at the same time bring the playfulness or alternative tracks in as something obvious, naturally that regularly happens in meetings with children, youngsters and their carers, so it doesn't become something that is experienced as extremely special. We don't want them to start to think of themselves as if they are such 'a special case' that needs such 'special methods' to be helped. It is neither hocus pocus, in which we have special knowledge or an all-seeing eye that can discover things that others can't notice. We have to be transparent about our intentions and hopes, the possibilities it holds. We can refer to the knowledge we have already collected with other children and families in walking these pathways.

We also have to reassure parents and carers that it isn't about creating a special, exceptional or exclusive relationship with the child in which we are able to realise where parents or carers failed. When the proposed playful directions and ways are too far away from the ways of their usual doing or being and remove or estrange them from their family, community or culture, we have to put it away and find more appropriate points of entry and pathways. Just like playfulness and creativity isn't a goal in itself. Our therapeutic journey remains a serious business, although when a smile may appear or there is room for a sparkle of humour, this means there is a crack in the darkness through which the light can come in.

Weaving networks of resilience

In recent years network-oriented working has skyrocketed. The idea 'It takes a village to raise a child' became very popular and it is nowadays taken-for-granted that everyone benefits from a network as it can be very helpful and supportive. Many therapeutic approaches in the context of adverse childhood experiences state the importance of a network (Jakob, 2011; Lang & McAdam, 2001; Madsen, 2014). Minuchin et al. (1998) claimed that 'networking' is the core of care as families can't function without networks, so we need to help families as widely as possible. Also Walsh (2007) emphasises that people need relational lifelines so they can go on after loss and trauma. This can be family members, people from the networks or community.

Minuchin (1967) argued to see the family as a resource for cure of the child instead of a source of pathology. I think this claim can be enlarged in many directions. Not only the family can be a valuable resource but many different people and networks can be engaged as resources. But even more important is not to invite or 'use' the network just to 'cure the child' because in this way we immediately frame the child as a passive victim or sick person who has to be cured. Lang and McAdam (2001) state the importance of networks of care instead of cure. These networks can form a protective shield (Richardson et al., 2016), a protective coat (Splingaer, 2020) and a ring of confidence (Guishard-Pine et al., 2007). Perry (2017, p. 280) even speaks of a 'therapeutic web of relationships' that can be created. While Madigan and Epston (1998) plead for communities of concern where networks of clients can provide consultation, information, support, etc.

Creating networks for the child can be expanded to creating networks for the people involved. One of my colleagues, Willem Beckers (2016), also states the importance of organising networks of support for the parents, carers and professionals working in these contexts. '*It takes a village to support the parents (carers) to raise a child*' is an idea to bear in mind when developing these networks in the therapeutic process. 'Fostering good relationships', enhancing a sense of partnership and relational agency in the network of parents, carers and professionals can create a 'protective shield' from unnecessary deterioration of the child's problems (Richardson et al., 2016).

The (family) relationships are sometimes so under pressure, rejected or cut off that the network is very thin or ends up in the same diabolical spirals over and over again. As the child as well as the parents, family or carers often get isolated in context of adversity, we often need to work together to (re-)build networks.

Certainly, when family relationships are injured, many constraints to (re)connect can get in the way. Children as well as family members will need support in overcoming these constraints (Jakob, 2011). We will have to examine together which networks and connections can be supportive and maybe restored but also which relationships can't be restored or have to be put 'on hold'.

In these multi-stressed contexts, networks are often introduced and engaged for the benefit of the child. Ideas of care can put us quickly into action: we try to map children's and families' networks and mobilise the appropriate network of support or care. Although these are valuable steps and interventions, troublesome effects can be created and opportunities missed. We run the risk that everyone is mobilised in functioning for the child, talking and organising 'over' the head of the child and sometimes slipping into 'pep talk' or unsolicited, well-intended advice. We don't conceive of the child as an active participant in this networking process, but mainly as needing support and help (Lobatto, 2021). The bidirectionality of relationships becomes obscured (De Mol & Buysse, 2008).

Focusing on reciprocity can have mutual valuable effects. '*It also takes children to raise a village*' can be a refreshing addition. When children are invited as co-directors in this 'networking', they can regain 'a sense of relational agency'. Certainly, when they start to notice that they still make a difference in the life of their parents, family, carers, peer group, the child as well as the network can (re-) experience that they matter to each other. Even alternative, meaningful ways of relinking can emerge. Resilience processes can be enhanced as well as a sense of relational agency for all the people involved. When children and their carers notice that they can act in a meaningful way to contribute to the lives of people in their network and community (De Mol et al., 2018) the first seeds can be planted to enhance a sense of being socially embedded and a sense of belonging.

If we want to take the possibilities and resources of collective weaving networks seriously we have to be flexible and playful in our therapeutic meetings. We need to bring in family members or their voices (even fathers, mothers or siblings who disappeared from sight), just as we must make room for carers, peers, professionals and community members. We are interested in a wide variety of network partners and many ways of involving them. Members of the network can fulfil different roles, positions and functions at different times. We can invite them live as well as imaginary. We can even think of populating our therapy room with people who are no longer alive but can offer support, inspiration or advice. Teddy bears, dolls, rock stars and football players can offer guidance through difficult times. Sermijn (2020) even uses symbolic witnesses when gathering a network of people is not feasible. We can let them participate in our conversations and explorations or let them join as witnesses of our discoveries.

In these ways we open up the therapy room for the outside world as no child is an island (Vermeire, 2020). Although this doesn't mean that the safety walls of the therapy room aren't important and should be handled with care. The child, as active participant, is and remains the co-director in our weaving of networks, of course in an ongoing dialogue with the people involved. Together we can reflect on which family members, neighbours, peers, teachers, soccer coaches or professionals involved are most relevant at each stage or moment in the therapeutic process and in which way each one can contribute to, and take part in, our collective weaving of resilience. The commitment and insight of all people involved can be used. Below is an incomplete list of good reasons and possibilities to engage significant people and networks in the flesh or as imaginary figures:

- Not only the child is 'working' on the problems but everyone involved is. They can become collaborative partners in the therapeutic process. In doing so we resist individualising the problem and we understand resilience processes as enhancing collective agency.
- Collecting from the start the different concerns and perspectives on the problems so we are able to develop a broader vision on what is going on. It makes room for multiple perspectives and polyphony.
- It allows for the development of a shared language and the social sharing of experiences, emotions, involvements, stories and meaning in ever widening circles. So, acknowledgement of experiences, stories, responses, skills and knowledge becomes possible.
- It can offer a serious antidote to feelings of loneliness, alienation and being worthless by enhancing a sense of mattering, belonging and solidarity. The child can feel noticed as their stories can be told and listened to by the significant people in their lives. These people can get a better or richer understanding of the child's adversities, responses and maybe the child themselves. They can respond in ways that makes the child feel stronger.
- New ways of collaboration, talking and sharing and new ways of relating to one another can be introduced so new relational dances can be enhanced. It opens the possibility of sharing meaningful new experiences and to new actions.
- The discoveries, new insights or meaning developed in the therapeutic process can be held and carried collectively. It can facilitate the transfer to daily life and important life domains. They can act in mutual support in daily life so long-term transformation can be developed.
- Sometimes significant people or networks can be invited as witnesses, supporters, inspirators, advisors and even operate as co-therapists or co-counsellors. They can offer comfort, protection, care or a shelter for one another.
- Some people in the network can operate as guardians of (life)stories in the past, present and maybe for the future.
- Through this whole process networks of resilience are developed that can be supportive in the future once care systems are no longer involved.
- …

Chapter 3

First meetings

At the start of our therapeutic journey children are often not eager to talk about the difficulties, the pain or the fear. An important goal of our therapies is to create a safe haven for children to speak, play and reflect without marginalising their voice or forcing them to talk. In this chapter I address the many possibilities as well as disadvantages of 'talking', encompassing both silence and speech as expressing relational involvement. We engage in different actions. We create a platform from which we can explore the difficulties and traumatic experiences together by searching for safe stories and collecting a 'team of support and solidarity' for our conversations. We explore ways of speaking about 'painful experiences and their effects' with children and youngsters in ways that are manageable and that allow parents or people significantly involved to join the conversations as witnesses or co-researchers from the very outset. We unravel the different stories in the 'trauma' story and explore which stories open doors to what kind of territories and which ones are helpful for the moment in the conversation and in the process. From the beginning it can be important to break through the child's experiences of alienation and stigmatisation and find different, more appropriate ways to respond to the child and these stories. The therapeutic scope is broadened to encompass peers, networks and wider communities, not only the child, or the child and its primary carer. This approach takes into account that it not only 'repositions' or 'moves' the child 'towards new experiences, meanings and actions', but that everyone is involved.

Intake as re-connection and re(dis)covery

The concept 'intake' or first conversation is informed by many professional discourses on the requirements of good, correct and professional acting (Madigan, 2011; White, 2004). It is a commonly accepted idea that a first conversation is about collecting information about the details, the course and history of the difficulties. It is not only about gaining information, but also explaining the treatment process, and verifying whether the client is motivated or fits into the criteria of our care (Madsen, 2007). At the same time, while working through these *to do's*, you also try to set up a collaboration.

DOI: 10.4324/9781003167860-4

The way in which the child, young person or their parents participate in the initial discussions with a professional is also partly shaped by ideas and beliefs about how one should behave, or talk, or how one should present oneself as a 'good client'. *Maybe it is better to show your best side and appear engaged and motivated or maybe you should be 'on your guard' and pretend everything is fine or ...*

Traditionally we consider the intake as 'the preparation' for the 'real work'. This often means that an obvious pattern unfolds. Certainly, in contexts where youngsters or families have already had several 'intakes' it has become a taken-for-granted ritual as part of the process. Some youngsters or families can predict our questions and we seem to know what they will answer before they do. Our curiosity and a not-knowing stance disappear (Anderson & Gerhart, 2007).

Such taken-for-granted ideas can put us unintentionally in an expert position by which the client can feel interrogated, controlled or analysed (Vermeire & Sermijn, 2017). Expressions, actions and stories of clients get interpreted and understood within the frameworks of our psychological theories or scientific findings (Madsen, 2009; White, 2004) whereby the child or their family risks losing ownership of their stories. However, we want to realise that their contribution and knowledge is just as essential to the success of our therapeutic journey (Jørring, 2022).

If we don't want our conversations from the very outset to be framed in single, limiting directions, it can be important to invite in children, youngsters and their family or carers even before the first meeting in a way that makes a difference from previous experiences and maybe is a bit irreverent towards some taken-for-granted ways of doing therapy or 'performing' intakes. Can we welcome the child and the significant people, honour their efforts to find solutions or ways out and make them curious about our upcoming meeting? Can we introduce some playfulness and let them know we will not be 'just talking' or 'just problem talking'? Perhaps more importantly, can we address children as active participants and already encourage their participation in the upcoming meeting, especially since it is generally not the children's idea to come to therapy? To do so it will be important to carefully negotiate with the parents or carers who will invite the child, how they will be invited and what they will be told about the reasons this therapy or counselling is believed to be important or helpful.

By developing a collaborative working relationship from the very start, we try to honour the parents' and carers' relational involvement in contacting us, and trusting us. An important step in this process is that we listen to their knowledge when considering how to start our journey and that we always respect their position in relation to the child. A telephone call before the first meeting in which we discuss how to organise this meeting can for instance make a huge difference for the upcoming process. We can suggest different conversational settings each with their constraints and opportunities for them and the child and invite them to reflect upon what can be the most fruitful direction to take. In doing so, we begin, from the very first moment, a collaborative alliance in which the parent or carer is a valued partner and co-researcher. We believe caring for carers from the start is a means of caring for the child. The outcome of this negotiating is not known beforehand.

Do you think we can start our conversations together or would you prefer a separate conversation with you as parents first? Could it be valuable or necessary for you as parents to have the opportunity to tell what happened from your perspective before we invite your child to therapy? Do you think it would be a good idea to talk to your son alone from the first moment? Or would it be helpful for him that you are around and that you introduce him to me? What would be a welcome and motivating introduction? Sometimes the presence of involved third parties closes doors and young people experience this as too intrusive. How would you assess this? Do you have any idea how this young person will experience your presence? Do you have any idea what coming for talks might mean for your child? Would it be a relief, or a burden? Or might coming to therapy make them feel even more like they are the problem? Could being in therapy perpetuate the idea that it is their fault and they should work on it?

All these questions also have the ambition to make visible and assess together what kind of meanings and what kind of conversations can, and probably will, be created by choosing certain conversational settings. A discussion about particular familial and cultural ideas about including children in conversations or speaking alone with children can be important as meanings in the broader social and cultural contexts will influence the meanings created in the conversational setting. After these negotiations and reflections, sometimes sending a letter, an email or short phone call to the child can open doors to start our journey.

Dear Yusuf (age 9),

Next Monday we have planned a meeting together with your mum. I heard that you are a dinosaur expert. Could you bring some of your favourite dinosaurs? And I have no idea who are the important people in your life so if you want to bring some pictures of them, these are certainly welcome, as well as your cuddly bear or pets (if they are too big, please bring a picture of them ☺).

To be honest, I am a bit nervous to meet you. I am curious about what you want to talk about. Your mother told me that there are some worries that are bothering you and her. She hopes that together we can find some ways to make things feel less heavy and that things become better between you. (Maybe there are already some things you tried to do about it? Have you found some small tricks in the past that made problems feel less heavy?)

I just want you to know that I have color pencils, clay and other craft material in my room. There is even a supersonic digital flip chart to help us explore and understand what is bothering you and your mum.

Looking forward to welcome you. If you like I also can introduce you to our house cat.

Warmly,
Sabine

By already offering some questions before the meeting, the child and their family or carers get a first notion about what and how we are going to talk and reflect, but also that their voice and their stories will matter just like their input about the directions we will be taking together. As such our collaboration and journey has already made a start.

By doing so, we inscribe ourselves in a tradition within systemic therapy and narrative therapy. Epston (2017) listed some pre-session questions that can help people to shift into paying attention to their abilities, skills and accomplishments and how to use these in relation to the current problem they are experiencing. Young (2011) emphasised the importance of pre-session questionnaires in walk-in clinics to set the stage for conversations that strive to understand the problem and to find hope, new ideas and knowledges about how to proceed. Fredman (2014) encouraged the therapist or counsellor to engage in a pre-session reflection guided by questions such as *'How would this child and family feel when coming for this meeting?'*, *'What would this child appreciate that at least I notice?'* And *'What posture or attitude can bring the stories and perspective of the child into the room?'* All these steps can contribute to the creation of an invitational, playful and collaborative first meeting.

Depending on what questions we ask and what fields we explore in our first conversations, certain aspects and stories of the person, their family, relationships and lives will emerge and others will sink into the background. If we ask mainly about the problems or traumatic experiences we invite problem or victim stories into the room. The point of entries that we take also influence what stories and narratives will be co-constructed. It is important for the therapist as well as for the child and the significant people to invite a multiplicity of differentiated, nuanced, multilayered and richly described stories in our first meetings so the child and their family or carers can appear and perform in a multiplicity of contexts and landscapes of identities. This goes hand in hand with the idea of situating the problems, obstacles, painful experiences from the very beginning within both the local and wider context and within networks of ongoing mutual influencing relationships. Instead of just focusing on the child or the problems, while trying to define the problems we have to widen the scope for ourselves as well as for the child and everyone involved. Children prefer to be listened to with a focus on their strengths. They are very sensitive to being labelled, judged negatively or reprimanded. The role of the therapist is very important in this respect (Moore & Bruna Seu, 2011), also in creating 'a sense of mattering' (Madsen et al., 2021).

From the very beginning we aim to become a companion on a journey through their lives and relationships. We create a context in which they are invited to share *their* kaleidoscope of stories in ways that suit them, that make them curious about different, sometimes forgotten aspects of their lives, stimulate them to reflect on them, which can initiate transformative processes. Visiting and exploring problem areas, as well as not yet mined areas or alternative stories, can open new perspectives, re-connecting them with what is meaningful or valuable to them and to the important people in their lives. But in order to facilitate the telling of multiple stories and to become curious again we first need to create safe grounds.

Doing safety

Many children and youngsters step into the room accompanied by hesitations and suspicion. If we don't want to get into the grip of this suspicion, feelings of unsafety or overwhelming emotions, we noted earlier that we have to find a river-bank position and create a platform from which we can start our journey. The other requirement is that the child or youngster has to become an active participant.

When children and their carers are seated, I often introduce 'red cards'. As soon as I navigate in a direction that the child, youngster or carer don't want to go, or ask questions they don't want to answer, they can use 'a red card'. This means we can collaborate in finding useful and safe enough questions regarding interesting territories of life to explore together. Each session we start the conversation with reflections on the letter I wrote after the previous session. 'What was interesting, helpful and brings them a step further? What do they want to explore further and what do they want to hold on to?'

As referring explicitly to 'safety' can invite even more 'hesitation' or 'suspicion' in the room, the main focus will be on 'doing and creating safety together' in order to hopefully become trustful in relation to each other throughout our journey. I consider collaboration and 'doing safety' as ongoing processes. Bring the child's or young person's knowledge of safety and 'doing safety' to the foreground can be very helpful. It is equally important to want to get to know them against the background of different areas of their life and not just from a background of problems or trauma.

I meet Yusuf together with his mum in the waiting room. He drags a bag with dinosaurs with him. Once seated in the therapy room I ask him to share his knowledge about the dinosaurs. After introducing me to the Tyrannosaurus rex and some other carnivores, he picks up the Parasaurolophus with its giant horn. He explains that they use this horn to communicate. So I wonder what this communication is about?

- *Oh, when there is danger, the boss can blow through his horn and warn the whole family. So everyone can hide in time!*
- *Do you also know what the good 'hiding' places or hiding strategies are for the Parasaurolophus?*

He looks at me full of amazement 'Do you really have no idea?' ... There were caves so they could escape from the T-Rex and especially the children had secret hiding spots.

- *Can I be that curious and ask you if you have hiding places at home? Or favourite places? Places of comfort? Would you be so kind to take me to your home and draw a plan of the apartment?*

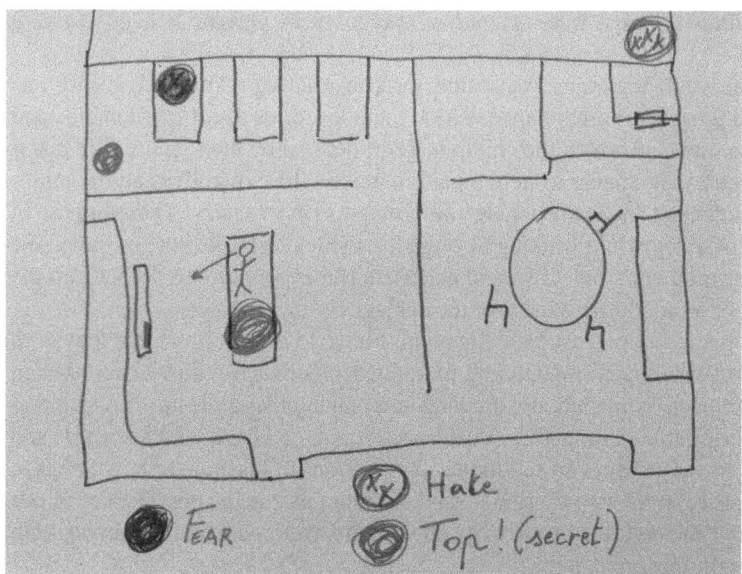

Figure 3.1 Map of a house. Photograph by the author.

Yusuf draws enthusiastically his personal, favourite place: sitting/laying on the couch where he watches his favourite television program 'Lego Ninjago'. His bedroom seems to be a complicated place. In the corner of the room he made a small cave that offers a lot of comfort but he can never be sure nothing will be stolen from his cave because he shares his bedroom with his little brothers. In the evening the nightmares and bad thoughts are coming. At these times, his bedroom becomes a place of fear. When I ask if there are also places of hate he looks from the corner of his eyes at his mum, hesitates and mumbles 'the storage room at the basement'. As I notice this can open a painful direction in the conversation, I check if it is okay with him to talk about this place maybe another time or does he want to go on? He seems relieved and whispers 'Another time'. I repeat he can make use of the 'red cards' as much as he likes.

After showing me around several places I ask if he could take me through a day in his life. Together with the help of his mum we draw the whole building and neighbourhood. We start early Monday morning when he lays in his bed waiting for his mum to tickle him awake. The irritation of the nightmares fades away by tickling but the stress about his dad is always around. Could he give this early morning stress a score from 1 to 10? He replies: Two!

Step by step we walk together with his mum through his day and his life and try to listen carefully to the different aspects of his life. I become a guest in his life and relationships; I meet his school friends, the funny school bus driver who always winks when he steps in, his judo coach, etc. and I learn that he appreciates honesty, hates promises and loves to become a Lego Ninjago Warrior.

From the very beginning we search for constructive relationships, safe territories and territories of resilience, which include stories about life domains and relational contexts in which the children aren't defined by their painful life histories but where they appear as active participants in their own lives and relationships. This doesn't mean we ignore the problems or obstacles. These appear in the course of a day while walking through his life and we take note of them. We can at every moment slow down and negotiate if they want to go deeper into the difficulties or would rather postpone the subject.

While I get to know Yusuf and his mum, I have to bear in mind that they both also start to get to know me. Getting to know each other is a mutual act with an important impact. While talking, drawing and playing they taste how I respond to what they bring into our meeting. Yusuf discovers how I cope with his words and stories and how I position myself to the contributions of his mum or how I engage her in the process. So step by step he and his mum assess the possibilities of our meetings and decide if they want to go on with me. Our cooperation is an ongoing process of mutual attunement.

Widening the scope

In our conversations the visible actions and observable interaction patterns and the way stories are told risk becoming the one single explanation for the problems. Problems as well as explanations risk becoming situated *within* the child, *within* the family, *within* their communication and interaction patterns or *within* the traumatic experiences. Often children and significant people involved enter the session with such reductionist, solidified conclusions about the problems and what causes them. If we collude with this viewpoint we risk not being able to ask anything new or bring anything new to the conversation.

Therefore, we have to undertake special actions to keep a broader view of the problems, the child, the family and the network. After all, in the background, many people, groups, institutions and communities engage in conversations with and about these children. And they speak from a certain position, a certain perspective, that is embedded in social and cultural contexts, sometimes privileged, sometimes disadvantaged. Actively making these networks visible in our conversations proved to be a serious antidote to the tendency to focus exclusively on what is already in the foreground (Vermeire & Van den Berge, 2021).

Just like Yana is introducing her cuddly bear 'Little Orange', Esma presents her grandparents and talks about Wendy and the football team KAA Ghent or Xander shares his knowledge about how to take care of his mum, I ask Yusuf if he can introduce me to the significant people in his life.

We agree it would be a real challenge to collect everyone important on the table as dinosaurs. He takes this task very seriously and deliberates which dino he will take for each person. An extra-large diplodocus for his mum and two smaller

*ones for his little brothers are put on the table. Finally, he takes a small diplodo-
cus for himself. When I explore what made him doubt, he explains that he might
become like his dad if he keeps on being so angry. As his dad was very violent at
times and died a year ago from an overdose, he had chosen the T-Rex to represent him. He doesn't want to become like his dad and he definitely doesn't want
the T-Rex on the table. So, I ask where he wants us to put the T-Rex? Outside the
door? In the closet is fine with him. For the other family members, schoolfriends,
etc., he picks all kinds of animals, figures and material.*

By inviting children and young people to build up their network of relationships materially and playfully, they become in charge of what they want to show
or share with us. More importantly, their focus (as well as ours) moves away from
themselves towards the networks they are embedded in. This can be done by using
small pieces of paper, post-its, all kinds of animal toys or other small objects that
they choose (Vermeire, 2019). They can even draw it on the whiteboard. Our
questions can guide them to 're-member' (White, 2007) the networks and relations they are engaged in.

*Once we have collected all these people I ask him if he can position them around
him at a distance or in a way that feels appropriate to him. Maybe he wants to
add some symbols, some special lines or colors. As his paternal grandparents still
live in Somalia he puts them in the corner of the room. Together with his mum he
folds a small airplane and draws a tear on the wings of the airplane. He thinks his
grandparents must be very sad because his dad left them to come to Belgium, and
later became addicted and eventually died. The tears are also a bit his sadness
because he never saw them in real life. I notice that his mum is surprised by this
story. She replies she didn't know that he sometimes thought of his grandparents.*

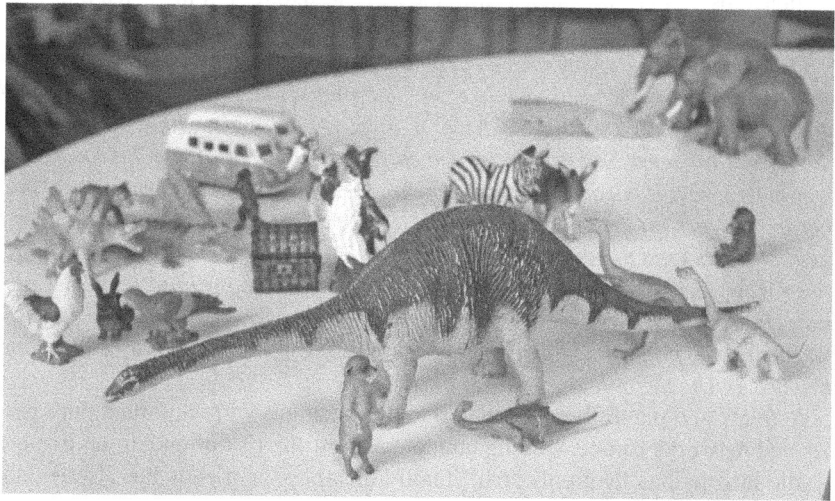

Figure 3.2 Dinosaurs and other animal figures on a table. Photograph by the author.

While journeying through these networks of relationships, some 'unsaid', forgotten or alternative stories become visible and shared. We also enlarge our focus from 'intimate relationships' to the many influencing relationships and broader contexts (Burnham, 2009).

Making visible that they have to manage daily life in a small apartment, in a neighborhood where in the playgrounds youngsters are often dealing drugs also makes the social difficulties Yusuf has to deal with visible, as well as the obstacles and constraints to parenthood for mother. It provides an opportunity for the mother to share her concerns about these social difficulties in relation to her son. Just as Yusuf can explain to us that inviting classmates to come and play in the flat is not an option.

A team of support

Children often aren't eager to speak with an adult they don't know. It can be helpful to invite the people they still trust or rely on. This relates to the idea that if problems and difficulties are to be understood in a multitude of relationships and contexts, the voices of important people must be taken into account. Maybe there are much more interesting experts and advisors in the life of the child or the family whose knowledge is much more appropriate, reliable and inspirational. So we have to 'populate' our conversations.

Unfortunately, often the histories of these children are characterised by experiences of alienation or dis-connection from the significant people in their life. So reconvening people who have made, and can still make, a difference, and can help us to create a multi-voiced conversation, is an important intervention. Once we loitered around in their local and social contexts and we made their networks of relationships visible, we can ask who they would like to join their 'team of support', live or imaginary, for the upcoming conversations.

I ask Yusuf while looking around at all the people collected in front of us who he would like to join our meetings, 'live' or 'imaginary', and who he believes could offer support in case we need advice or inspiration, or get stuck. Immediately he looks at his mum and asks me if she can stay. He even falls on his knees and begs her to stay. It becomes clear that he understood he had to come 'alone' into therapy to work on the problems and his aggression. On the face of his mother I see that she is glad to hear that her son wants her in his 'team'.

Looking further around he wants his hamster, Timon, because he knows him best. He is as crazy as Timon in the Lion King. He asks hesitantly if his grandparents can be present now and then because he has some questions for them and they are maybe the only ones who know the answers?

Actively and playfully populating our conversations with important third parties and networks can be a strong antidote against the risk of ending up in mere dyadic interactions. Not only 'real' family members or friends but also cuddly bears (like Yana and her Little Orange), pets, inspiring pop stars or famous sports players can become a member. Instead of being seized by the urge to explain and

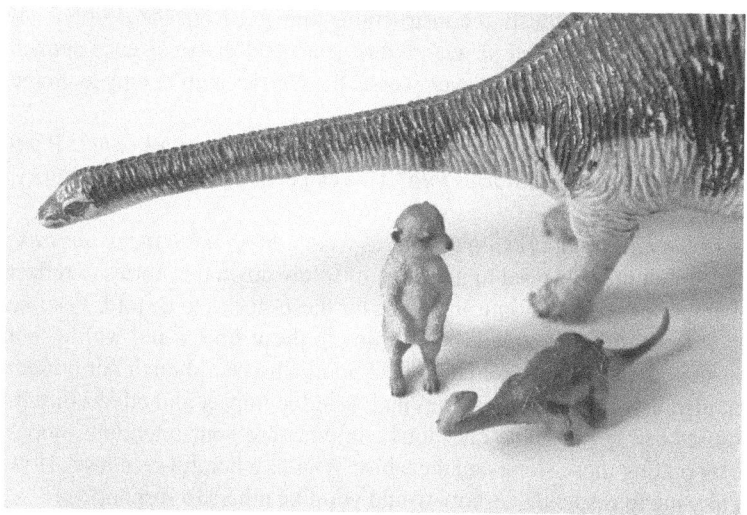

Figure 3.3 Two dinosaur figures and a meerkat on a table. Photograph by the author.

to worry, we can slow down the conversation and, in an imaginative way, invite one of these members, for example, by giving that person a chair. We explore *who* could offer *what kind of* support and we reflect on who should be invited at what moment or for what issues (Vermeire & Van den Berge, 2021). Reynolds (2011) also emphasises the importance to think about ways to people-the-room with folks, even people who are not alive, who will nurture them, support them, remind them of their ethics, call them to account, and work in complex and imperfect alliances with them.

This support and solidarity team can also contribute in creating a riverbank position from which we can talk and reflect about the painful experiences or traumatic histories and its effects. Parents or carers can also be invited to introduce their 'team of support and solidarity' during difficult times.

Yusuf's mum talks about a friend when she was a little girl and that she hasn't seen for a long time. They used to play and sing together. That friend would understand the hardships she and Yusuf had endured in recent years.

'Talking about our talks'

It is always a surprise how children, youngsters and the people that accompany them will present themselves, what will be told and how it will be told. Some children have their heart on their tongue, others try to hide themselves, just shrug their shoulders and keep silent. Some have impressive stories and others are silenced by the people that bring them to these conversations. Some drop a small story that contains a huge message and others just bring 'a good news show'. Sometimes they just follow duty-consciously the instructions they got from the people con-cerned, '*You can tell everything, it will relieve you*', and discover once spoken they can't take their words back and even worse, the worries aren't stopped. Some children hesitate and keep hesitating.

What will my mum think about this or how will this therapist think of me? What will happen with my words and stories told? This can evoke feelings of insecurity, doubt and self-blame.

This means *we have to address, from the very beginning, the issue of our talking together.* Sometimes we need to interrupt and slow down the stories to reflect together whether this is a good time and place for these stories to be told. Just like it is important to negotiate who will be listening to these stories and with whom they will be shared afterwards. We can reflect upon who is, although not present in the room, also listening to these stories and what the impact and effects of telling these stories can be. Possible questions are: what are your intentions, hopes and wishes by putting these stories on the table? What is a helpful response? How would you like me to respond? Or how would you like others to respond?

Some children in painful contexts bring incredible, fantastic or tough stories, some even tell stories about themselves, others or their life that are labelled by the people concerned as 'pathological lies'.

- *Esma told at school that her dad has an important job and an impressive villa in Turkey. Each summer she leaves for two months to live with him. He treats her as a princess and overloads her with presents. Her school teacher and grandparents are very worried about those 'lies' she tells at school. Her friends are just impressed.*
- *Steff (16 years) tries to convince me that he was the head of the gang and that all his friends would give their lives for him although he has been in a youth home for months without any visit or contact.*

How can we deal with what these children say? If we take these messages as containing information, this information clearly is wrong, which means they are simply lying, or not telling the truth. In order to find a way out, it can be helpful to take a look at language. Although our traditional understanding of language is that it describes or mirrors reality (Gergen, 1999), different perspectives have been developed. The anthropologist Malinowski (1923), for instance, observed that what is probably the most important function of language or conversation is not so much the transmission of information as rather the experience of a kind of togetherness, or connectedness (he coined the term 'phatic communion'). The later Wittgenstein (1953) replaced the idea that words are reflections of an inner or outer reality with the idea of 'meaning is use', which means that words derive their meaning from the language games in which people participate. In the same vein Rober (2002) articulated the idea that words are tools that people use to live together with some understanding and dignity. Such a take on language can help us to be open to a 'social truth' instead of only being interested in the 'real truth'.

It allows us to consider such questions as 'What are their hopes when telling these stories?' 'Can we understand these big stories or "lies" as utterances of relational, social involvement and so as invitations or efforts in a web of interconnectedness?' 'What kind of connection are they hoping for? Where or with whom do they want to belong?'

- *Exploring with Esma what she is hoping for by telling these stories about her dad, we discover she just wants to be 'normal' like all the other children of her class. They go on a 'normal' holiday, they spend 'normal' weekends with their 'normal' parents and just do 'normal' activities. You can't stand with your friends at the playground without any interesting story.*
- *Steff tells after a while he feels himself as 'trash'. Until now, he didn't accomplish a thing. On the contrary, he ruined everything.*

Sometimes children just drop little stories of frustration, troubles or disadvantages while checking how we and other participants in the meeting respond to these stories of harassment or trouble. They often investigate whether we are able to receive or bear such stories without reducing the complexity or jumping into simple solutions before they share something that is really painful or traumatic. Anderson and Goolishian (1988) draw our attention to the stories that are not yet told in therapy and focused on the process of expanding and saying the 'unsaid'.

Rober et al. (2006) analysed in a first session in family therapy how the storytelling of a highly charged and delicate topic like domestic violence actually developed. The researchers saw how in the back-and-forth process between voices of hesitation and voices of reassurance, the participants weigh the level of safety in the session. The family talked first about violence between toys and told narratives about violence between children before narratives between adults and between adults and children came into the conversation. By accepting this interplay between hesitation and reassurance it can gradually become possible to talk about more delicate, problematic experiences.

If we follow a more postmodern view on language, we should also keep in mind that our words are not 'innocent'. They have real psychological and bodily effects on the other person. We can see them as touches that can comfort, support but also hurt. We cannot predict in advance and from the outside what they will bring about. Certain words or sayings are loaded with meanings and can easily trigger painful histories. In the context of abuse of children, for example, conversations about father and mother in the classroom can be very disturbing. Children may suddenly stiffen, jump up or sometimes clown around. This can happen very quickly without us having a clue of what is happening.

Possibilities and disadvantages of keeping silent and speaking

Many children or youngsters are often not convinced that speaking can be helpful and that therapy is the right thing to do for them. On the contrary, they often experienced that speaking leads to more trouble and that adults aren't always reliable.

Some of these children already have a long history of keeping silent. They have experienced that when they tried to talk about the difficulties it turned out bad, so they fear the consequences. In some families it is common sense not to talk about difficulties. Children are made to understand that you do not hang out your dirty laundry in public. Just like taboos in their cultures can make it unthinkable to talk about certain themes. Cornfeld (2018) shows how silence sometimes can be woven into religious and family culture so the individual's journey can linger in despair and suffering. Keeping silent can indicate relational impasses and also the fear of stigma can contribute to the silence (Weingarten, 2003). The fear of their friends and others finding out, linked with a sense that they will then cease to be considered worthy of care and support, silences many children (Mullender et al., 2002).

It makes a difference if children don't have the words or ways to express what is on their minds or if keeping silent became an act of relational or social involvement. It is most painful when the person who caused the damage has forbidden them to speak or denies what happened. It can increase the self-accusations or make them distrust their own experiences (Sheinberg & Fraenkel, 2001). The child may also be afraid of not being taken seriously or of not being heard. It is important to keep this in mind as we know that a critical variable in determining the severity and duration of symptoms in contexts of maltreatment appears to be the way in which the family and environment responds to the abuse (Mullender et al., 2002).

The stories that children bring, or don't bring to the meeting or hesitate about shouldn't be disconnected from the contexts in which they are told. We can't be blind to the impact of speaking in the moment itself, after the conversation and the possible effects and meanings that can be generated out of this speaking. Talking and being 'open' is taken for granted for many professionals but not for the children and families we are working with. As long as the child keeps silent, they keep a sense of being in charge. They can have a sense of being in control of the stories about what happened, about others, themselves.

Although when children begin to speak, it opens the possibility that they can be heard and be taken seriously. Their hard work and responses can be noticed. The experiences, the effects and the stories and meanings generated out of these experiences can be explored, contextualised and shared. Maybe acknowledgement for the suffering becomes possible while private, single stories and meanings about the experiences can be revised based on sharing so new, alternative meaning and actions are developed.

Utterances of relational involvements

Speaking and keeping silent can both be acts of relational engagement that can serve many purposes. Caring for family members, protecting them, not burdening them, preventing things from getting worse. They want to be loyal to their family and not put them in an embarrassing position. They want to avoid threatening the integrity of the family (Rober, 2014). They often hope to create better prospects for their parents, siblings and family.

Tina kept the sexual abuse by her father hidden for years. At the age of 17, she started to suspect that maybe her younger sister, Shirley (14), also was sexually abused. The fear pierced her to her heart thinking that maybe her youngest half-sister (8), could be the next victim. After weeks of hesitation she talked with the school psychologist and after the disclosure her father was immediately removed from the house. Her mum collapsed and indicated she couldn't speak at this stage. In spite of this, she supported the idea to send her daughters to therapy.

Silence is often lonely, invisible hard work on the part of the child, just as speaking can take a lot of courage to step over the threshold. Similarly, hesitation can take a lot of energy. It can be very supportive to notice these efforts, and to help them notice who is also, apart from ourselves as counsellors, noticing and maybe even appreciating their relational commitment. We need to negotiate about what, when and in whose presence we are going to talk and, above all, for what purpose. By first accepting the child's silence, the therapist can then make some space for reflecting on the meaning of this silence through a subtle and careful dialogue with the family members (Van Parys et al., 2014). As Mullender et al. (2002) found in questioning these children: they have to feel they have permission to talk about the difficulties and need to be reassured that this is neither just being disloyal to their family nor something that negatively reflects on themselves and their worth. The conversation they take part in has to be conceived as a collaborative, dialogical process accomplished by all participants, including the therapist and the voices of significant people who are not present.

Paraphrasing Lang and McAdam (2003), we can say that both 'speech' and 'silence' are like drops of grammar containing an ocean of meanings that we can explore with children and young people. During this exploration, we try to make their relational involvements, values and commitments visible, both to themselves and to other important people.

When Tina comes for conversations she harms herself and doesn't know if it was 'a good thing' to disclose the abuse. We invite her sister, Shirley, to the conversation to explore together what stories and meanings are linked with keeping silent in the previous period for each of them. Together with Tina I use a linguagram to create a web of meaning (Lang & McAdam, 2003). In the meantime Shirley witnesses the words and sentences that appear on the whiteboard. The writings on the whiteboard make clear that for Tina keeping silent is linked with a lot of concerns about her family especially her mum and sisters but also with the fear of getting removed. It becomes visible that she hoped to keep the family together by keeping silent. Also the unpredictability and not knowing what would come prevented her from speaking.

Shirley responds that she had no idea of all these concerns and would like to know some more about it. She often thought Tina was just dominating everyone.

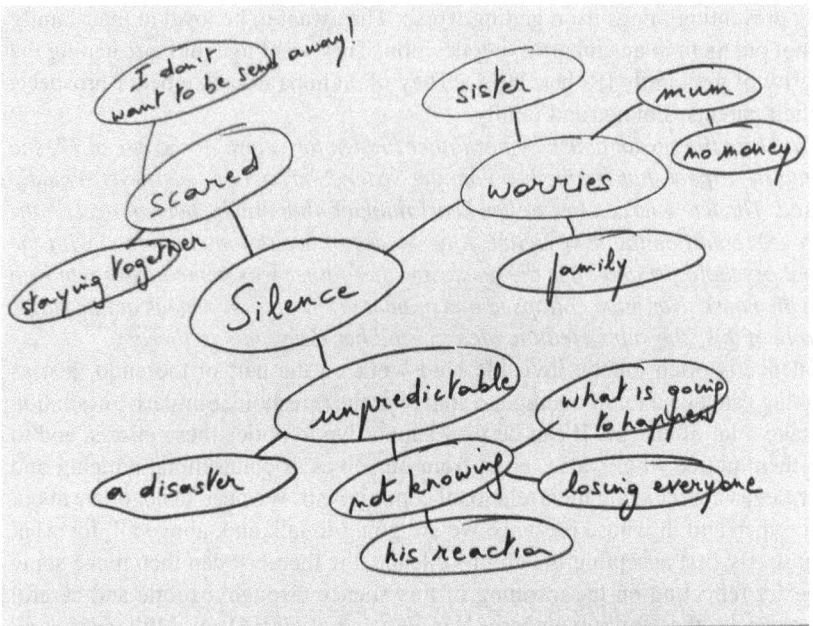

Figure 3.4 Word web around silence (scared, worries). Photograph by the author.

As she until then didn't talk about what happened, she makes clear she still doesn't want to talk about the abuse but is willing to make also a similar drawing about 'keeping silent'. Both similar and different words appear quickly on the board. Shirley says that keeping silent had much to do with her thinking 'It's my fault', 'I had to be smarter', 'I had to be able to avoid this'. She started to lie about what happened to her mum and once she started lying she got the feeling she couldn't step back. Her fear had a lot to do with what other people might think. She didn't want to be seen as a stupid child and she tried to protect her family by keeping silent.

By separating speaking and listening and by making words and meanings visible on the whiteboard we open space for a collective reflecting process. This way of talking and sharing didn't resolve all the problems but made it possible to make their relational involvements visible and mutually acknowledge their efforts. Some shared values and commitments were brought forth. They also collected language to start a dialogue with their mum in a manageable way.

What do we need to talk about?

Once we have created safe ground as a platform or riverbank we can look at the struggles in the here and now or at what happened in the past. We can invite them to explore the worries, difficulties, disadvantages or obstacles in their lives.

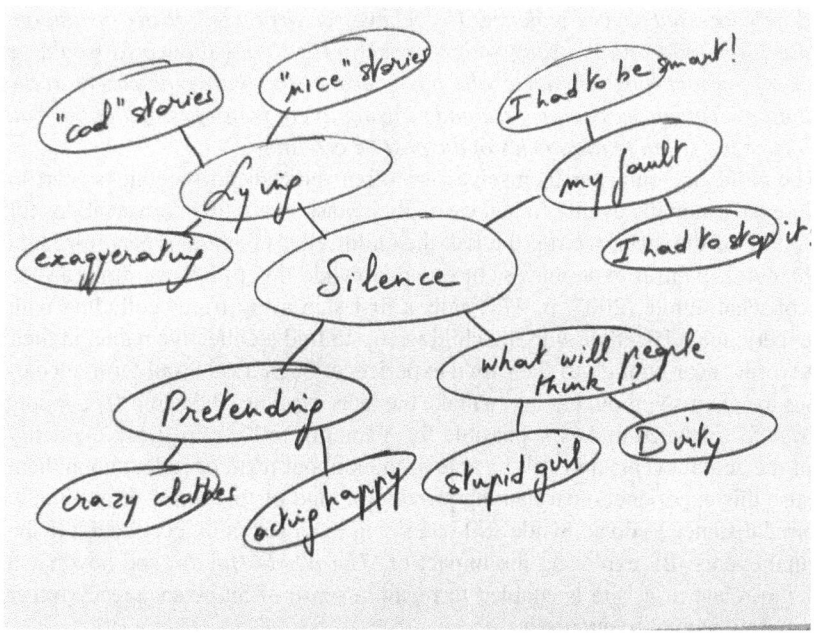

Figure 3.5 Word web around silence (2) (lying, pretending). Photograph by the author.

Parents, carers and sometimes the child or youngster themselves are often eager to talk first of all about the problematic behaviour or relational problems, the overwhelming, uncontrolled emotions or body reactions that dominate their life or relationship. Often these problems are put on the table to be examined closely. The panic attacks have to be stopped, the anger and quarrels must disappear, the self-harming and nightmares need to be resolved. Rober (2014) suggests focusing on the concerns and worries and not the problem behaviour or the so called 'problem'. What parents or carers consider to be the greatest concerns or problem may differ from what actually occupies the child, just like there may be different ideas about the main cause of the problems. Sometimes painful experiences from the past become the exclusive explanation for everything that goes wrong, while others steadfastly refuse to make precisely this connection. So sometimes there is the idea that the child needs to speak as quickly as possible about the traumatic experiences in the hope this will bring relief and the events can be processed. In other situations people who are directly affected by the harassing actions consider talking about these previous events as offering an 'excuse' for this 'behaviour' and so they don't think it is a good idea to make room for conversations about these experiences.

Thomas (16) is placed in a secure juvenile institution after a handbag rob-bery, with a friend, of an old woman. He had been living for more than four years mainly on the street. His parents are both drug addicted and unavailable. As a child he witnessed severe violence. He behaves as depressed at the institution, often refuses food and is losing weight quickly. He claims the world would be better off without him. His uncle who has guardianship warns the carers in the institution. 'This depression is fake and refusing to eat is just manipulation! You had better not listen to the stories of the past he is telling'.

The child or youngster themselves are often reluctant to recount or start to explore the traumatic events. When we explicitly ask in our first conversations for a retelling of the facts, we run the risk the child relives them and gets re-caught in shameful, painful experiences. In order to evade this pitfall we draw on the idea of what White (2007, p. 275) calls a first step away from 'colluding with the experience'. Together with the child we try to find a collective name, in their own words, near enough to their own experience. Such a catch-all term encompasses the events without having to make the facts explicit. The name '*The Whole Hassle*' for instance makes it possible for Yana not to have to speak explicitly about the actual events and still be able to think about them or reflect upon them because this experience-near naming provides a kind of 'platform' or minimally required distance to do so, while still remaining in close bodily connection to the original events. By exploring the impact of '*The Whole Hassle*' and how Yana wants to relate to it, she is enabled to regain a sense of influence/agency rather than merely having to endure it.

In the conversation with Yusuf and his mum I ask after our first explorations if we need to talk first of all about the stress in his life, the quarrels with his mum, the death of his dad or the things that happened in the past with his dad or still something else. I am curious to know what occupies him most and what he finds most important to talk about here and now.

While I present this list I notice that Yusuf turns his head and looks down the moment I talk about his father and what happened. Keeping in mind that he already indicated that talking about the storage room in the basement in relation with his father wasn't a good idea, I ask him if talking about his father and the past is a difficult thing to do? He nods.

I propose to put 'the things that happened' in a small box and while proposing I take a collection of boxes out of my drawer and put them on the table. I invite him to choose one of the boxes.

S: *Is it okay with you to put these painful things in it and keep the box closed for as long as you think this is necessary?*

   He looks at his mum. She nods encouragingly. He replies: 'How can we do this? Is this really possible?' At the same time he picks up a box and looks at it in detail.

S: *I am not completely sure, but we could give it a try? How would you like to call this box or what is in the box?*

Y: *'The Dark Stuff'.*

Y: *Can we write 'The Dark Stuff' on a paper and put it in the box?*

   He immediately takes a piece of paper, draws a skull, writes 'Danger' underneath the skull and puts the paper in the box.

S: Will I keep the box with the Dark Stuff here with me or is there someone else you want to take care of this box?

Y: Just leave it here (again he looks at his mum and she nods approvingly).

S: Can I ask later on some questions about how you managed to keep going on despite this Dark Stuff?

...

S: Shall we now start our investigation of the nightmares or do you prefer to explore the quarrels or what about the school issues? What do you think your mum would like us to explore first? Or is there still any other concern we didn't talk about yet?

There is often a hierarchy and cluster of disadvantages and adversities. By ordering them and examining how they are possibly connected we make them at the same time visible and take them seriously. We can negotiate to talk first about the painful experiences in the past or start our explorations with the difficulties that push and pull in the here and now.

When we put our focus on the traumatic experiences it can also be helpful to distinguish between inquiring about the *effects* of the trauma on the young person's life and their *responses* to the events (Yuen, 2007; Wade, 1997). If we limit ourselves to asking about effects, we risk getting more victim stories in the room. On the other hand it can also open the opportunity to acknowledge the pain and suffering, or contextualise the distress and share it with others. Yuen (2009) distinguishes between such questions as '*How did you feel?*', '*How did it affect you?*' and questions as '*How did you respond? What did you do or try to do?*' Both directions can be valuable depending on where we are situated in the therapeutic process and what already has been expressed in language by the child and the people involved, noticed, shared and acknowledged and has been made sense of – at least partially.

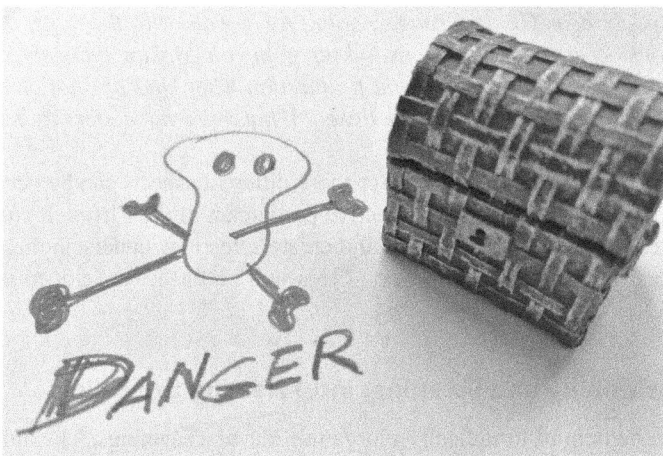

Figure 3.6 Treasury with drawing of a skull. Photograph by the author.

Making responses visible is in line with White's (2006) way of working. He invites young people to name the steps and actions they take, as responses to the trauma. The underlying idea is that children and young people always make attempts to prevent the trauma to which they are exposed. When preventing the trauma is impossible, they take steps to modify the trauma or to change the effects of it on their lives (White, 2006c). Even in the face of the most dramatic events, steps are taken to protect or preserve what they consider 'valuable'. Making these responses visible can invite alternative stories and meanings about what happened, their lives, their relations and about themselves.

An important aspect here is that some responses are highly visible both during the events and after the painful experiences (shouting, screaming, running away, nightmares, crying, self-harming or drug use), while other responses are physically invisible (a small gesture, escaping mentally, brooding, holding on to a thought or having a poker face). However, even these responses mean that the child in question has done, or is doing, something and is more than just a passive receiver. Wade (1997) emphasises when open defiance is impractical or too dangerous resistance is expressed indirectly and on a micro-level of social interaction. The smallest responses can be meaningful and can create ripples (Yuen, 2009).

In the case of children and young people, involved bystanders often do not notice these responses and the accompanying involvements, nor acknowledge the young people's efforts (White, 2006a). When we ask children themselves what they did in those difficult circumstances, the answer is often 'nothing'. They themselves do not notice their actions either. Although they were not able to stop or prevent the abuse there are many small acts to discover: ways of protecting or cherishing what is precious to them, acts of caring, skills of living or acts of resistance (Yuen, 2007; Wade, 1997).

When I asked Yana for the first time what she had done in relation to 'The Whole Hassle' she had no clue. She had forgotten that once she even packed her suitcase and wanted to leave the foster home. Her crying in her bedroom, seeking comfort in her cuddly bear 'Little Orange', going for a walk with the dogs, or fretting can be considered as small actions to keep going on. Making these small actions visible can become a starting point to question what kind of relational involvements, intentions, hopes, wishes are linked. What and who matters to her or what does she want to keep precious?

Making room in our first conversations for these different aspects can be very helpful in letting the child re-appear as an active participant of their lives. It can open, from the very start, new perspectives and create some new understandings on what happened, their life and themselves. (This will be further developed in Chapters 4 and 5.)

Radical re-positioning and listening: interviewing the child

Sometimes it can be helpful to radically reorganise our first meetings. The aim is then to centre, from the very beginning, the voice and perspective of the child or youngster. This also allows room for the development of a multiplicity of stories with layered meanings and experiences while weaving threads of (re)connections with what and even more importantly, who matters. This is especially the case when we notice that the child or youngster has not often experienced being listened to, or being supported, or being taken seriously during the previous years.

Proceeding in this manner often increases a sense of agency, a sense of coherence and a sense of belonging from the very start. We create a context in which we invite the young person to talk about their life path so far, the problems, obstacles and limitations they have encountered and the steps they have taken. We do this in the form of an interview. The interview takes place in the presence of the people they regard as important people in their lives and they like to be present. Also the people who will be working with them the upcoming period are invited.

Rinske is 15. She is referred by the youth court. She ended up for two weeks in a crisis unit. After an escalation of violence with her father, she was thrown out of the house. Her little sister died when Rinske was six and her mother died when she was ten. Both parents struggled with addiction problems. For the moment Rinske refuses to attend school. She wants nothing more in this life and can't stop crying. The past years different forms of help were offered and many professionals were involved but it didn't bring any change in the situation.

Together with her individual mentor, family counsellor and case manager she comes in for a 'biographical' interview as a kind of alternative intake. Her auntie and her best friend are also present at her request. As Rinske is willing to come for this conversation and she even invited important people to be present, I assumed she had some stories she wanted to share and that there were still tiny glimmers of hope for her life.

Within this interview context we both take a novel position: we meet as 'interviewer', with therapeutic skills and 'interviewee', with a bumpy life path. This can decrease the power imbalance inherent in child–professional relationships and allows us to park our eagerness to take care, help or give advice. Also future professionals, family members involved, carers or friends receive an invitation: they are asked to listen to the interview from an (outsider) witness position. Separating listening and speaking opens space for reflecting processes and to park their own perspective. The whole interview is recorded so we can offer the tape afterwards to the youngster. This creates an additional framework of being listened to and taken seriously.

I ask Rinske what is important to know about her life and to talk about to make this interview as good and valuable as possible. She answers immediately while tears roll over her cheeks: 'The death of my mum and little sister'. I ask if it is okay to explore together what these deaths mean to her while I hand over a handkerchief. I also ask permission to add two chairs next to her for them. A little smile appears for the first time on her face.

We create a context in which these youngsters are immediately put to work by inviting them to tell their stories. They are stimulated to reflect on different aspects of their lives, which can initiate transformative processes. White (2007) suggested to investigate the problems from a shared position of *cool engagement*. So, I just connect indirectly with the tears and the sadness by offering a handkerchief and invite her to tell me a bit more about what bothers her most.

Rinske tells she always misses her little sister and mum: morning, evening, afternoon ... She hates that she has no memories of her sister and hardly any of her mum. While crying she sighs that she can't let them go. I ask her: 'Where do the ideas come from that you have to let them go?' Apparently her father has removed all their belongings after the death of her mum. It was too painful and so he hoped she could let them go. Curiously I ask if she agrees with these ideas. To which she firmly says she does not share his ideas. We talk together about which connections with her mother and sister she refuses to give up.

From the very beginning we can notice some dominant knowledges and practices of our culture and connect them with one's experiences and problems. In the story of Rinske, I could even ask how she positions herself towards some of these ideas and practices.

Unexplored areas and forgotten stories

We first invite the youngster to become curious about the different aspects of their own lives by walking around together in the many areas, relationships and stories of their life. This 'loitering around' can bring to the foreground richer descriptions and stories about their lives, relationships and identity, and this happens in the presence of different witnesses. We have to bring them into the past landscapes of action and relationships then and there to be able to re-find experiences and stories that have been covered by the painful experiences. Forgotten, subjugated stories are awakened to re-discover important aspects and enhance re-connection. By bringing different memories into mind, these memories can help build a sense that there is hope.

As Rinske says she remembers nothing about her little sister I invite her to recollect together some stories about her little sister and mum. I ask if her little sister had a cuddly bear.

R: Her hospital bed was full!
S: Was there one that stuck out?
R: A kitten with pink spots.
S: Where did it come from?
*R: From the hospital store. I actually wanted it, but didn't get it from daddy, so
    my sister asked it for me.*
S: Does this mean that you were very important to your sister?
R: Yes.
S: Does it also mean that she was a caring person?
S: Have you gone looking for that cuddly toy yet?
R: Yes, on Google images, but I didn't find the same one ...

A small fragment of the letter Rinske received after the interview shows how the conversation continued.

Rinske, your little sister called you 'Jinse' because she couldn't pronounce the 'r'. Bit by bit memories came back. If she could hear that you know all those small things, you thought she would appreciate this and find it very nice. We came to the conclusion that you always carry her with you. We made also a supposition: 'How would your little sister like that her sister carries her with her?' You answered: 'Remembering her and my mum like I used to do and still be able to laugh (also mum would want this)'.

Before zooming in on the difficulties, it is helpful to highlight a number of safe territories. Rinske appears here for herself, the witnesses and myself as an involved, caring person who wants to maintain the connection with her sister. These territories work as a safe haven from which we can look at the problems or life obstacles and reflect on them without being absorbed by them. Going into these territories also helps the interviewer to see and address the client as much more than a 'problem child' or 'victim'.

A manageable way of speaking

Talking directly about the death of Rinske's sister and mother can provoke tears and inconsolable grief. If this is the case, it often does not help and may cause Rinske to stop talking and reflecting. Asking children or youngsters to retell what happened in the same old ways as they have done maybe a thousand times to themselves (and maybe to others) risks reproducing the painful experiences or trauma and create even more solidified stories. When these experiences are accompanied by too overwhelming pain, disgust, fear, shame, etc., we can propose to put 'the violence', 'the painful experiences', 'the whole hassle' for the time being in a container, a box or a sealed envelope that cannot be opened without their permission.

The process of supporting children and young people often starts with putting the power of naming problems and worries back into the hands of the child and their families and communities. Rather than re-visiting the traumatic experiences or painful histories we can invite the children or youngsters to name the pain in an experience-near way, or to cast the problem in an appropriate image (Vermeire et al., 2018). In this process we collaboratively identify the issues that need to be addressed in order to gain a clear as well as a rich description. There are many ways to go about this. Next to verbally articulating the problems in an experience-near way, staying close to the language they normally use, we can for instance draw the problems on the whiteboard or on a piece of paper. By using clay, we can literally put the effects of the painful experiences, instead of the 'problem child', on the examination table. These are all instances of externalising conversations (White, 2007).

The rotten feeling

We sometimes ask children to search for an object that feels appropriate to their experiences (Russian dolls, cars, Skylanders, dinosaurs, Duplo, …). Rumbling

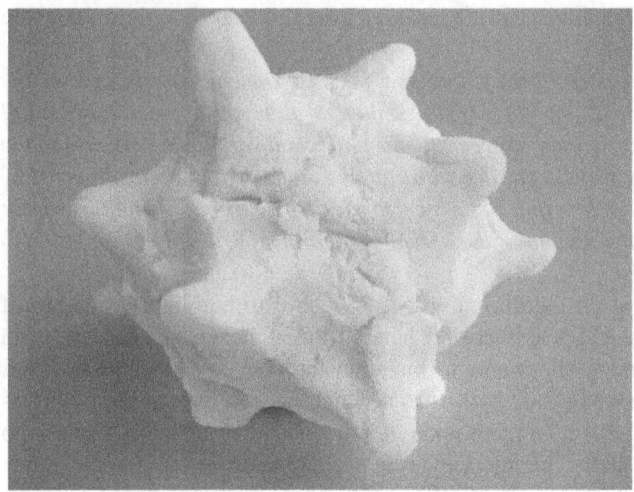

Figure 3.7 Pink ball of clay. Photograph by the author.

in the play toy boxes they can choose an object that fits. Even searching images on the internet opens surprising possibilities. Parents and other family members attending the interview can be invited to help the child, or to find a suitable image.

We do not engage with their experiences and emotions directly to begin with. Instead, we invite both the child and his/her carers onto a safe platform from which they can look at their difficulties without becoming emotionally overwhelmed. By inviting the children or youngsters to cast the difficulties in images, we create a common language.

R: It hurts so much to miss them and I always have to hide that pain. But this is no longer possible. I have to cry all day long and feel bad.
S: Can I ask some maybe crazy questions?
R (stops crying and looks up curiously).
S: How big are the pain and the sadness? Is this pain larger than this room? Could we contain it in this room?
R: You can't put it in this room. It feels like a granite rock.
S: Has this granite rock a specific colour?
R: Black!
S: That black granite rock has been there since your sister died and has grown bigger since mum died?
R: Yes, I used to be able to leave it in my room, but now I have to carry it everywhere. It sticks to me and won't let go of me.
S: How would you call this granite rock of pain?
R: The Pain of Missing

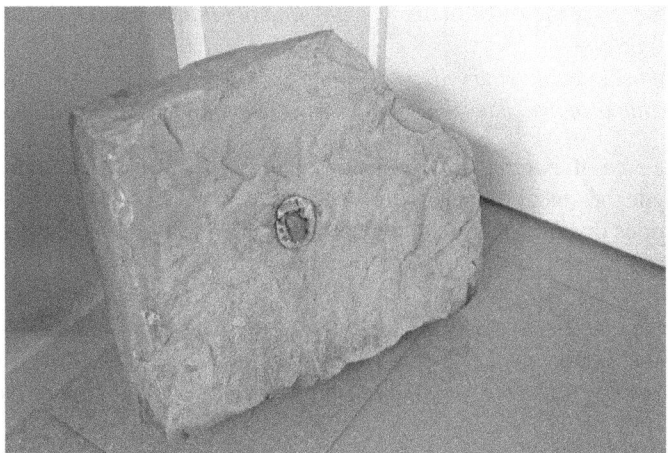

Figure 3.8 Granite rock. Photograph by the author.

'The pain of missing'

These descriptions of their worries and dilemmas often bear witness to a large resourcefulness and creativity and open doors to new ways of exploring things. This naming can be a whole sentence or description '*the sneaky monster with the critical voice*', '*the whole hassle*', an exclamation '*The Bwuuuurgh thing*' or even a character '*Monsieur Anger*', etc. It is not about finding the right problem or the right naming. It can just be a provisional naming developing or changing during our research. When they can't grab a name we can sometimes offer examples that others used or evoke the image by inviting all their senses: how does it smell, taste, sound, look like or feel if you could touch it? Once we have a 'container' for their experiences we can ask questions that investigate these externalised problems. This means assessing the problem together in a way that feels manageable.

S: *What does that granite rock do to your relationships? Does it nibble at your dreams? (while I put a black block on the table and together looking at the block).*

R: *I don't have any more dreams.*

S: *Did The Pain of Missing also crawl into your body?*

 ...

S: *What would you prefer to do with the rock, The Pain of Missing (while taking the block on the table in my hands and offering it to Rinske)?*

R (*after reflecting deeply*): *As far as possible. In the corner of the room.*

S: *It can stay in the room?*

R: *Yes. That pain doesn't have to disappear completely from my life. It's about my mum and my sister... I don't want to forget them. I want to be able to put the*

> rock in the corner of the room in the morning and not think about it all day.
> I still want to be myself.
> S: What does that mean being yourself?
> R: Someone who thinks of her sister and mum but still can laugh and enjoy things.

In addition to the area of externalised problems and alternative stories, it is also important to include the voices of meaningful people in the interview. This means that we ask questions that imaginatively 'populate' the interview or allow important people to participate in our explorations.

Her auntie and some other people frequently say to Rinske that she has a 'character', just like her mum. Together we explore what these people mean by that and what this possibly could mean for her mum. Then we look at her mum's chair and reflect on what she might say and what advice she would give in the current situation.

Ways of responding

Many children and youngsters are sent to therapy because the people involved are worried, notice the suffering, feel helpless or got stuck in relation to the child and don't know how to go on themselves. This means that these significant people developed a perspective of the child, of themselves, of the problems of the child and of the cause of these problems which proved to be unhelpful. Sometimes the child became 'a traumatised child', 'an unwilling child', 'insecurely attached child' that needs to be helped or changed. From the very start we try to widen these perspectives by letting the child share a kaleidoscope of stories. We invite them to tell alternative stories, to share initiatives they have taken. We unravel their understandings of the problems, we facilitate a rich and multilayered sense of experiences, actions, emotions and problems. This opens the possibility for the people present to see the child and what occupies their minds in a much richer picture. This requires us to structure our conversation in ways that are different from the ways we usually have conversations with each other (Freedman, 2014). One way to achieve this is by inviting the people involved into a witness position providing clear instructions and transparency about our hopes and ambitions in doing so.

Future professionals as witnesses

During the interview with Rinske future care workers were asked from the beginning to listen to her story in a different way than they are used to. After the interview, they were asked the following questions as 'outsider witnesses' (White, 2007):

1. Was there a word, phrase, theme, expression … that caught your attention, that surprised, touched, intrigued you or made you think?
2. Did during Rinske's telling a particular image came to your mind?

3. Was there anything told that resonates with your own work, life? Where did this telling bring you in your own life or relationships?
4. What do you take away for your own life, relationships, etc.? Did you hear anything you want to reflect on later? Does Rinske's telling inspire you in any way? Is there anything said that you want to hold on to, or that inspires you for tomorrow?

The family worker says how she has been touched by the pain of missing and by how hard Rinske works to keep giving her mum and sister a place. She sees Rinske as a little hamster in her lair, constantly trying to keep them alive. The story brought the family worker to her own childhood and the divorce of her parents. The temporary loss of one of her parents every week was terrible to her. She takes the strength of Rinske with her to remember in hard times, as well as her power to keep looking for ways to keep a loved one with you and at the same time not let the suffering take over your life.

This outsider witness gathering (White, 2007) structures the telling and retelling of clients' experiences and stories. It opens the possibility to understand the youngsters and their story in their own words and helps to acknowledge the youngster's local knowledge, skills and wisdom. Professionals and caregivers need to park their 'professional view' for a moment and, above all, listen to what touches them or attracts their attention. They move from a more 'analytical, inquisitive, expert' chair to an 'affected, moved person' chair. Here, a few social and professional discourses emerge that often make listening to and answering the questions for these witnesses a challenge, such as 'you keep private and professional worlds separate', 'you don't show your emotional feelings', 'you don't expose yourself', etc. It requires an effort from the interviewer to help caregivers cross thresholds by explicitly inviting them to contribute their stories that resonate with those of the youngster.

Rinske's mentor is touched by the theme of loss and hesitates about where this theme takes him in his own life. I note that it may feel a bit strange to tell something about his own life here, but ask if he can give us a small piece of story after all. He tells us about his grandfather, who was suddenly gone after a heart attack. He was never talked about again. He now realises how terrible he found this silence as a child.

Parents, family members and friends as witnesses

Not only can the future care workers be present at this first interview, but also the relatives or friends the client would like to invite. It often remains a challenge to invite parents, siblings or partners to listen and speak in a way that focuses on the child's story. It is not about 'is the child telling the truth?' or 'is the young person doing well?'. What parents say and do is also informed by social discourses: 'A parent tries to protect their child from disadvantages', 'a parent knows what occupies their children's mind (they know the "emotional inside" of the child) and so has to explain to the therapist what the real problem is'. They can also be focused on 'what says the child about me?' So there is always the risk they will interfere during the interview. We must first acknowledge that we are asking something difficult of them as parent, as aunt or friend. The social instructions as a family member or involved insider make it tempting to react or correct the young person during the interview. We have to explain that we hope they will be able to 'listen differently' (Freedman, 2014).

The person in charge of the crisis unit where Rinske is staying sends an email to warn that her aunt will constantly interrupt the interview and overload Rinske with good advice on how to take back control of her life.

Before we start with Rinske's interview, I take the time to thank the witnesses for coming and emphasise that we are together to listen to Rinske's story. I explain how important it is that what Rinske will tell us will be taken seriously. Next, I address myself to her aunt and mention that she is in one of the more difficult positions because I assume that as an aunt she is very involved and concerned. We discuss what can help her to listen carefully to what touches her and to keep track of what she wants to say after the interview. If it all gets too much for her, she will give a signal and go outside for a few minutes.

Investing time in explaining and recognising the difficulties or pitfalls helps create a good listening context and a valuable testimony. It makes family members or other loved ones sometimes put in even more effort and stick to the instructions when difficult topics are discussed. When you notice that people really can't keep listening, you can point them to the beforehand agreed way out.

Auntie is particularly touched by the way Rinske honours her mother (and sister). The story about the hugs moves her. She takes with her the idea that you're only really dead when everyone has forgotten you. She is reassured that this will never happen to Rinske.

Myerhoff (2007) emphasises that telling stories out loud in the presence of witnesses is more than an announcement. It is an event in which the listener is more than a passive receiver. The listener can also change by listening. White (2004) shows how the position of outsider witness can bring the listener to new or forgotten places or opens up new paths. At the same time, by sharing and retelling, youngster and witness can become connected.

Planning and documenting our collaborative journey

'The harvest' of our meeting

At the end of our first conversation, together we (the child, people present and the therapist) review what has been spoken about, became visible or was discovered or created. We collect what has to be kept in mind, the main worries and obstacles and what has to be further explored or developed. We negotiate about what is important for the child and others involved to be documented and maybe shared with others. We take pictures of what was co-created and suggest to write it all down in a letter or a document in a way that feels suitable to them so they can re-read it. The practice of documenting helps to retain certain words, sentences, statements or ideas (White & Epston, 1990) and to strengthen the collaboration between the child, family and therapist.

The interview with Rinske is filmed. About a week later, she receives the film and a letter with her story told also including the reflections of the witnesses. She can re-read the interview or watch it again and listen to it again. By mirroring the words and meaning co-created, she feels and realises what she was saying and what she has uttered becomes more lasting (Epston & White, 1992). Capturing the interview in a letter also has the advantage that it can be shared with others. Some family members or friends who were not present can watch the film afterwards and still give their reflections. Rinske visits her father a few weeks later with the recorded film and asks him to look at it together with her.

When the child or youngster agrees, the carers or future professionals who were present during this first meeting will also receive a copy of the letter. This telling and passing on immediately creates a collaborative relationship and connection between them. It is a stepping stone for the route the client will take together with the carers.

If we want to install a strong culture of feedback, especially in contexts of adversity, we also have to check how the child and the people involved experienced this first meeting and whether we are on track for a collaborative journey. Questions like 'Did you feel listened to?' 'Did everyone have the experience of being noticed and being heard about what is worrying them?' 'Was our way of talking and working together appropriate?' (Duncan et al., 2010) and maybe most importantly, *'Is there already something we talked about or discovered together that brings something new or that surprises you? Are you still in the same place as at the beginning of our meeting or was there something new or different? Were there small discoveries? Did you discover anything helpful?'* As Duncan et al. (2010) indicate that the most important change in the therapeutic process happens in the first three sessions, it is valuable to check where we are in our journey and what works well from the perspective of the clients in order to become 'a collaborative learning community'.

These first conversations gave us an idea of themes that are important to the child and their family. We discussed their main worries, some responses they found, which skills and local knowledges they developed through life, etc. Common grounds, connectedness and togetherness became visible and felt, as well as unique perspectives, personal stories, wishes or hopes of the child, parents, carers and networks. These different aspects can form an interesting entry point to discuss and agree on our next steps to take.

Rinske and her mentor decide to place a heavy granite rock in her room symbolising 'the pain of missing'. They will have daily conversation about this rock, its effects and how she deals with it. Together with her aunt and Rinske, the family worker suggests to collect valuable memories that Rinske can cherish and that maybe counterbalance the pain of missing. During the interview, Rinske expressed concerns about some unresolved issues that she would like to ask her father about in the future, but she feels this will require some preparation.

Subsequently, we must collaboratively agree on the course to take in the thera-peutic process and how we will proceed. We will have to negotiate what needs to be done, who will be involved, and what our goal will be in a recursive process (Sheinberg & True, 2008).

At the end of the first meeting with Yusuf and his mother, we discuss which con-cerns and obstacles need to be further investigated and what especially requires our attention during our next meetings. Yusuf says he would like to have less quarrels with his friends at school and it would make a difference to him if his best friend could pass by now and then to play with him. He also likes to talk some more about his grandparents who live in Somalia. His mum emphasises that the quarrels at home have to stop and she thinks it would be helpful for Yusuf if the nightmares were less frightening. Asking his mum if she wants something particularly for herself, she answers: 'Peace of mind! I would like to know that everything will be all right. I often think I had to leave his dad much earlier'.

Conversational settings

At the end of our first meeting(s) we have to re-negotiate and re-decide how we will further organise our conversational setting and how exactly the significant people (professional as well as non-professional) will be involved. Who will be present in our meetings, in which role, in what position and for what purpose? Which information will be shared with whom, in what way and for what purpose? If we centre the child's stories and perspective, in which conversational settings will the child be listened to, understood, supported and taken seriously?

Our conversational setting choice for the therapeutic journey covers a broad range: speaking with the child alone, with the parents or carers separately, speak-ing all together, inviting people of the network (professional or non-professional). Each choice creates a context in which certain meanings can emerge and others fade into the background. Choosing a particular setting influences the process of meaning-making and therefore the therapeutic process. Our first conversation(s) already gave us an idea of what can and what cannot be spoken of, discussed and explored in the presence of parents, carers or other important people. They informed us about what setting can be helpful in enhancing change or the devel-opment of richer stories, or the creating of new meaning or finding new ways of relating. We also need to explore and observe carefully which meanings are gen-erated when we speak with the child alone, with their parents or carers, with peo-ple involved (friends, teacher, …). This counts not just for the child themselves but also for all the people involved as each context of speaking is permeable and interwoven in a complex process of influences (Van Daele, 2014).

Some parents and youngsters insist on coming with the whole family because they want to emphasise they belong together, are very close and have no secrets for each other. Other family members want to stay in the room so they can clearly hear what the child tells about them, the family or the problems. They some-times hope to finally get some all-encompassing insights about the child. Some understand their presence as their 'duty' to help the child explain all kinds of issues to the therapist. From the perspective of the child or youngster they can appreciate the presence of the parents or carer or network and experience it as a real support. It can create a sense of being 'together' on this therapeutic journey. Although for some children, it will make them play 'safe' and prevents them from sharing stories.

Yusuf and his mum agree that it was a good conversation. Yusuf told a few things he never told before and his mum also heard some new aspects about his struggles. Both have the impression that they worked hard together and Yusuf gives his mum 11 points out of 10 for helping him finding some answers and developing an image for the nightmares. Both he and his mother decide they want to talk further together.

When speaking, exploring and developing new perspectives goes fluently and each of the participants agree with the common goals and themes to talk about, we can go on all together. Although it can be interesting to keep the door open for separate conversations when felt necessary by one of the participants (the child, the parents/carers as well as the therapist). In contexts of violence, traumatic experiences, radical responses, there can be subjects that are first better discussed with the child alone or with the parents or carers alone (Sheinberg & Fraenkel, 2001). Some subjects can evoke shame or blaming in the room and children or parents can unintentionally disadvantage each other while expressing their experiences, worries or perspectives on the problems.

Sometimes children nor parents or carers want to burden their loved ones with their stories of suffering. Sometimes they have no clue how the people involved will respond to their stories or disclosures so they want first to explore this in individual conversations or without the co-actors in the stories of suffering. Their lives can be such an emotional rollercoaster that they need time and space to find ways to deal with it in the privacy of the therapy room and regain a little bit of sense of control before sharing certain stories with others.

Rinske was clear about inviting her father to the interview: if he would be present, she wouldn't say a word. In our negotiation about how to proceed she maintains this position and does not consider it necessary to involve him. 'He is too unpredictable and can ruin everything. He would probably minimise the things I say'. In questioning if and maybe how we keep him informed, she shrugs her shoulders and replies: 'I'll think about it but for now we do nothing'. So it was rather surprising that a few weeks later she went to her father and they watched the recorded interview together.

Sometimes parents, carers or referrers keep insisting that you speak to the child alone as a therapist-expert. The first meeting they consider as introduction, to inform the therapist and clarify the right perspectives and directions to take. After this step the real work has to be started and the child or youngster needs to process the traumatic experiences. In these contexts the child can understand the choice for an individual conversational setting as *'The therapist agrees with my parents or carers. I am the cause of all these troubles. I have to work hard and change'*.

On other occasions the child experiences the opportunity of individual conversations as a kind of acknowledgement of their worries and the painful things that have happened in their life. It can evoke a feeling of being taken seriously. The therapy can become a safe space to explore and share what is bothering them. Choosing individual conversations doesn't absolve us, as systemic therapists, from the negotiation of how to involve or inform the significant people.

Leaving parents or carers out of the meetings can give them the impression that they are considered incompetent or even seen as the cause of the problems by the therapist. This can enhance their sense of failing. For other parents or carers, choosing for individual conversations connects with social instructions that as good parents or carers you have to find the best help and expertise you can get for your child. By bringing the child to therapy they 'act' as good parents.

The remark of Yusuf's mum 'I had to leave his dad much earlier' becomes a stepping stone to check with his mum if she would like, besides the conversations with Yusuf and herself, to also have some conversations separately about her worries as a mother and how to go on after all these painful experiences. She sighs and replies that this might be helpful. Now, she sometimes has the feeling her thoughts are running in circles. While talking about this, Yusuf is attentively listening. So I turn myself in his direction and ask what he thinks about me having some conversations with his mum besides our collective meetings. As he stands up, steps towards his mother and rubs her back, he says he thinks this is a good idea. He also replies that his mum has to take care of him all by herself and that this is quite hard.

Speaking with parents or carers alone can open the possibilities of reflecting with them about their worries as parents or educators as the child can make a big call on them in many ways. Feelings of helplessness or exhaustion in parents and carers are constantly lurking around the corner. We can then make room to find ways to understand and respond to the problematic actions of the child and strengthen their parenthood. We will, however, need to be vigilant and careful not to give the impression that we consider parents or other carers as the problem or the cause of the problem. It has been remarked that family therapists who work intergenerationally sometimes seem to assume that the problems of the child must be caused by early (traumatic) experiences of the parents (Rober, 2014). Such a viewpoint risks being experienced as blaming and a sense of relational agency can get lost. We prefer to invite parents and other educators in a collaborative partnership so we can re-discover their knowledge and competencies in doing good parenthood in relationship with their child.

A background of painful life events or traumatic experiences and fixed interaction patterns can turn speaking all together into a real burden. The child's ways of protecting themselves or responding to perceived insecurity, but also the ways of responding by the parents or carers, can become activated immediately. The space for speaking and listening differently can be very limited as it happens almost automatically. It sometimes seems as if their bodies all together start to speak for themselves. The child and people involved, each one gets overwhelmed by the disadvantages and their own struggles. So even when everyone agrees to keep on talking together we will need to structure our meetings that something new or different can emerge and each one can become a co-researcher in our journey (see the story of Rinske). Just like new, more helpful ways of relating and connecting can be evoked while their mutual sense of relational agency expands (see Chapters 5 and 6).

A playful seriousness in the process of choosing the next conversational setting including the possibility of inviting relevant people (a teacher, grandparents, a Rabbi or Iman, a friend from school) can be considered a powerful intervention that makes room for alternative meanings and novel relational dances. Inviting significant people from the network, furthermore, keeps the multiple connections in which the child and family are embedded visible and lively.

Once safe grounds, a team of support, a rich exploration of disadvantages, worries, relational involvements, hopes and wishes are established, what follows in this book can be considered a rhizomatic web, that allows the reader, as a clinician, to engage in therapeutic ways and several entry points that are finely attuned to the always unique situations of our clients (Deleuze & Guattari, 2013; Sermijn & Loots, 2015). In other words, the order of the following chapters should not be taken as an indication of the correct sequence of steps or phases in the therapy.

Chapter 4

The tentacles of trauma and adversity

Children who experienced trauma, violence or painful life histories often get caught up in difficulties, become overwhelmed by painful emotions and their bodies are in the grip of distress. 'Problematic behaviour', 'self-harming' or uncontrollable bodily reactions can become omnipresent. These jamming tentacles often enhance negative identity and life conclusions and the loss of any sense of agency. These children get stuck in solidified meanings of being 'worthless'. Toxic guilt and shame are often present, just like several other painful feelings and convictions. In this chapter, I will focus on these often individualised and decontextualised struggles and confusions and explore some playful therapeutic possibilities of contextualising and making meanings fluid again. Rutten (1999) shows that the chain of resilient outcome is enhanced if there is a cognitive and affective processing of experiences. While zooming in and unravelling the traumatic experiences and their tentacles, we try to rediscover what and who is still valuable and matters to the child, always in a web of communicative, relational and contextual influences. Through this process of rediscovering a sense of agency and mattering, we invite the family and networks, live or imaginary, into the room as co-researchers. We hope that perspectives can shift a little, meanings become less solidified and possibly some alternative ideas and stories will emerge. In doing so, hopefully this opens possibilities for new meaning and action. As change comes more over time than overnight, I consider all these playful entry points and unravelling as possible steps to develop a broader, more differentiated and layered view of painful life histories and their impact.

Creating a context for sharing stories

Starting from the notion that children, youngsters and their families, carers or network during the periods when they were subjected to abuse or trauma often had no sense of power or choice, just felt 'trapped' and often still have no sense of agency, we have to be aware during our questioning and journey that there exists a risk that such experiences are reproduced. As in these contexts adults often decide what is best for the child or youngster, we have to make room for the child's voice and their accounts of what happened and what may still be going on. We need to

DOI: 10.4324/9781003167860-5

take into account the relations of power that, although often invisible, are at work when it comes to issues as to which stories can be told or will be listened to, who is authorised to tell them and how they are supposed to be told.

Because we consider children and youngsters as full agents (Cooklin, 2001; De Mol et al, 2018), we choose to consult them(selves) about the painful aspects of their lives. We do this in ways that help them articulate more clearly what preoccupies them, what their worries are, which disadvantages they experienced. We inquire about their relational involvements, their intentions and values but also about how other people respond(ed).

Often therapists (Chapter 3) notice that children are reluctant to speak of their experiences of trauma as they don't want to become trapped in the immediacy of these experiences. Likewise, it is important not to let them give expression to their experiences in ways that contribute to a reinforcement of the single stories and negative conclusions they often hold about their identities, relationships or their lives. Otherwise, this can easily invite and enhance shame, vulnerability or desolation in our conversations. We need to keep in mind that the way we talk and interact will have an effect on the child's self-understandings and experiences.

Iris, 11 years old, is placed in a children's home after years of living with her mum and several partners. The house and family life was dominated by domestic violence, one of the partners sexually abused Iris and her mum stepped out of life a year ago. She found her mum hanging in the stairwell hall. Carers at the children's home are very worried and send her for conversations so she hopefully can have someone to talk with in order to process the traumatic experiences. At the weekends she stays with her uncle and auntie. They are afraid she is going the same way as her mother. She is kicking and bossing around in the children's group. At school she often gets into trouble and is seen as a manipulator. She pulls out her eyebrows and has a bald spot at the back of her head from pulling out her hair. Bedwetting happens every night.

During our first conversations she refuses to talk about her worries and troubles because, as she repeats several times, 'It is the carers who have a problem, not me! You can't imagine how stupid they are just like the children at school'. She tries to reassure me and emphasises 'I can manage my life myself, I don't need anybody!' Although she shouts loudly that she doesn't need to be in therapy, she keeps on coming to 'chat' with me and inventing cooking recipes in the toy kitchen. We spend a lot of time in creating safe ground and collecting a team of support. We even agree on a secret code when questions became too intrusive, feel inappropriate or go in a direction she doesn't want to go. As soon as she starts to talk about the weather, like 'Oh, the sun is shining!' Or 'I think it is going to rain', I have to change subject or I must prepare some dinner for her in the toy kitchen. These small negotiations give her the direction of our journey and contribute to the first steps of re-experiencing a sense of agency.

At the end of our fourth session, she remarks that actually she is angry and frustrated but nobody will ever understand. I ask her if I can consider 'being angry' as a kind of protest to make clear to people what she does not agree with.

Did anyone ever notice how hard she worked during the previous years to keep on going? First, she curiously lifts her head and later with a little bit of pride in her voice she asks: 'Do you think you can discover my secret weapons to survive?'

S: *Are you into a challenge? Would it be an idea for our next meeting: you per-form a puppet show of the past years of your life in the puppet theatre and I try to discover your secret weapons and survival skills?*

Iris earlier on in the therapy chose to do puppet performances about school related incidents. This choice of hers helped me acknowledge the importance of story development while making influencing contexts visible through action and activity. I hoped puppetry could once more be an appropriate way to share some of her even more painful experiences but also to explore her responses in a meticulous manner.

In therapy we need to take care to create a context in which what might be called 'psychological and emotional' safety is ascertained for the child (Rober, 1999; White, 2006). It has been noticed that the re-positioning of the child in a way that helps them to take some distance, or to find material that mediate between themselves and their stories can be very helpful in creating such a context. For instance, Denborough (2008) pointed out that adults who went through difficult times as kids were speaking of themselves in the third person (*what 'kids' went through ...*). Using a non-individualistic voice offered them a possibility to distance themselves and at the same time to relate to a collective of other children. White (2007) used what he referred to as 'stuffed colleagues', namely cuddly bears, etc., as spokesperson for the children, youngsters and the family. They seemed to be very helpful to distance them from the immediacy of their experiences. They became a third-party present at the meetings where the spokesperson could be interviewed instead of the child directly and the puppet or cuddly bear could check back with the child if things were understood in the right way or represented correctly.

Rucinska & Reijmers (2014) emphasise how play and objects can be used to elaborate the therapeutic dialogue. While engaged in action, the playing adds as well as reinforces narratives. More specifically, a puppet performance can be particularly helpful to situate feelings, like the anger and frustrations of Iris, into a sequence of actions, a storyline. Since contexts, actions and meaning are inseparable, different stories, alternative and multi-layered contexts can potentially emerge through this puppetry. The child can act and experience from different relationships and contexts. It can help the child to move from the *known and familiar* single, reduced, pathologising stories to *what is possible to know* by developing, through the play, richer understandings, multiple meanings and new steps to go on (White, 2007). The puppetry can be considered as a dialogue that enables the creation of new meaning (Rucinska & Reijmers, 2014). As the child can freely choose which role they will perform, and in what way they will do this, they can engage in what Holzman (2009, p. 19) referred to as 'creating who you are by performing who you are not'.

I (with a big smile answering my proposal): Oh! Yes! I take the Koala Bear for my mum and I will be the Big White Rabbit.
S: Would it be helpful to have some other people watching the puppet show and help me discover?
I: Who are you thinking of?
S: Any idea who would be interested in this or maybe surprised noticing your hard working or your skills? Is there someone you would like to share this with?
I: Laetitia, my mentor, she is really worried about me.
S: What are you hoping for when she is watching the puppet show?
I: That she knows I will manage. I want her to believe in me.
S: Someone else that could benefit from this performance?
I: My uncle and auntie. I think they know only half of what happened.

We have to carefully prepare where, how and in whose presence this will take place. Just like we try to grab what their purposes, wishes and hopes are by sharing these stories. This puppet performance can offer possibilities not only to give voice to their experiences but also to share and richly acknowledge the effects of the painful life events. Carefully and collectively listening for multiple accounts of these experiences can change some of their perspectives. We try to find practices that can honour the special skills and coping ways that made it possible to navigate through the dark hours into the present (White, 2006c). As many acts of children aren't noticed it is important that not only I, as a therapist, or the child themselves start to notice these small actions of living, small actions to keep going on, etc., and the multiplicity of stories. Also, significant people who are part of their world can start to see and understand the child in a much richer web of crisscrossing influences and maybe reach more differentiated and nuanced conclusions. This means we always try to approach children from a stance of dignity in the sense that we take all their experiences seriously (Reynolds, 2020).

At the beginning of our journey there has been a conversation with Iris's uncle, auntie and professionals involved where mutual concerns were shared and an agreement on collaboration was established. Our 'team of support' was very willing to attend the puppet show.

The puppet show: re(dis)covering a sense of agency

At our next meeting Iris appears well dressed, just as her special guests. We instruct her mentor as well as her uncle and auntie to look and listen in a special way. I explicitly ask them to pay particular attention to, and make note of, survival skills and possible secret weapons during the performance. After the puppet show, Iris will question them as quizmaster. They can earn five points for each skill discovered.

Iris disappears behind the puppet screen and introduces the different puppets of the play and who they represent.

I: Welcome to this performance! This is Big White Rabbit also known as Iris, who will be the leading lady. We also have Koala (mum), Roaring Lion (father), Stupid Kenny (one of the ex-partners of mum), ...

S: Dear Rabbit, can I interrupt for a moment? Are there some special things we have to know about these puppets before we start?

I (jumping with her face from behind the screen): Silence please... everything will become clear within a few minutes.

I prefer to approach children as the owners of their experiences and stories. Iris for instance often hadn't had a sense of power, control or choice during the many moments of abuse. That's why I want her to be the director of the play as I hope that this will facilitate a sense of agency. I don't want Iris to just 'reproduce' through the puppetry the same single stories or reinforce the dominant meanings that inform her actions nor revisiting the sites of abuse and trauma. Just like I have to be aware of the risk of getting imprisoned by the painful events myself or into the grip of rigid, fixed interpretations of actions that take place in front of my eyes in the puppet play. I need an openness and attentiveness for what the child brings into the performance and listen carefully to each moment to moment offering. Occasionally, I ask permission to interrupt the play and ask questions when things are unclear, make me curious and would like to know more. We will need to find a way to co-monitor if we are still on track. I hope to endorse a process-oriented interaction between Iris and myself, between Iris and/or the different puppets and between Iris, the people involved, the puppets and myself.

I do not consider this performance as just 'a representation of what happened' but rather as a personal story told from an insider's perspective. What at first sight appears to be no more than one single story in fact contains many small, differentiated, alternative stories filled with multi-layered meanings depending on which contexts are in the foreground. A representation furthermore would leave everything as it 'is', while performing their story for an audience generates new understandings and meanings. The audience is not just a neutral spectator of these stories, but actually help to create these new, alternative meanings by offering questions, making remarks, being surprised, laughing, sharing reflections and by simply being there.

The puppet show starts with a lovely scene of Koala and Roaring Lion embracing each other and looking at new born White Rabbit in a cradle. Pretty soon a quarrel starts between Koala and Roaring Lion. They shout all kinds of accusations at each other.

S: Is this happening in the apartment of White Rabbit's mum? How old are you at that moment, White Rabbit?

Surprisingly a lovely princess puppet pops up, singing and dancing and giving White Rabbit a kiss on the forehead. It turns out to be her half-sister (14 years older than Iris who at the age of 17 and a half left the household without leaving a trace). Princess answers my questions and tries to calm down Roaring Lion and Koala in the puppet theatre. When asking to stop screaming at each other doesn't make a difference she throws a vase on the ground. Roaring Lion takes Princess up and throws her out of the house. White Rabbit starts to cry loudly. A bit later Koala throws Roaring Lion out of the house, yelling 'I am angry, I am angry!'

S: *Is Koala angry because Princess was thrown out?*
> *Puppet Koala answers still with angry voice: 'Yes, but also because everyone hurts me. No one is to be trusted!'*
S: *And the crying of White Rabbit? What is this about?*
> *White Rabbit jumps out of the cradle and says with a baby voice 'I am missing Princess'.*

Iris is not just the director but also the puppeteer of the performance. This means she becomes the animator, instructor and manipulator of the puppets. She decides what will be 'performed', shared and told by whom. At the same time, she can hide behind the screen which prevents her from being 'watched' directly and offers a sense of safety and an antidote to a sense of vulnerability. It is White Rabbit who says she is missing Princess, not Iris. While speaking through the puppets, she can explore how other puppets in the play might have experienced the different situations, what they might feel, think, etc. In this way a more embodied experience is created. The different actions, feelings, thoughts can be noticed and examined for their importance to themselves and significant others. Iris can verbalise and share her understandings and meanings given to the actions of Koala/her mum.

She can play with different roles and positions like 'Iris as client', 'Iris playing Iris as White Rabbit', 'Iris speaking as her mum' or 'Iris as director or puppeteer who lets others perform'. We move into an ongoing playful negotiation with me as therapist, as spectator, as interviewer of the puppets, of Iris, of Iris speaking up for her mum and so on. As such she cannot only explore roles and positions but also what can be said, shared, noticed and acknowledged. Initially my questions aren't addressing the child in a direct sense but through the puppets. This can work as some 'filter' and space between the child and the questions but some moments later it can be that Iris pops up from behind the screen and responds herself to my question. Even 'the audience' can get a new role during the performance.

At a certain point Iris is short of hands and asks her mentor to join her behind the screen. She gives instructions to her mentor with which puppets she has to play and what they have to do, say and in what kind of way.

At that moment it becomes really a collective project. Together now they engage in what we consider a dynamic, relational, communicative and embodied practice in which the child can share their worries, their disadvantages and sufferings as well as their relational involvements, commitments and efforts to sustain or their attempts to persevere and re-investigate interpretations and stories developed. We consider dealing with trauma as a relational and social process.

Later on in the performance, after several new partners of Koala appearing and many quarrels and beatings between them, White Rabbit addresses the public and warns them of something bad to come.

Koala mutters to herself, steps on the stairs to the roof of the building and speaks to us 'That's enough! I'm going to jump down!' Koala falls down with a scream 'Aaaaarrrgghhh!' A puppet yells 'A woman on the street!' and an ambulance comes 'WEE-oww-WEE-oww'! A few moments later Koala is in hospital with broken bones. She whispers: 'White Rabbit must not know what happened. Shh'.

Meanwhile, White Rabbit comes in the hospital room, flies into Koala's arms and asks: 'Mummy, what happened?' She responds: 'I was cleaning the windows and fell down. You'd better stay with uncle and auntie until I am cured. Everything will be all right'. White Rabbit embraces her mum with great affection and makes a lot of promises about behaving well, helping her uncle and auntie as much as she can and always thinking of her mum.

S: Dear White Rabbit, can I ask something?
    Curious, White Rabbit looks up.
S: Did you know from the start that it wasn't an accident?
    White Rabbit nods firmly.
S: Does this mean that you always had pricked up ears and kept an eye on
    everything?
    White Rabbit nods again.
S: Does this mean that Iris is a rather smart girl, that you can't fool her?
    *Iris's face appears in the puppet theatre and together with White Rabbit
    she nods at the audience while whispering a bit mysteriously 'very smart...'.*
S: Did she pretend to believe her mum?
I: Yes, of course. Her mum had enough on her mind already.
S: Does this mean White Rabbit is not only smart but also tried to take care of her
    mum? Or how do I have to understand this?
I: Not to burden her with stupid things, it was better to overload her with happy
    words.

We intervene with questions in order to link the things that happen, feelings and actions with local and broader contexts and meanings. Each of the puppet's actions can be understood within a relational and contextual web of involvements just like each response can be linked with disadvantages, intentions, values, beliefs, wishes, hopes. Instead of just listening to what happens, we engage actively (and responsibly) in a process of co-creating alternative, new perspectives and understandings.

As therapist it is also my responsibility to keep the other spectators and listeners in mind, for they too will be touched by what is being performed. I don't want the audience to get stuck in single interpretations of Iris's life, or in simplified or negative identity conclusions about some puppets/actors or in feeling more pity for Iris. At that point the performance would just become a confirmation of her being a victim or of as auntie told me once 'I fear she is a bird to the cat'. By interrogating the puppets and making them more richly describe their actions and expressions, we can try to make visible what would normally escape the gaze of family members, carers and professionals. I want them to stick to the viewing and listening instruction given at the start of the performance so something new can be discovered. I am constantly trying to keep in mind that this performance is situated within a network of relationships (Wilson, 2007). What I hope and strive for is that the network can become a learning community through the process of this performance.

During the puppet show some more painful moments pass by interspersed with some bright spots, like the dancing camp and the cooking moments with Koala and auntie. Each time I ask some questions that can shed light on the small actions of White Rabbit during the quarrels and fights and on how she kept going on in moments of loneliness, fear, anger or sadness without minimalising or ignoring the disadvantages she experienced. I also ask questions that meticulously illuminate all kinds of aspects and contexts that possibly matter.

We get to know that the death of her favourite dog was a very painful moment, a turning point. He was beaten by Kenny. I ask White Rabbit how she would name this moment. White Rabbit calls it 'The moment hope disappeared' and explains to the audience that she changed into an angry rabbit, snarling around and biting everyone who stood in her way.

S: Dear White Rabbit, can I ask one more question about the snarling and biting?

I ask this because moment by moment I want to check in with Iris if we are still on track and if she wants to go in that direction. I want to give her an active role in monitoring the effects of our work together.

WR (while snarling and biting): Give it a try! As long as it isn't a stupid question!
S: Was the snarling and biting mainly at others like children at school, your mum, Kenny or also at yourself?
WR (yelling and slapping herself in the puppet theatre): Yes! Yes! Yes! Silly White Rabbit!
S: Can you help me understand why White Rabbit became silly?
WR: She couldn't protect Rocky (her dog). She promised to protect Rocky always!
S: Is 'protecting and caring for' an important mission of White Rabbit?
    ...
    The period stupid Kenny did the evil things towards her became the moment 'catastrophe' fell on her head and made White Rabbit dirty. Iris, as director, decides that this part of the story will be continued another time.

The performance creates a distance between the child-as-a-performer and the child-being-in-the-experience. It gives her the opportunity to shift roles and positions as she pleases. In the puppetry we get to see 'language in action', a term used by Wilson (2007), which evokes also the idea of the movement of thoughts and words. Through the performance naming 'traumatic, painful or shocking experiences' in an experience-near way becomes possible and we can have a closer look at the impact. While the performance is developing, the child can notice their own small actions and discover that they have ideas, knowledges and responses to certain experiences. We can explore their expressions of experiences and the meanings that went along with this. They can reconnect with values that are important to them. They can even re-evaluate their relationship to these experiences and position themselves differently to the problems.

We arrive in the performance again at a point where White Rabbit warns the audience: 'Something bad will happen again'. White Rabbit is visiting her mother and before leaving for the children's home, she says goodbye at length. Koala promises to pick her up next weekend. White Rabbit repeats about 20 times while hugging and kissing her mum: 'I love you' and 'Until next week'.

Once left, Koala murmurs 'I give up. I'm going to hang myself'. Meanwhile, White Rabbit is doing her homework and gets a lump in her throat. Koala is hanging in the corner of the puppet theatre.

I ask White Rabbit, still coughing, if she had a premonition that Mummy was going to die. Iris reappears and nods instead of White Rabbit.

...

She also asks the audience if we want to know how it ends. She adds that she is going to skip the moment she found her mum. Everyone agrees. She disappears again behind the screen.

White Rabbit is in her bedroom writing a letter. She reads aloud what she is writing.

'Dear mum, I miss you for ever and ever. I love you for ever and ever! A million kisses, White Rabbit'.

White Rabbit takes a second piece of paper and pretends to be writing: 'Dear Uncle and Auntie, I love to be with you. Please can I stay with you all the time, for ever and ever. I promise to behave well, obey always and be sturdy. I won't bother you. A million kisses, White Rabbit'.

Immediately after this reading, Iris jumps from behind the puppet theatre with a big smile on her face saying 'And they all lived long and happy. The end!'. She bows and looks expectantly.

Responses to the performance

In the contexts of a puppet performance, a theatre play, a film premiere, it is customary for the audience to applaud. We express our appreciation for the show, the director, the actors, etc. When we are deeply moved by what has been staged, we even give a standing ovation.

Yet despite the expectant looks of Iris, hesitation is noticeable in myself as well as in Laetitia and her aunt and uncle. None of us wants to applaud the horrors and the injustice told in the story. Nor does a one-tune praising of White Rabbit feel appropriate. However, Iris brought a unique, personal performance. How can we honour this in an appropriate way and show our gratitude for what she offered us?

Reflecting on this issue brings me back to a training week on 'Narrative Therapy and Community Work with children and families in the context of trauma' in Kigali, Rwanda. After each presentation of trainees' projects, often filled with horrible stories, traumatic experiences and situated in conditions of social or institutional injustice, there was a short negotiation with the group about what form of appreciation they wanted to give to express the richness this story brought them. There were maybe ten kinds of applause that were always followed by singing or dancing together. It really felt as an act of relating, responding, honouring and at the same time 'doing hope together'. Each day a 'morale' was chosen from the group, i.e., a group member who had the responsibility to take care of this. This practice was also inspired by Mukamana (2020), who invited one member to fulfil the role of 'morale' in her team of professionals working with survivors of genocide. The team members were often themselves affected by the traumatic experiences in Rwanda and by involving song, dance and humour a sense of taking care of each other was evoked. The way people involved and communities relate and respond to the stories told will mutually influence the relationships and self-esteem of the child.

Feeling Iris's yearning eyes burning on my retina, I tell her: 'I would like to give an applause with a lot of fireworks for all this incredible knowledge you gave me. I would also like to stamp loudly with my feet for the courage you found to share this with us and even whistle on my fingers for performing with such a dignity. Still, I am hesitating because, for sure, I don't want to applaud the violence, abuse or injustice. Neither do I want to applaud the distress and suffering caused by all these painful events. So which kind of applause feels appropriate to you? She straightens her back and proudly says 'All of those you said first!'

Together with Laetitia, Uncle and Auntie, we start a concert of applause and reflect further on how to respond to the stories of suffering and the many voices that speak in it.

Not only 'puppet shows' but all kinds of 'playful performances' can open dialogues about the adversities. Depending on what fits for the child, the family or carers and the social-cultural context, we can step into a TV show, a theatre play, a musical, etc.

The quiz as a context of acknowledgement

The idea of a 'puppet show' started with a kind of challenge and the purpose of discovering Iris's survival skills and secret weapons during difficult times. But the process isn't finished yet. Iris will be curious about what has been heard and may be discovered. The active participation of an audience can be a powerful practice of acknowledgement (White, 2006, p. 33). I hope through a quiz we can make visible a broad range of relational efforts, skills and local knowledges to go on during these difficult times and indirectly create a context of acknowledgement for the disadvantages, sufferings and responses.

As a quiz master, Iris holds the reins of the quiz. The answers to the quiz questions are not about judgements of these skills and knowledges neither is it about approval or applause. The pressure, burden or disadvantages experienced by the child up to now become visible and nameable. It gains a right to exist in the social world. We mainly hope that what often remains unnoticed can become noticed, and, in a broader sense, a sense of 'being noticed' can be reached, as many of these children no longer experience making even a small difference in this world. The quiz offers a framework and structures the setting in ways that can be helpful for the participants of the quiz to adhere to the instructions. As I want Iris also to be the audience of the discoveries shared, I negotiate with her if I can be the co-presenter who now and then asks some questions of the participants. She agrees as long as I also answer her questions.

Once the quiz stage is arranged, Iris pretends to take a microphone in her hands and steps towards Laetitia, her mentor. With 'a quiz master's voice' she asks: 'What kind of survival skills did you see in the first part of the puppet show (the part with the yelling and fighting)? With this question you can win five points!'

Laetitia: 'I noticed that you could hide under your blankets. You could shield yourself from the terrible things. You could also comfort yourself with songs and dances'.

Iris interrupted and said with a lot of enthusiasm in her voice: 'Five points! Congratulations!' She brings the microphone in the direction of her uncle and asks if he has something to add also for five points.

Uncle: 'I was impressed with how you tried to keep a close eye on everything'.

S (I interfere because I want the discoveries to be very particular so Iris can notice there has been very careful listening to her performance): 'Can you give some specific moments you noticed this?'

Her uncle gives a few examples and Iris responds with 'Just like Sherlock Holmes!' and walks around as if with a magnifying glass in her hand she is searching in the corners of the room. She returns to the participants and the quiz goes on.

...

The audience is not just 'a spectator' or 'listener' of a performance or a puppet show. Each of them is a relationally involved member who is 'moved' by the stories performed and probably 'moved' by small shifts in their perspective and modes of understanding.

While the quiz goes on, I also ask the participants whether they take something away for themselves from this performance. Is there something they will think about, something that will possibly still occupy them or something that will incite them to something new? I ask Iris if she wants to give points for the answers given. She proposes to offer ten points for each interesting answer.

Auntie: 'I learnt now how important Iris's sister is although she hasn't seen her for ages. I also will bear in mind how hard Iris tried to take care of her mum and maybe how she feels abandoned by many people. I remember how angry I was when my sister (Iris's mum) stepped out of life. It makes me also think how we can be more supportive in different ways.

Through this playful telling, sharing and re-telling movement is induced, movement of actions, feelings, thoughts but also of perspectives and meanings (White, 2007; Freedman & Combs, 2002).

In this sense the puppet show and the quiz can become processes of social sharing that open new pathways, reconnect the members of the network with each other and enhance resilience processes. I would like to emphasise that such initiated processes and created ripples or shifts do not bring about revolutionary changes as what is developed in our therapy room always has to stand the many dialogues in the outside world and children don't live in one context but in a multiplicity of contexts. What became visible in our talking and searching can quickly fade back into the background in other contexts. What was discovered in the therapy room can be subscribed, contradicted or undermined in the many ongoing dialogues outside. I just consider them as valuable openings, steps in re-experiencing a sense of agency and finding ways to go on.

Ordering the messy stuff into a story

A few weeks after the puppet show and the quiz Iris comes for a conversation. With sadness in her voice she tells me she became very angry at the children's home. The Snarling-and-Biting was all around. The situation became worse and finally she pulled out a big tuft of hair in the evening. Her head was bleeding. She is afraid of becoming as crazy as her mum. While bringing this story, the therapy room gets filled with bodily reactions and emotions. Her head hangs down and in the corner of her eyes a small tear appears. Hopelessness is all too present.

I wonder what could be a good step to go on. Often these children get stuck in a mixture of bodily reactions, emotions, actions and thoughts without experiencing any sense of agency. Many utterances by children who experienced adversity can easily be seen as consequences of the trauma or sometimes even the opposite while the previous adversities just get neglected. These children are described as 'full of anger', 'struggling with an inconsolable sadness', 'being depressed', 'deeply damaged' and they begin to understand themselves in these ways. Often dominant social instructions seem to imply they have to learn to regulate these emotions, control their bodies, thinking in the right way and learn to talk about these feelings in an appropriate way to overcome the traumatic experiences.

These bodily reactions, emotions, actions and thoughts often become one big mixed soup in which children have the experience of spinning around and around (thanks to Iris for the image). Emotions are mostly accompanied by bodily reactions (e.g., snarling and biting), actions (pulling her hair) and thoughts (I'm becoming as crazy as my mum). In line with Holzman (2009), Fredman

(2004), Gergen (1999), we believe there is no hard cognitive/emotion divide, nor a thought/reaction divide and so on. If we would step into this kind of binary thinking, we would risk to disconnect mind and body. For Holzman (2009), inspired by the work of Vygotsky, cognitions and emotions are like two sides of the same coin, standing in a kind of dialectical relationship, rather than being separate phenomena. Notwithstanding bodily (re)actions, emotions and thoughts are to be understood as embodied actions interwoven with each other, it can be worthwhile to distinguish them and to explore with the child and people involved how they influence each other in specific relations and contexts, hoping to regain a sense of agency. Also, it can be interesting to listen carefully if the child is mainly talking in emotion language or thoughts, or to notice that it is rather the body that speaks so we can connect to their language.

Emotions, thoughts as well as our body experiences aren't to be conceived as isolated entities, but are part and parcel of particular situations and can be considered as utterances within a complex relational and contextual web of influences and stories.

The vortex of emotions, thoughts, bodily experiences risks making no sense to bystanders nor to the children themselves as they get disconnected from the many interpersonal exchanges in the here and now or of the past and from relational and social contexts in which they are rooted. The way we understand our bodily (re)actions, emotions will guide our interpretations, thoughts and actions, which in turn will influence our emotions, etc. in an ongoing recursive meaning-making process. Just like Iris, as more and more she starts to understand her anger and the actions that go hand in hand with this anger, like pulling her hair or shaking on her legs, she sees this as proof she is becoming as crazy as her mum. The anger, not being able to 'control' her body and her self-harming actions acquire more and more the meaning that she is crazy, not only to herself but also to others. These embodied reactions become more and more decontextualised and individualised. *Iris gets instructions from her peers and carers to go in therapy to learn to be 'normal'.*

Emotion, cognition and body are also never separated from culture, politics and ethics (Bruner, 1990; Denborough, 2019). In these specific contexts of adversities, a child gets disconnected and experiences are no longer shared in a common language. So how can we facilitate these communication processes and engage in participatory sense-making (De Jaegher & Di Paolo, 2007)?

We need to punctuate (Watzlawick et al., 1967) this chaotic interplay in order to help make sense of it. Fredman (2004) has developed some very thoughtful ways to facilitate the ordering of all this messy stuff into a story. Such stories typically have a point of departure within the real events of children's lives that are populated with real people, with their inevitable misunderstandings and moments of alienation. We can explore together, meticulously, the contexts in which this diversity of feelings, thoughts and actions take place. In doing so they can get a new weight or size and open sometimes new, alternative identity conclusions (Decraemer, 2021). We can ask questions that invite amplification of answers so that the experiences generated have a past and a future, become connected with certain characters, become situated within contexts and gain meaning (Freedman & Combs, 1993).

As Iris was, first of all, mainly talking about the snarling and biting, we started our research at that point. *I ask Iris if she can help me understand what happened at the children's home that made 'The Snarling-and-Biting' rush in.* I asked her to make in clay any emotion, thought or body experience that pops up in the unfolding story and give them a name. *Could we make a kind of cartoon and step by step, image by image, picture what was influencing and playing a part? Could we try to grab what was good food for the Anger, 'Snarling-and-Biting' and what kind of Anger it particularly was?*

'I was standing in the kitchen when two girls were staring at me. I was sure they were gossiping about me. Before, they had asked stupid questions about my mother and made silly remarks. I got fully absorbed by these girls and their gossiping. My eyes just stared at them and started to fire. My whole body got warm. Having the feeling I am not ok is a perfect moment for the bright red Pick-A-Fight-Monster with her glaring eyes and unhappy mouth to come. She has a mohawk that screams: No one can touch me! She explodes inside my body and my heart really thumps. She wakes the Blah Blah Blah Monster. In no time, the snarling and biting at them begins'

Children can experience all kinds of (bodily) sensations, not really knowing how to make sense of them. As Shotter (2010) reminds us interacting is always embodied. What happens in contexts of adversity 'moves' their bodies. These affects are often unfixed, unstructured and non-linguistic. By inviting them to articulate these sensations, we transport them as it were, to the social domain of language. The social sharing of emotions, in language, allows them to exist in the social world (De Mol & Rimé, 2017).

By asking children to shape the different experiences in clay, we collect a series of images and objects that can be understood as 'affordances', i.e., possibilities

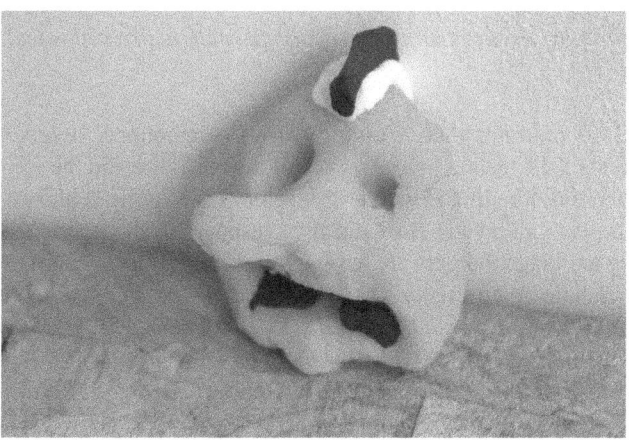

Figure 4.1 Red head of clay. Photograph by the author.

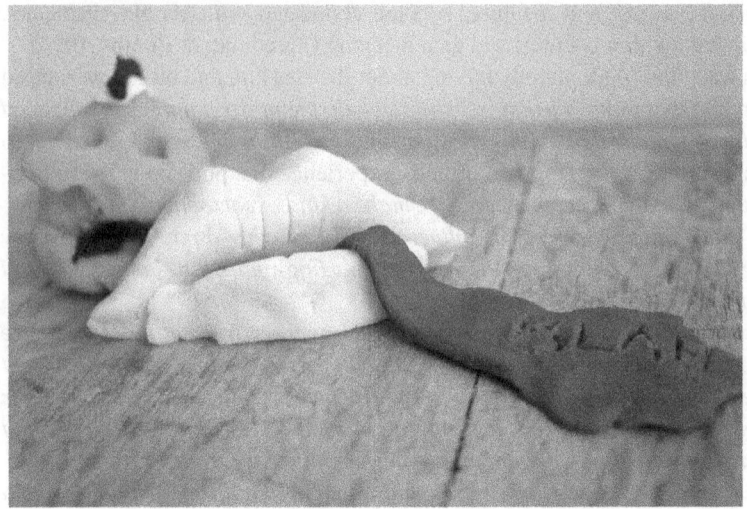

Figure 4.2 Lips with blue tongue in clay. Photograph by the author.

for action (Holzman, 2009) and not just 'representations of their inner world'. We can start to walk around them and open a dialogue about the shape, the colour, the form and how different aspects are related, different feelings linked. We can move the clay figures in a way which can evoke bodily and emotional changes and enhance fluidity of meaning (Rucinska & Reijmers, 2014).

I: The Pick-A-Fight-Monster is red because I am sure my head turns completely red at such a moment.

S: If I could look into the mouth of this Pick-A-Fight-Monster any idea what I would discover?

I (taking the clay figure from the table and looking into the mouth, in a soft voice): Stop hurting me.

Fredman (2004, p. 112) indicates that 'weaving stories of emotions' involves inviting people to situate their feeling in a sequence of actions (How did the feeling come about? When did it begin? How did it develop?) and in the context of interactions (Who else was involved? How did they respond?). Through externalising and picturing an image, borders are assigned to emotions that otherwise would have an all-encompassing presence.

When the Blah Blah Blah Monster showed up, Laetitia (the mentor) said: 'Stop it or go to your room' ... Sometimes the monster makes me roll my eyes. At that moment, the girls and Laetitia too were gripped by the Pick-A-Fight-Monster. Everyone around me got infected. The Explosion Thing smashed everything. I stamped my feet on the stairs, slammed the bedroom door and was hiding my face under my pillow.

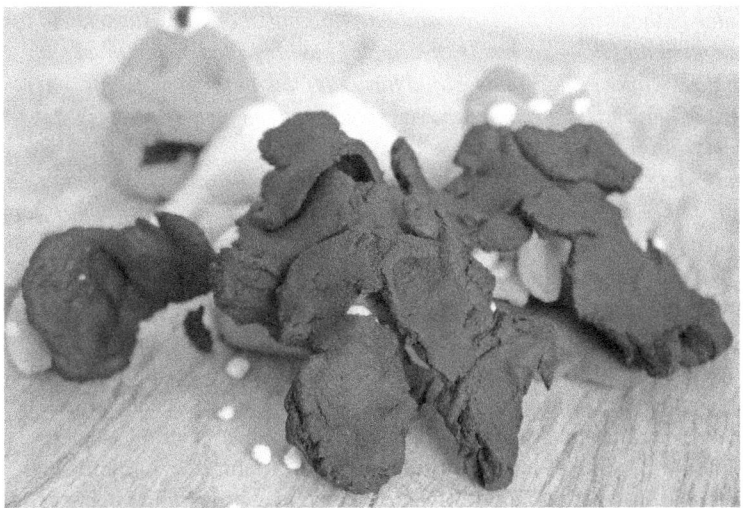

Figure 4.6 Clay figures covered by black clay. Photograph by the author.

As these emotions as embodied actions are situated in relational and social contexts they can always be considered as utterances of being touched, or moved. This experience of being deeply touched calls for a contextualisation within relational and social involvements. In these children's stories we first need to listen very thoughtfully and in detail to the experiences of disadvantage, pain and suffering these children had to endure. We can try to unravel in what kind of relational involvements they are touched, and how disadvantages reveal what they give value to in life.

Iris responds to my questions by explaining that she hates people being so unfair. With a big sigh she asks why people are hurting each other so badly. I don't give in to my urge to start explaining, and instead recognise that she values 'not hurting each other in relationships'. I ask her what efforts she has made to prevent people from hurting each other. Can she share what is maybe the most painful 'hurting' in her life until now?

As we conceive of emotions as complex multi-layered phenomena, White's (2006) 'double listening' practices are a helpful means to re-sense a grip on them. Besides inquiring about experiences of disadvantage and suffering, we can indeed also attune to intentions, expectations, values, wishes, hopes, principles and commitments in these relations and contexts that are less obviously visible. Expressing emotions can be considered as taking a personal, relational, ethical stance in a particular social context. This means we can also listen/be on the lookout for social issues linked with these emotions (Denborough, 2019). Thus, these emotions can be understood as relational and contextual responses, as a means of reaching out to others and as invitations for social action (Fredman, 2004; Lang & McAdam, 2001; Vermeire, 2020).

A bit later in the conversation, Iris and I are talking about how she tried to take care of her mum and how she has the feeling of having failed as her mum stepped out of life. So, I wonder if her mum would have noticed all these moments of trying to take care of her and if there were maybe some small moments or acts that might have made a difference to her mum.

Suddenly she remembers a moment at night, her mother crawled into her single bed, probably after yet another fight with Kenny. Iris told her mum a funny story about a little girl. Her mum had to laugh and took her closely in her arms whispering in her ear 'You are my little treasure'.

While exploring and reflecting together on these emotions, thoughts, actions and interpersonal relations these emotions are not 'resolved' but still they undergo changes. New meanings, just like new self-descriptions, descriptions of others and life events emerge during the process. It is not clear beforehand which new meanings will emerge and how they will do so. They rather emerge during a step-by-step ongoing process of mutual responding. This requires, each time again, a careful listening to what the child brings to the conversation while being on the lookout for openings to richer descriptions and meaning development. We need to carefully consider which contexts we bring to the foreground and in what way. This is the responsibility of the therapist or counsellor. Pearce and Cronen (1980) emphasised the contextual determination of communication. As children live in different contexts, we can ask questions that open doors to less dominant or less defining, destructive contexts. Illuminating alternative contexts can open broader perspectives, generate new meanings and actions. Since we as therapists or counsellors don't collaborate with the child in an isolated bubble, these shifting meanings and changing hierarchy of contexts can, outside of our conversation, easily become reclaimed by dominant contexts, reinforcing single stories or wiping out emerged new meanings.

A few weeks later, Iris has a conversation with the student counsellor at school. He explained to her that children don't have to take care of their parents. She is obviously a child of parents with a mental illness and she has to learn to stand up for herself in an appropriate manner. When I meet her shortly after this conversation, she asks if it's true and if I too believe she took bad care of her mother.

Interpersonal interactions are ongoing recursive processes that generate meanings over and over again. This makes it important to bear in mind, during these conversations, the continuous influence of important people and contexts. Exploring these bodily reactions, emotions, thoughts and multiplicity of contexts in collaboration with, and in the presence of, significant people, loved ones or representatives of their communities can be a strong antidote against the individualisation of experiences. Since these are vulnerable stories, the child can also prefer to first explore all these aspects individually in the safety and privacy of the therapy room before all these voices and contexts literally speak together (see also Chapters 2 and 5).

Do horses hurt themselves?

As Iris pulls out her eyebrows and has a bald spot on the back of her head from pulling her hair out, these actions have become more and more signs to her of being crazy just like her mum. After developing different foundations for richer understandings, discovering multi-layered meanings and sharing, she asks what I think about these crazy things she is doing.

Children and youngsters who experienced violence, abuse or trauma like Iris are often not only kicking against others or 'the world', but also against 'themselves', or so it seems. These (self)destructive or (self)abusive acts tend to create a sense of urgency in the people who care about them. The abusive actions, the violence enacted upon them, being left alone, can become seen as a proof of being worthless, that they are not worth caring for or even that it is their fault. Notwithstanding the many efforts to stand their ground, to stop the abuse, keep their families afloat or care for their loved ones, these efforts did not bring about what was hoped for. On top of that, their responses and actions such as thrashing around, hurting themselves, just as their interpersonal frictions and struggles seem to confirm these modes of understanding. They spin around in circles. They also get caught up in unhelpful relational dances with the people involved. Carers often try to control these actions and expect these children to learn to control themselves. This often prompts 'more of the same'.

Talking directly about the self-harming or their sense of worthlessness is often not possible without tumbling into the same stories. Relying on the idea that the detour is often the shortest way, we need to find ways to open dialogues and reflection without creating a sense of 'forcing' them to speak or confess.

Katinka (13 years) is coming for conversations. The carers of the children's home are very worried. She has cut herself again in her arms and thighs after a phone call with her mother telling her she can't come home for the weekend (for the sixth time in a row). The carers sent an email asking me to talk about this self-harming. It has to stop! She is infecting the group! In our previous meetings we talked about her fascination for horses and her assisting at the riding school so I asked to bring some pictures of these horses.

After our conversation I wrote the following letter to her:

Dear Katinka,

It was incredibly hot last Tuesday. Still, you had found the courage to put on the riding boots and show me all that you have already gathered about horses. Your mum once made a promise to go horseback riding with you at the end of the vacation but you don't believe her any longer. You're tired of all these unfulfilled promises. Meanwhile you know people aren't to be trusted.

In between I told you that Justine sent an email informing me that you had 'cut' or 'scratched' your arms again. I asked what I should call this anyway? You preferred not to talk about it all. It happened already a few days ago and according to you it was 'over'.

We spent the rest of the time studying the world of horses. We took a picture of you with all your 'horse treasures'. In the riding school there are still a few horses that you remember from the old days like Gabbar. This means Strong and Pride. He has a special place in your heart. When you told me a bit about his story I wondered if horses can give comfort. You were very sure of that. While writing this down, I wonder if you also know how to comfort horses?

Consulting Doctor Google ☺, we discovered that horses don't need much sleep. You think the ears and the eyes are the cutest. And the best features are that they are very reliable from an early age. By that you mean that they never abandon you and they are certainly not traitors! (They will never just swap you for another owner). A foal is usually born at night and they usually take the father away. We tried to figure out what it might have to do with them taking away the father.

A horse is not only a good comforter but you can also confide secrets to it. You were clear: horses are more trustworthy than people. They are also very honest about what they like or not. I also wondered what happens when a mare can't take good care of her foal. You figured out that's when the foal is taken away too. You showed me that you can feel when a horse is sad. You can tell by the position of the ears (also a little by the tail and head). It makes a difference if the ears are forward, backward, sideways or spinning around ...this can all mean something different. For example, backwards can mean being angry or cranky. (In your case, this doesn't show up so well on the ears ... they are well hidden behind your hair)

Finally, we also wondered if horses would hurt themselves when they are angry, sad or being hurt. You were initially very convinced: no. Through some further searching on the internet we found out that sometimes they bite themselves, buck, rub or make strange noises when they are not feeling well. Together we had some further thoughts about 'what could happen in the life of a horse that could help us understand horses hurt themselves' but also about how we could understand this 'harming themselves'.

The best approach for these horses, according to you, was:

A friendly approach! Speaking with friendly words and in friendly tones. You have to give the animal enough attention as well as 'freedom'. With that you meant 'not to be on top of it right away'. You should not immediately start to punish. Such an animal needs good care, if you don't want it to happen again. It needs to know you really appreciate it by this permanently giving enough attention (though not too much).

When I asked if these were also guidelines for you, you shrugged and with some sparkling light in your eyes you said: 'You could give it a try ...'

Later on, when you are an adult, you would love to buy a horse! Brown with white spots and black are your favourite colours.

Katinka, I hope I didn't forget important things in this letter. If I have written things down wrongly or misunderstood anything, please let me know! At the end of our meeting you said you would consider to let the carers also read this letter. I am quite curious if you did so.

Looking forward to see you next week. Maybe there are some new horse stories to share.

Warm wishes! Sabine

While exploring this animal world together, Katinka can share and make visible, to me as well as to herself, her acquired knowledge and skills about horses, about caring and comforting others and herself, about sharing confidentialities, the importance of trust and being trustful, etc. Indirectly, we may notice violated values, significant loss, unspoken longings and unravel what multiple meanings are given to the painful events in her life. While talking, searching and reflecting, discoveries in the world of horses can unfold new understandings but also contain ideas of possible helpful responses that are appropriate for Katinka. Sharing the letter with her mentor at the children's home connected them also in an alternative way. It opened new conversations about important themes in Katinka's life. Our ambition isn't to 'instruct' the carers in how to handle Katinka but rather to initiate new interaction and dialogues.

By talking in our next meetings about what 'hurting' horses, 'ill-treatment' of horses, 'violence' towards horses means and what are conditions for 'taking good care' of horses, it became possible to talk about the complexity of 'caring' and its many interpersonal and contextual influences. This offered a stepping stone to reflect upon some of the things that happened in her home in the past. When difficulties are too close to the skin or beliefs are unshakeable, we can explore them in completely different contexts in the hope of revisiting certain ideas or discovering new angles. Meanings then can become fluid again. To Katinka, looking from a relational context of care in the world of horses, some new understandings emerged. The caning was not merely something she just deserved because of being too noisy but could also be seen as 'bad treatment', just like the ice-cold bathing sessions became named as 'poor upbringing' instead of 'learning to be strong in life'. Naming the painful, traumatic things that happened as 'bad treatment', 'poor upbringing', 'violence' or 'abuse' can offer a new context in which children can develop new understandings about these events, their responses, about their relationships, themselves and others. This can help them find new ways to relate and position oneself towards these events.

While watching an instruction movie together on the internet titled 'How to train a horse' Katinka remarks: 'When horses are trained badly, they protest and become rebellious. Do you think I am rebellious? Maybe I have to say 'no' to a few things'.

After these 'horse conversations' not all the problems were 'resolved', neither was the pain and sadness about her home situation gone but the self-harming decreased. I was informed that Katinka entered into calmer waters at the children's home.

Brewing stories: imagine the unthinkable

For children, after traumatic experiences, the confrontation with certain contexts can be so intrusive that it overwhelms them. They seem to relive certain aspects of previous experiences. Their bodies start trembling, they end up in a tunnel vision or seem riveted to the ground. Their attempts to do something disappear into thin air or lead to the extension of problems. Also, all the efforts of the people nearby seem to cause more of the same. Moreover, this experience often recursively becomes the context for the next, similar situation. We increasingly get a story of personal failure in which all avenues towards a solution are cut off. Even reflecting or talking about it becomes a 'no go'.

During a ball game on the playground, a couple of sturdy guys from another class stormed at Robin (age seven). A pile of reproaches was hurled at his head and the 'captain' beat him up. Robin was left alone. It wasn't the first time that he was bullied but this time it went completely out of hand. School tried to deal with what happened as well as possible. Punishments were handed out, apologies offered, class friends had discussions about how they wanted to relate to one another and sent heart-warming invitations to Robin. But despite all these efforts Robin refuses to go to the playground. Only accompanied by his father or stepmother he goes to class. Other places are 'no go'. The subject cannot be discussed with him. He immediately puts his hands over his ears and starts to yell and scream. His parents, school, etc. tried all kinds of things to convince him. The situation is no longer tenable for his parents and school.

Asking questions or trying to examine the situation together is no option and does not provide new ideas. It often leads to further confrontation, deadlock and the conversation comes to a halt when children make statements such as 'I can't do it anyway' or 'It's impossible ...' They often cannot hear the advice or suggestions of the people involved. A particular difficulty is that giving advice may imply the suggestion that the problem can be solved if only enough effort is made, or if one is clever or strong enough. Bystanders offer solutions that they think will benefit the child, and that they believe will meet their needs. Such advice determines how the child should act in the given circumstances, but ignores the fact that the child cannot imagine exactly that. In their eyes, the problem is something they cannot change, they cannot do anything about. More and more the child is in danger of appearing as a failure in his own eyes and in the eyes of third parties. Any self-recriminations on the part of the child at this point can increase their hopelessness (Smith & Nylund, 1997, p. 22). Wilson

(1998, p. 118) suggests that if a child will not (or cannot) answer your questions, stop asking them.

A direct, structured approach to the difficulties does not provide relief for Robin. On the contrary, it generates more of the same. Varela (1999) speaks of 'breakdowns' when 'our world collapses', and we have no clue how to go about things. When something unexpected happens or when we enter a 'new, unknown' world, we may discover that we simply do not have any behaviour at our disposal. Our self-evident knowledge is no longer sufficient. We don't know 'how to go on' anymore.

As we need to leave the well-trodden paths, we can try to create new openings by 'story brewing' together, based on imagined 'breakdowns', or seemingly insoluble challenges. It can often become a resource of inspiration to deal with real-life problems. Entering together with children into a fictive, magical world might generate ideas about how to go on. It also opens 'a zone of calmness' where children are no longer overwhelmed by the events but can be present with their distress (Pederson, 2015; Weingarten, 2003).

I present Robin a difficult, fictional problem for which a story must be 'brewed'. Tomorrow we must transfer five wild, aggressive animals from the village of Kwanabu to the village of Altze. In doing so, we must cross a large mountain range with narrow mountain paths and incredibly deep gorges. Once over the mountain range we will have to cross a swirling river and if we survive this, we still have to pass a ghost village before reaching Altze. The animals are a roaring lion, a hungry crocodile, a snake, an elephant and an eagle.

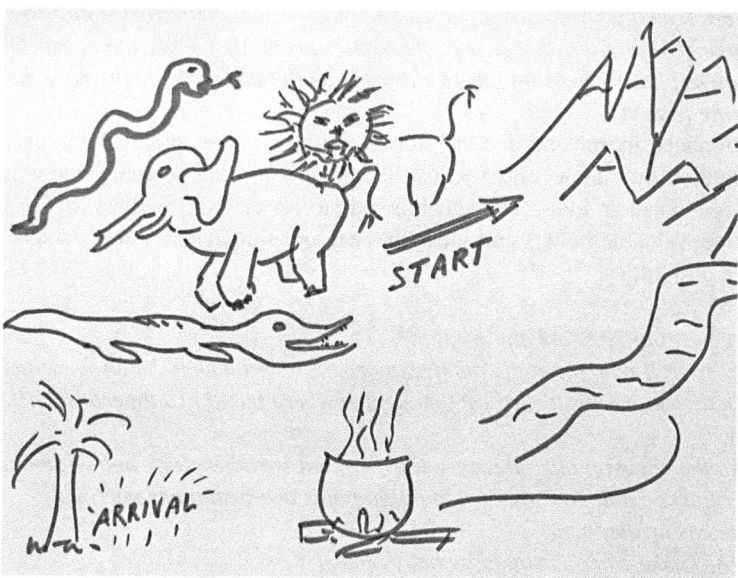

Figure 4.7 Drawing of animals, mountains and cooking pot. Photograph by the author.

Phenomenologist philosopher Samuel Todes (2001) remarked how we, as human beings, are 'capable of transforming ourselves at will from an active observer to a productive creator of our own imagination, and back again'. As such 'we *are* our ability to transform ourselves reversibly between these two forms of ourselves' (132, *italics in original*). Werner (quoted in Breeuwsma, 1993) refers to creative scientists and artists who, precisely from the ability to see the world 'magically', manage to find solutions for their intellectual problems and come to artistic creations. Moreover, the world of the child is filled with uncontrollable situations both large and small, so that they must frequently resort to magical transformations. Breeuwsma (1993) considers magical thinking to be a constructive, imaginative activity that plays an important role in the organisation of knowledge about social reality. Magical thinking and logical thinking can find themselves side by side in this process, mutually influencing each other.

By entering a world of imagination, the child can immediately experience a sense of agency. Turning to imagined situations in a safe therapeutic context can prove very helpful as imagined breakdowns need not be accompanied by a loss of a sense of agency and also because a sense of agency appears more easily in fantasy. Children's fantasy always draws on what they have actually experienced, interpersonal exchanges and on the social discourses they 'inhabit'. The exercising of fantasy can in turn inspire real-life situations in the future.

Together with Robin, I make a sketch of the course to be followed on a flipover. He draws a long snake and adds 'It's poisonous and can sneak in anywhere. The crocodile has an armour that no dagger or arrow can hurt him and the elephant can carry more than a million pounds ...' Some animals get big teeth. In the drawing they look aggressive. When I ask if the teeth only look dangerous or actually are dangerous, he replies promptly: 'Only the crocodile can bite you to pieces. The lion has to show his teeth because he is the king, but sometimes he is sweet'.

The introduced ingredients for the stories can be a metaphor for the experienced difficulties but not necessarily, just like the mission can be connected with the challenges in their lives. The self-brewed stories contain feelings, actions, ways to cope, valuable beliefs and ideas that can open interesting, new perspectives on the difficulties.

S: *How are we going to start our mission?*
R: *Oh, just ... we'll send the eagle out to explore the environment. It can see which path in the mountains is the best to take and where possibly dangerous tracks can be.*
S: *And also the widest paths? Because the elephant is rather thick and wide and he too must be able to cross it. Mountain paths are sometimes narrow.*
R: *How thick is an elephant?*
S: *I think the snake can go around its belly once.*
R: *Then the snake must go along in the eagle's beak to go and see if it is a good path.*

S: A brilliant idea! Then we'll put the snake on the path and we'll know.
R: It's okay. We can leave!
S: Does anyone have acrophobia?
R: What is that?

> *After my explanation, Robin says he understands: 'It's like in the movie of Ice Age'. We suspect that the crocodile might be afraid of heights and decide to blindfold her and tie her to the elephant's back. It even seems interesting to tie the crocodile's mouth shut at the same time. Imagine if she starts to bite out of fright. A number of other difficulties are discussed such as: 'What if it starts to storm in the mountains?' or 'What if the path is crumbling?' each time coming up with alternatives.*

> *Arriving at the swirling river, the crocodile is sent to explore where the fewest swirls are and where the river is narrowest. The elephant yanks out a few trees and a raft is built.*

> *...*

S: Ouch! We're getting into a whirlpool!
R: Throw the snake like a rope. ...
S: Oh yes, and winding it around a tree!
R: Yes, she is long enough anyway.
S: Whew! Saved.
R: The elephant is a little drunk of being on the wobbly water.
>   *... We are approaching the ghost village.*
R: The snake can sneak up to them quietly and put them to sleep with its eyes (as in Mowgli).
S: So that they don't see that we are passing?
R: Yes!
S: And if one does wake up?
R: Then we sing a lullaby so they fall back asleep.

> *Finally, after many twists and turns, side roads and detours, we reach our destination where a big feast is held.*

Brewing such stories together is an exciting, enjoyable and above all challenging adventure with often profound effects. We step into 'embodied doing' and interacting processes not knowing what will emerge. A multitude of actions and possibilities can unfold in creating the story. The child reappears in our exploration together as a person with ideas and potentials, someone with whom it is fun making stories, coming up with magical solutions and devising seemingly impossible constructions. We can relate in a different way and park the pressure of 'fixing' the 'real' problem. Even humour can enter our conversations and bring about a sense of lightness. As they make an incredible effort the burdens and difficulties of the characters in the story become visible, are named and possible solutions figured out. So, it is still a 'serious job' that has to be done.

The main goal is neither the construction of a beautiful or fascinating story nor finding the right way out of the problems. While brewing stories together, we keep a close eye on the child. Are we still co-researchers on a therapeutic journey? It is a constant mutual tuning in on the concrete content of the story, but also of our collaborative relationship whereby we take into account the multiple contexts of the child. Within the stories and our 'brewing' together, we can connect and tune in to different levels of influence that also matter in their real world of experience. In the story we can address many relational issues, the disadvantages, frictions, obstacles and emotions involved in multi-stress contexts. There is room for exploring and experimenting with different ways of dealing with these issues and for discovering along the way variants or new ways of dealing with challenges. At the same time the stories offer reflections about who they are, what they can do, how they think or feel, etc. but also about how all this is linked with others and social situations. It can open certain new perspectives and limit others.

In the story, the unthinkable becomes thinkable and a sense of agency begins to nestle, just like hope can come in.

After having created this story, I ask if this 'brewed story' could contain ideas for their situation, the constraints or problems in their daily contexts. This is in line with the work of Nyirinkwaya (2020) who challenges and connects children through games and afterwards reflects with them on what kind of skills, knowledge and collective actions were useful. By making a link with their everyday world I am taking a risk. If they start to experience this activity as a 'set up game' and feel they are being lured into a trap, our joint search and the accompanying reflections stop. So a direct link is neither desirable nor necessary. In such cases I prefer to leave the storytelling for what it is. Sometimes they come back to it later. Sometimes I notice that a child starts to use some ideas without having made things explicit. As remarked earlier, a one-to-one relationship with the 'real' breakdown situation is not always required to regain a sense of agency. Moreover, it should always be borne in mind that it is more often than not impossible to pinpoint exactly what brought about the therapeutic effects.

In Robin's case I do choose to make the transition to his daily life. It is not clear in advance what parts of the story will be useful, or can be transferred or applied. Ideas are worked out together, and I can only illuminate certain elements, but the child decides whether it is inspiring or not. During the storytelling process a pile of possibilities may unfold, but it is eventually the child itself that must see and experience them as possibilities.

S: *You suggested sending the eagle out on an exploratory mission to find the safest way. On the playground, have you ever sent someone on such a mission? Or is this a crazy idea?*

R: *Who then?*

S: *I don't know. Who would be the most suitable person? Who has eagle-eyes? An eagle can see a lot from the air that we couldn't see from the ground.*

R: *The teachers don't see everything. The supervisor walks around and my teacher is in the classroom sometimes writing things on the board during playtime.*

S: If we made an aerial photograph of the playground like we did in the story, what would be important to notice? What is bothering you the most?

R: The big Turkish boys. They are the boss on the playground and decide on everything. The teachers do not notice this or say 'just go and play somewhere else'. (Eighty percent of his school is populated with children with Turkish and Moroccan roots of second and third migration.)

Soon we are exploring together how things work at the playground. This was hardly conceivable before our story making and evoked only resistance at the time. Instead of focusing on what became named as Robin's 'individual problem', we start to explore the many interactions and the social world in the playground. We bear in mind the complexity and the many influencing aspects. It has been remarked that the cracks in our communities, or the lack of solutions for problems inherent to living together, can be heard moaning in individuals' accounts of life. This reflection of the social in the personal is often not immediately visible. Violence can be considered a social problem (Omer, 2004; White, 2006; Jenkins, 2009), but it is a challenge to let the social issues surface when contextualising difficulties experienced on a personal or an interpersonal level. Nevertheless, this can create opportunities for children and young people to reconnect with a team of solidarity (Reynolds, 2020).

S: In our story, we sought help from the other animals. Do you remember? We tied the crocodile on the elephant's back and we swung the snake like a rope ... Do you have any idea what a classmate could help us with? Are there any children who have special skills that would make a difference? Or children who have special ways to respond to these boys?

All these questions can also be seen as an invitation to look around and explore his social world.

...

S: We also used materials like tree trunks to build a raft. Do you need equipment to go on the playground?

R (laconic): An electricity machine!

S (amazed): An electricity machine?

R: Yes, to get rid of these stupid boys when they come closer.

S: Oh, you mean a sort of remote control that will prick them if they come too close. How close they may come? What is this all about?

R: Ten metres! Big boys like them think they are allowed to play the boss over little kids. Someone has to stop them.

...

S: You said the lion showed his teeth just because he was the king. He wasn't such an evil one, was he? Are there any children at school who look tough but are not? By the way, what is all this hassle at the playground about?

While changing some perspectives and creating new meaning, we puzzle out all the possibilities and write them down on a sheet so that we don't forget them. We agree that next time, we will look together at what we should investigate some more, maybe can do in 'real' life or would be worthwhile to give it a try. But maybe even more important, we talk about who also has to be informed about our discoveries and can be engaged in our quest.

Constructing stories is only one possible pathway in our journey with children. It is not a miracle or magic bullet for breaking impasses. If it were, it would be a disqualification of the efforts of parents, carers or other people involved. They have already tried many things before the child came to therapy or counselling. That is why it is important to brief them regularly about our 'work together'. What we have 'discovered' or 'invented' together, must also connect with their daily world and they can be called in as 'helpers', members of our team of solidarity.

Robin's parents are invited. Robin and I have made a plan in advance about what and how different issues will be discussed with them. The 'mission map' is put in the middle and Robin proudly shares the brewed story. Then I ask his parents if they have any idea what we have learnt from this story. Father looks surprised and mother smiles. Robin cannot wait for their answers and comes up with the second map, the playground drawn in the middle. After further clarification father makes the following suggestion: 'Maybe together, we can keep an eye on the playground from the top floor of the school building ...'

Also later on, Robin and his father informed the teacher and classmates got involved.

During our explorations and talking we fostered collective care, put our shoulders under it 'together' and created partnerships. We stepped away from Robin's individual 'assignment' to get over the traumatic experiences. Through creating the possibility of sharing experiences, stories and ideas in an alternative way, we also found more collective responses. Although difficulties and hardship also concern social issues in which we have not immediately reached 'solutions on a social level', this doesn't mean we can't stand in solidarity.

Trapped in feelings of guilt

As the many stories we have presented so far have shown, beliefs or feelings of guilt, and all kinds of embodied expressions of these, are often explicitly present in contexts of violence, abuse and trauma. In Yana's story (see introduction), she said even literally: '*It's my fault. I had to communicate more in the foster family*'. Iris, too, became convinced that she had to take better care of her mother, so that she would not have walked out of life. Children and youngsters in these contexts often tried to figure out how such disasters could happen and often came to single, linear-causal explanations and negative conclusions about themselves in which the complexity, a web of continuously influencing exchanges and power relations, seems to be out of sight. These conclusions are also informed by many social ideas and narratives about what they must be able to do, say or realise in these contexts and shaped in dialogues filled with all kinds of interpersonal and social perspectives about their actions, responses, etc.

Tina (see Chapter 3) kept silent for years about the sexual abuse of her father. At the age of 16 she met a boy with whom she fell in love. He took her to all kinds of parties and she stayed away for nights. When he broke up the relationship, she used drugs for a period and had sex with different men. In the meanwhile, she remained silent about what was happening at home. A lot of people became angry at her, were disappointed and tried in many ways to convince her to stop this derailing behaviour. In that same period her mum got more and more depressive moods which Tina was held responsible for by the family.

Her father insisted that she better keep silent about what happened because she allegedly had provoked it. It was part of their 'special bond'. Even more, as her little half-sister has an incurable disease and if Tina would talk about their 'special relationship' with others, her father might be sent away and there would be too little money to pay for all the medical expenses. After Tina discovered her father doing the same to her sister and was afraid the same might happen to her half-sister, she revealed the abuse. Everybody was perplexed and outraged but could not understand why she had not told it earlier. This was one of the things that made feelings of guilt grow.

These children and youngsters can get stuck in tightening spirals of feeling guilty. Their responses often aren't noticed as efforts to keep on going, to escape painful experiences or as relational involvements. These children or youngsters are often called to account for their actions and asked to behave differently. People ask questions like 'Why are you acting like this?', 'Why did you keep silent?' This doesn't bring new answers but often feeds their belief that they are an important cause of the problem, responded in the wrong way or that they are guilty of how things turned out.

When Tina emphasises that it is her fault that things have gone so wrong in the family, I do not want to give in to the urge to explain that it is not her fault. But when she adds: 'How could I have been so stupid to keep silent for so long? Does this mean that my father was right: that I provoked this, that I encouraged this special relationship?', I feel the compulsion getting stronger to reassure her that it is not her fault.

From a kind of commitment as therapist or counsellor but also as significant others the urgency to relieve the child or youngster from these self-accusations can be huge. Sometimes I can hear myself start to 'preach' and explain 'it isn't your fault'. Once I have started, I even try to make clear to them that they have nothing to do with it. The guilt lies entirely with the other person who did harm. At such a moment I also get trapped in single explanations and reduced stories. The complexity, the entanglement of many mutual influencing contexts and relationships over time disappear from my sight too. Often these 'lectures' appear to make no difference to the experiences and convictions of the child or youngster. On the contrary, we risk getting into a 'truth battle' and deny their experience of being part of this complexity as well as their efforts to make a difference and try to turn things in other directions.

As a point of entry, I propose we take their experiences and conclusions of being guilty seriously. Without entering into a discussion of whether these conclusions are correct, we can ask if it, in their experience, is rather a feeling of guilt, a conviction, a truth, a certainty, etc., and become interested in how they came to these conclusions. I want to develop together with them alternative perspectives, richer understandings of what happened, situated in multi-layered landscapes of meaning and maybe find a new stance towards what happened or towards the persons who enacted the violence.

S: *Can I ask you something? Is this sentence 'It is my fault' a feeling, a conviction, a conclusion, ... or how do I have to understand this?*

T: *It is something that is howling around in my head all the time!*

S: *Oh! So this howling around all the time 'It is my fault', can you remember when this became very present for the first time?*

T: *Shortly after the first time my father came to my bedroom and the tickling was no longer tickling.*

S: *How would you call these things that happened and invited the 'howling around in your head'?*

T: *The black spot things. The tickling was normally big fun. We laughed and rolled over the bed but then ... I had to be able to say 'Stop, this is no longer fun' but I kept my mouth shut ... I kept silent for years. I should have told it to my mum immediately. ... I wasn't honest with her. I really disappointed her. I let my family down.*

S: *Can you tell a bit more about this 'howling around in your head that it's your fault'? For whom or what were you working so hard in your mind?*

T (first looks up a bit surprised): *Don't know ... it had really a hold on me all the time.*

S: *What exactly had a hold on you? What were you hoping for or trying to find solutions for?*

T: *How to stop it ... not offending my father ... not losing my sisters. It became one messy thing in my head.*

S: *What was harmed so badly? Can you still grab what was your biggest concern at the time?*

    ...

Feeling guilty can be considered as an ethical emotion that shows that they are concerned, that they do care about what happened, that they would like things to have gone in a different way and that they still hold on to important values. While exploring and illuminating their responses to the abuse or violence and connecting with context and meaning, the feelings of guilt can become nuanced and given relief. Richer descriptions and meanings of what this 'howling around in your head' and 'feeling guilty' can uncover what and who they find important and what they ethically stand for.

Step by step we try to reach a more accurate understanding of how and which of many small interpersonal events and exchanges created the contexts that lead the child to believe it is their fault. Many children and youngsters are looking at what happened through the eyes of now and here and with the knowledge and ideas of now and here at what happened then and there. They judge themselves, others involved and the situation from that perspective. Many people involved also tend to judge children's actions at that time through the knowledge and the lens of here and now.

Tina's mum repeatedly asked 'Why didn't you tell me what was happening? You know that you can tell me anything!' Also, one of Tina's boyfriends asked once in a drunken state: 'You never kicked him out of your bedroom or tried to keep the door closed? You are sure, you didn't like it?' This remark made her furious but at the same time, doubt about what happened and about what she had to be able to do, crept in as a fast-spreading poison.

Weingarten (2003) distinguishes between feeling guilty in the traffic of daily life and toxic guilt or shame that infiltrates all aspects of a person's life. Going back to then-and-there in a safe way and unravelling or making visible all kinds of overshadowed microprocesses and contexts that also had influence can broaden their view on what happened. On the one hand it can acknowledge the suffering of many acts of violence or abuse and their responses and at the same time situate them in a multiplicity of relational and social involvements, loyalties, particular situations, family habits and beliefs, etc.

Together we explore what 'tickling' meant before 'the black spot things' hap-pened. It was often a game in the family that started while watching TV, ever since she was a toddler. This could be with her mother or her father. It often started with poking someone in the side with a finger. It always brought excitement, fun and often ended in laughter. Her younger sister also took part in this game when she was a little older. Her father started doing this at bedtime when she was about eight years old. She remembers the moment when the tickling shifted to other places and she felt 'weird' afterwards.

I ask her if she, at the age of eight, could make sense of this shifting as until then this tickling seemed to be 'a family game'. Were there other moments that 'tickling' didn't have a sexual connotation? She immediately tells a story about tickling her grandmother behind her ears when she was little. Her grandmother always said it made her feel calm.

A bit later I ask what kind of meaning this tickling got after her father began tickling in other places. It became the warning for the black spot things. It also made her, for the first time, think she provoked it.

As we unravel different moments of tickling, the context shifts (cf. Pearce and Cronen, 1980) from 'a family game' over 'physical boundary crossing' to 'sexual abuse' and different meanings become visible and accessible; at the same time, the confusion, ambivalence, hesitation within this change of contexts begins to make sense to her.

When I ask who is responsible for what in what context, Tina still hesitates. She looks with questioning eyes: my father?

Within a multiplicity of influences also power relations can come to the fore. White (2006) emphasises the importance of establishing a political and contextual appreciation of a person's experience of abuse. It helps to undermine the self-blame and the shame. Bateson's (1979) often quoted 'difference that makes a difference' can also be of help here. We can invite the child or youngster to start to notice a difference in position, role, responsibility, knowledge, etc. in the relational interconnectedness. In contexts of violence and abuse children can get trapped in power relations and power dynamics. The person who enacts the violence or abuse is situated in a different position to the child or youngster. They have more or different access to, or possess more or different resources of, knowledge, power, words and language, money, material, etc. (Bourdieu, 1987).

Instead of 'explaining' all this to children or youngsters, we prefer to present them a series of questions that can reveal differences, above all differences in access to knowledge, strength, power, etc. In answering these questions, they can also develop a different understanding of the abuse, violence and their actions, even about themselves and the relationship (Denborough, 2008).

In our explorations Tina repeats suddenly: 'How could I be so stupid to believe that there would not be enough money for my sister's medical expenses if my dad had to leave the house?' I ask her if I can present her some questions to reflect upon and she nods.
S: When your father told these things how old were you?
T: Eleven or twelve.
S: How old was your father at that time?
T: Thirty-eight.
S: Who had at that time most knowledge about how our social security system works?
T: I didn't even knew that it existed.
S: Who has most knowledge about how our world works? A 12- or 38-year-old person?
T: Someone of 38.
Some other questions I asked were:How tall was your father at that time? Who had most physical strength at that time? But also: who has to know at that age and that position what is good or bad? Or what is allowed and not, just or wrong, ...?

These questions make power dynamics visible and can shift perspectives and meanings on what happened. We can also invite in our conversation all the voices circulating around 'what happened', around the 'black spot things' and people's thoughts, opinions and perspectives. Certainly, the voice of society or their community can open even more perspectives and new dialogues.

At some point Tina concludes: 'It is so unfair what he did'.

This new stance can also open doors to new actions. In the situation of Tina, it led to new conversations with her mum and sister.

Looking at then and there from alternative perspectives

Having a closer look at what happened or how things could happen, can always pull these children or youngsters back into the experiences of abuse and violence and just perpetuate their conclusions about themselves, others or their lives. They start to feel even more guilty. Freedman and Combs (1993, 1996) suggest re-authoring narratives of violence and abuse from alternative viewpoints.

- *If, as an adult you are now, you were to witness the abuse that you experienced, happening to someone else, how would you describe it? What would you name it? Who would you say was responsible for what happened?*
- *If I could look back through the past and see what happened to you, how do you think I would describe it?*
- *Which adult, who was in your life back then, but did not know what was happening, would have protected you had they known?*
- *...*

These questions can also be used to recognise acts of resistance or to draw distinctions between a child's stories and these viewpoints and to develop new descriptions. *Looking back, as an adult now, what do you notice that you couldn't notice then?*

White (1995) even suggests to look upon oneself and the situation from a position as the mother or father of this child. It can assist youngsters to develop a degree of discernment that can make it possible for them to distinguish those actions that are directed to them that are exploitative, abusive or neglectful in nature from those actions that are supportive, loving or caring in nature.

In the conversation with Tina I ask what Wolf, her dog, would have whispered in her ear to protect her against 'the black spot things' if he was knowing what was going on? And should he call it also 'the black spot things' or would he name it differently? What would he have appreciated that you tried to do? If you were the mum of this girl, what would you have done at that time to support her?

We can also explore what these new perspectives mean in relation to the emotions and effects of the abuse.

While reflecting further Tina says she feels angry but the self-doubt and sadness are still very present. She also remarks that maybe it is now a different kind of sadness.

Taking a stance: opening doors to new actions

We can actively engage children in exploring how traumatic experiences affect their lives and relationships. We can inquire whether or not they think that these effects are favourable. It is even possible to ask them to justify such evaluations. While we unravel all these bodily reactions, emotions, thoughts, etc., as they appear within contexts and relationships, we are also engaged in possible reinterpretations of their experiences and the unravelling of predominant and negative narratives or conclusions of identity that circulate about them and hold them captive (White, 2006).

While Tina and I spoke about the painful effects of the abuse and how it could happen, she made a drawing of the 'the black spot things'. It helped to focus our attention on the drawing and not have the effect of examining her. After exploring every nook and cranny during several meetings, I ask what she would like to do with 'the black spot things' and its effects. What place can it still take in her life or how does she want to relate to it?

Surprisingly, she answers resolutely: 'Back to sender!'

> *This makes me immediately wonder how 'Back to sender!' could look like. She herself suggests to put the drawing in an envelope and send it to the shelter where her father is staying.*

S: *What does this sending back mean to you? What is this choice or decision about?*

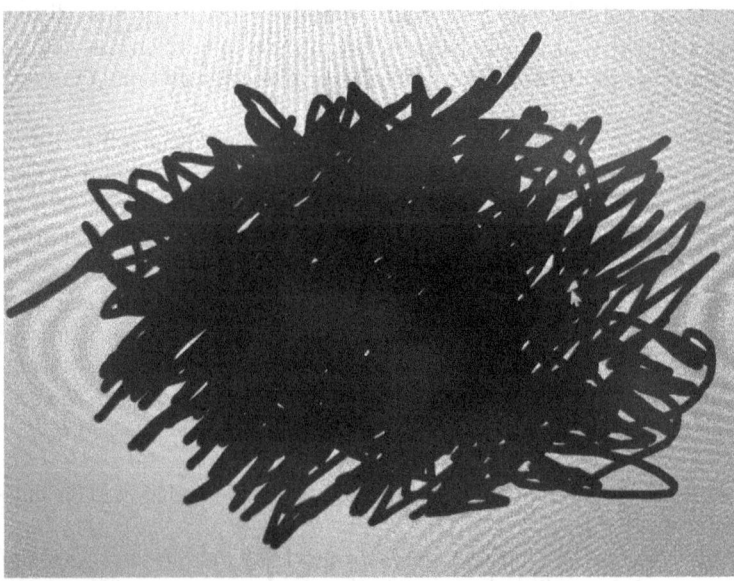

Figure 4.8 Drawing of black tangle. Photograph by the author.

T: I don't want to ruin my life by what he did. I want to go on with my life. I don't think I can call him 'father' any longer, although he also did some good things.

S: Do we need to put his name on the envelope and add a note with this drawing?

T: No, it doesn't matter if he knows from who this comes. I just want it to be with who it belongs to.

This repositioning and new choice goes hand in hand with re-gaining a sense of personal and relational agency and being reconnected with some important wishes and hopes for her life and what matters to her. It opens new perspectives and possible new actions.

A few weeks later she tells an astonishing story. She herself even seems still astonished about what she did. During the news on the radio, she heard yet another revelation about abuse in the church (this was very topical in Belgium at the time). She became so angry that she jumped on her bicycle, cycled to the other side of the city, entered the shelter where her father was staying, stood in front of him and shouted loudly 'asshole'. She turned around, walked out and stopped a few blocks away gasping for breath.

Together we explore, unravel and reflect upon this initiative: 'How can this be understood or be given meaning to?' and 'How would this be received by the various important people around you?'

Documents as consolidation

Step by step unravelling and exploring different understandings of the complexities of the painful experiences and effects can generate novel ideas and new ways to go on. But at the same time, they can quickly get recuperated by the daily interplay of many interpersonal exchanges, a multiplicity of contexts within which these children live and ever-present dominant discourses (Vermeire & van Hennik, 2017).

This also means that unique outcomes, initiatives, small actions that make a difference together with rediscovered values are vulnerable and easily disappear again. Hence the great importance of documenting them.

Listening to this astonishing initiative Tina has taken, I ask how she would describe this action.

T: It is as if I have climbed Mount Everest!

S: What is this 'climbing Mount Everest' all about? ... Do you think doing this was a good thing? ... What makes it possible for yourself, significant others, ...?

After exploring the different aspects, I ask if it would be a good idea to award a certificate for climbing Mount Everest and who might support all of this. Who would be interested in knowing this?

It is important to bear in mind that this meaning giving process doesn't happen in the isolation of our therapy room but is embedded in many ongoing dialogues in which Tina is involved and the broader context she is living in. So, besides asking how she would name this action and how we should understand this, I also ask if she shared this initiative with her loved ones. Does she have a notion of how this possibly was received by her mother, sister, friends and even maybe by her father? How would they understand this? Did she get some remarks, appreciations, etc.?

Children and youngsters can always unexpectedly engage in actions that we assess as containing a risk to their safety. Such actions are not particularly wished for or intended by us as therapists, as we can never be sure how third parties involved, in this case the father, will react, or how exchanges might perhaps lead to new abuse or violence. We can become rightfully worried. This is another good reason to deal with such actions first and foremost therapeutically, also because I believe that the way we try to consolidate the action can probably lessen the chances that impulsive or immediate (re)actions are repeated.

After hearing what Tina did, her mother first of all worried if she was okay but later on said she also was a bit proud of her daughter. She even remarked that she wished she was the one who had done this. Apparently, in her thoughts, she had already scolded him on several occasions.

Together, Tina and I make a certificate reflecting carefully about what to put on it. Tina liked it to be awarded in the presence of her sister and mother.

Certificate

For achieving

'A Mount Everest moment'

Hereby

Gathered courage en masse

Climbed Mount Everest figuratively

Said what needed to be said

Sent the black spot things back to sender

Proved that the Tina of last year is no longer the Tina of today

Made a scar out of an open wound

An important step to make it possible to get on with your life!

Awarded to Tina on ...,

Sabine Vermeire and The Team of Support

It is worth noting that consolidating practices such as, for example, a 'graduation ceremony' do not mean a 'happy ending' for the child or a definitive new attitude to the traumatic experiences and effects. Time and again, moments or events occur that can shake up discovered meanings and hard-won positions or ways of relating. It is best to see these initiatives and alternative stories as important steps in finding new ways forward, which need to be woven into the patchwork of life stories and which can make the dominant singular narratives less oppressive.

Chapter 5

Performing new relational narratives

Contexts of childhood adversities are often characterised by relational trauma. Important people in their life have hurt the child or were not experienced as present and supportive when needed. This means that feelings of suspicion, insecurity and painful memories got nestled in their relationships. Some children are not inclined to search for emotional support from people that are important to them as they can experience them as threatening and develop decidedly negative ideas about them. Other children cling desperately to adults, while still others are caught in all kinds of ambivalence. Therapeutically it is important to notice and acknowledge the pain of injured relationships and the many struggles that accompany them. We also need to focus on dealing with what have been called the ripple effects through relational networks (Walsh, 2007).

This chapter has one main focus: I hope to show how to make visible again that people still matter to each other and contribute in meaningful ways to the lives of others, increases *a sense of relational agency*, and paves the way for *the performance of new relational narratives*, on the spot. By widening our scope and engaging in conversations with peer groups and communities we can enhance *a sense of belonging* and strengthen processes of resilience within families and carers.

Entangled relationships

Since the age of nine Mauro (11) lives with his maternal grandparents in a small town. His father is in prison as he was involved in all kinds of drug trafficking. His mum became mentally challenged after an overdose three years ago and resides in a secure unit. For years there was domestic violence as well as social and financial problems. His older brother Rico (15) was also placed in kinship care with his grandparents but as he became more and more rebellious his grandparents couldn't handle him any longer. For the last few months he has lived in a youngsters' home. Grandparents blame father for mother's situation and feel very guilty themselves that they couldn't keep Rico at their home. Rico refuses to see them any longer. At the moment they are very worried about Mauro who developed several tics and makes uncontrolled face grimaces. He regularly hides

DOI: 10.4324/9781003167860-6

food in his room and he persistently lies about seemingly trivial things. They are convinced he does this intentionally because he is angry at them. In an attempt to have some control, they check all his assets on a daily basis. A few weeks ago it came to a physical pushing and pulling between grandfather and Mauro. Many subjects seem to be off-limits for discussion. Nobody trusts each other anymore. They come for conversations in the hope they can prevent Mauro also having to leave their home.

As discussed in Chapter 1, children, youngsters and their parents or carers can become entangled in all kinds of unhelpful relational dances, and other life domains and social relations can get infected by the problems. Rutter (1999) stresses that the reduction of negative chain reactions or an increase of positive chain reactions influences the extent to which the effects of adversity persist over time. He offered some interesting stepping stones for family therapists to enhance resilience processes as resilience may be strongly influenced by people's patterns of interpersonal relationships. Children with a background of violence, abuse or neglect often live in a world that they experience as threatening. Other people are perceived as fundamentally dangerous (Barrett et al., 1996), and relationships are not to be trusted. The steps they take evoke (re)actions from the people around them that only seem to make things worse. Parents and other carers experience a loss of control (Vermeire, 2020).

Losing a 'sense of relational agency' often boils down to resorting to coercive acts of influence, with parents, carers as well as children trying to control each other. These acts of control often have unintended alienating consequences within significant relationships (De Mol et al., 2018; Omer, 2004; Alon & Omer, 2006). As the grandparents start to check Mauro's bedroom, interrogate him, etc., and Mauro keeps his mouth shut more and more, hides all kinds of things, they become more and more stuck with each other. In their relational dances and interaction patterns they continuously construct meanings about each other, themselves, the problems and their lives that seem to go in a negative direction. The way each one involved will name or label the difficulties can evoke and reinforce a whole range of images, ideas and perspectives of the child as well as of their (grand)parents, carers and significant others (Vermeire, 2020). This also goes for the possibilities and impossibilities of their relationships with each other and with the outside world (Weingarten, 2003; Dallos, 2006). Children and their network risk getting stuck in 'negative identity and relationship conclusions', which consequently also limit their sense of agency (De Mol et al., 2018).

Mauro has been diagnosed with a 'reactive attachment disorder'. School and grandparents also want a diagnostic investigation into possible autism in the hope this will help them in finding solutions for the problems. The fear of the grandparents is that the genetic predetermination of his father and mother will cause him to evolve in the same direction, especially now that this has already happened to his older brother. Mauro is increasingly seen as destined to go wrong. Grandparents feel completely desperate and incapable. Mauro himself gets more and more disconnected from his grandparents, family, schoolfriends and experiences himself as a burden to everyone. He no longer experiences any grip on the problems and a sense of mattering seems completely lost.

Each one, in their efforts to cope, becomes increasingly entangled in patterns with often rejecting or ignoring effects that tend to separate them from each other. Their focus becomes mostly on 'what' and 'who' is the problem and in line with this 'what' and 'who' has to change. Mauro has to change, has to be treated and helped to change. Each step each one takes as efforts to change for the better, is informed by previous experiences, interpersonal understandings and many social and cultural instructions on how to be a good (grand)parent or (grand)child in these situations, how to deal with trauma and these painful family issues, etc. (Madsen, 2007). Once they get caught in these destructive spirals, the concerns, relational involvements and constructive contributions to each other's lives are obscured. So an important step in our therapeutic process is finding ways to stop these negative chain reactions and enhance their sense of agency and mattering by making them visible and tangible again.

Looking for common ground

During the first half hour, the conversation does not seem to go anywhere. Mauro refuses to sit down and keeps leaning against the wall, staring at the ceiling, half listening to the torrent of discomforts and complaints from his grandparents. The social worker from the foster care service desperately tries to soothe the grandparents and to bring out a few positive things about Mauro. Although sentences such as 'This ranting must stop' and 'This is not helpful' race through my head, I cannot find a starting point that will get another conversation going. Before I know it, I am part of this useless dance.

What (grand)parents or carers put on the table is an endless list of problems in relation to the child or youngster and of how hard they tried already to change the child's mind. This list is interspersed at length with massive examples. The traumatic past or attachment problems seem to have become the explanation par excellence for the difficulties and lead to the compelling conclusion that 'this problematic behaviour has to stop'. Often they hope I can make clear to the child that it cannot go on like this and that I can change the child or stop the problems. They no longer notice that their tirade makes the child cringe and drop out of the conversation. Just as the child no longer notices how frenetically their carers try to keep connection. Besides a child in need, I also meet (grand)parents/carers in need.

When I just try to stop these grandparents' 'ranting', this can easily be understood as calling them to order and in its effect it can be felt as not taking them seriously or not believing them. Before we know it we can end up in a dismissive struggle. To them, it may seem that I am putting the best interests of the child first. When I give (grand)parents all the space they need to express their worries and to explain what the child does wrong, I risk losing the child and the impression may arise that I am taking sides with them. So, instead of focusing on the often dramatic and problematic content of what grandparents bring to the conversations, I try to pick up their relational involvements and worries in this list of complaints (Rober, 2017; Vermeire, 2020).

Dear grandparents, may I interrupt you for a moment? All these examples and all these frustrations are these expressing how extremely concerned you both are in relation to Mauro? Do they also express something about how important he is to both of you and how hard you wish things to go well and differently between you all?

Both grandmother and grandfather sit back a little and take a deep breath. They nod in agreement. Out of the corner of my eye, I notice that Mauro, for the first time, curiously turns towards us.

Mauro, can I ask you, can you somewhat understand that your grandparents are concerned? Are their worries justified? Are there also some worries occupying your mind?

M (a bit acrid): Of course but they have to stop being on top of me.

In my questioning I am hoping to find some common ground from which we can start to talk and reflect together instead of being locked up in single monologues and just focusing on 'how to stop the problematic behaviour'. Instead of losing each other in different perspectives, stories and actions we are on the lookout for shared understandings. By bringing their mutual relational involvements and connected stories to the foreground we can maybe start an exploration of what is bothering each of them. In this exploration we may also find commonalities in the difficulties or problem definitions. Hopefully this can also invite (grand) parents or carers into a collective, alternative investigation of the perspective of the child and create new or alternative understandings. Recent scientific research shows how 'not understood behaviour' of (foster) children forms a big challenge to carers. It appears crucial when fostering traumatised children that carers have the ability to understand the child's experiences and emotions (Carolien Konijn, 2021).

In conversations we very quickly lose these common grounds and the focus goes easily to an examination of the individual person who seems to carry all the problems. Without interrupting our conversation, I write 'Shared Concerns' in large letters on the flipchart.

A collective investigation of relationships and social worlds

When one becomes an isolated agent in the family or in another close relationship, the estrangement from one's wishes, intentions, emotions and thoughts increases while the sense of relational agency decreases (De Mol et al., 2018). Although they are depending on the support that carers offer, children can still learn to give meaning to their own feelings and those of others, and generate stories from this (Dallos, 2006). That is why we, together with the significant people of their network, try to find and create a shared language, a common ground to reflect upon and to make sense of what happens or happened in their life.

In the family therapy room, there are some toys and on the wall are some drawings of other children, sometimes with messages to other therapy visitors. One protest poster grabs Mauro's attention. 'Parents have to stop quarrelling in the presence of a child', written by Chelsea, nine years old, whose parents are involved in a divorce with high conflict. While the tics are all around and he is still grimacing, Mauro asks who made it and why. Also grandparents' attention now goes to the drawing. After shortly giving some explanation about the drawing and Chelsea's intentions the following conversation starts:

S: Are there some things, just like Chelsea, you would like to stop, if you could? Some things that seem to ruin things? For Chelsea the quarrels evoked a lot of stress and it made people who are important to her become further away. Is there something that removes you from beloved people?

M (looking to the ground he mumbles): The question marks.

S: What do you mean by question marks? ... How should we imagine them? Big question marks? Various question marks? Dark question marks? Unresolvable question marks?

M (lifting his head, and throwing in verbal tics): Fire-red question marks, Argh! Orange question marks, Argh! Poisonous green question marks, Argh! Even exploding question marks!

S: How long are these question marks already present?

M: Since mum is in hospital, but also since dad is in prison and they became enormous when Rico left the house.

S: Where have they nestled themselves?

M: Mostly in my head but sometimes they are everywhere. No one can control them. They jump around all the time.

S (addressing grandparents): Did you have any clue Mauro had question marks occupying his head and life?

GF (grandfather): No, I didn't know but honestly, I am not surprised.

S: Oh, do you also have some question marks in your life as you say you aren't surprised.

GF: Of course. Doesn't everyone have question marks?

While further talking with grandfather, I ask Mauro to draw his question marks on the flip chart in the right colours. Did he know grandfather also had question marks? And what about grandmother and the foster care worker? Can we first start an investigation about Mauro's question marks (Figure 5.1).

Language creates personal and relational realities, and by giving words to the clients' 'insides' they acquire the right to exist within their social and relational world (Madsen, 2007). By collaborative searching and finding words for a person's worries, emotions, thoughts, etc., persons can feel what they feel. By exploring and developing collective language as co-researchers social sharing of

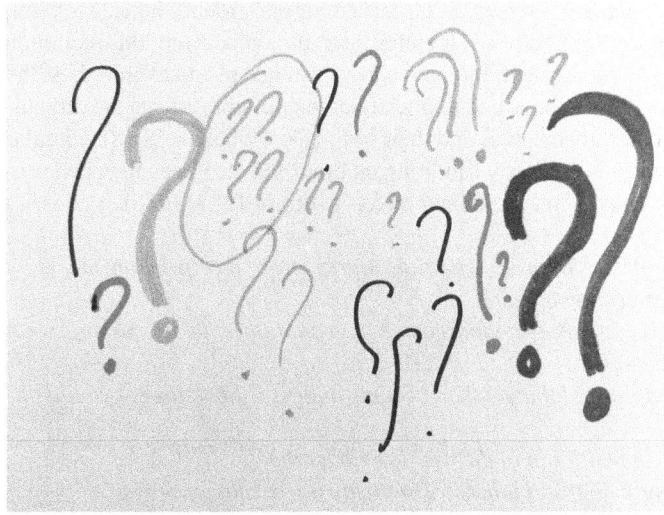

Figure 5.1 Collection of colourful question marks. Photograph by the author.

experiences can take place with the significant people in their life (De Mol & Rimé, 2017; Freedman & Combs, 2002).

Together we explore the question marks. What is good food for the question marks? When are they more or less present? Are some question marks more compelling than others? On the flip chart we add some more question marks that have a grip on Mauro and grandfather suggests to cluster them. Some question marks are about his brother, some about his mum, some about his dad, grandparents ... but some are also about the future in relation to himself: 'Will I also be sent away?', 'Am I abnormal?', 'Will this ever stop?', 'Am I so bad that nobody wants me?' At this very moment these last question marks hurt the most and we discover these make him very nervous and anxious.

Suddenly Mauro asks what the question marks of grandmother are about and what they look like.

GM: I am so worried about how we can make things better. What can we do to help you feel better is a big question mark! Day and night it fills my stomach.
S: Is this question mark also accompanied by nervousness and fear?

A recognition of feelings of being disadvantaged is facilitated between the child-(grand)parents-carers. By collective externalising, the hierarchies of worries and disadvantages can become visible but also the different ambivalences and dilemmas between family members as well as some common difficulties. It even makes it possible to explore whether some of the 'question marks' are linked with each other.

This collective naming creates a larger common ground between them. Acknowledgement of each other's feelings and thoughts from this common ground becomes possible while differences can be listened to and explored. At the same time it allows them to have a dialogue about the possible effects the difficulties have on each other, themselves and their lives (De Mol et al., 2018). Circular questioning in an externalised way can bring an order but also open new perspectives on the problems and their relational effects (Tomm, 1987, 1988).

S: What happens when Mauro's question marks meet the question marks of grandfather or grandmother?
    Mauro looks at his grandparents but grandfather insists asking what Mauro thinks.
M: Quarrels? Doing stupid things? You become angry. ... Sometimes I would like to disappear.
GF: I think we become a 'pain in the ass' for each other.
GM (looks scathingly at grandfather): 'Don't say it like that'.
GF: I think it's true.
M: The question marks get entangled.

And while drawing he proceeds:

M: It is like in Minecraft when the night comes. The night is full of zombies, witches, Endermen, skeletons, spiders and creepers. You have to make sure you are safe so nothing can happen to you. Sometimes I am afraid we will all change into zombies.

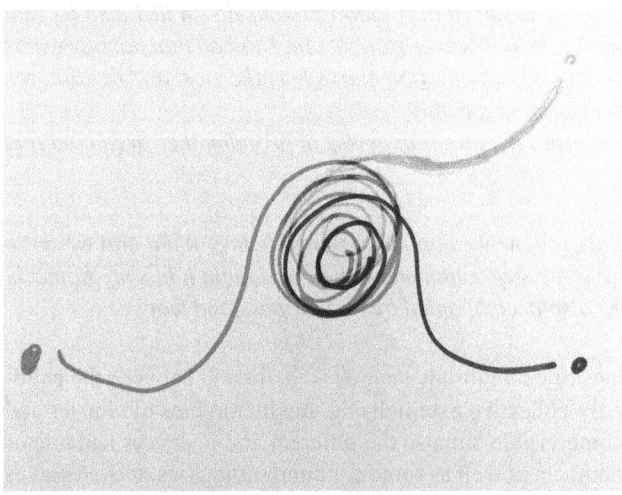

Figure 5.2 Three question marks entangled. Photograph by the author.

Everybody looks surprised. We all agree this is a scary idea and none of us want this to happen.

S: What kind of efforts have you done until now to deal with all these question marks or to keep the zombies, witches, etc. and fear at a distance?

Mauro explains that he created a special house under the ground in Minecraft that is perfectly safe and no one can destroy. A special friend from a previous school helped him to create this house. Grandfather remarks he has never seen this house. Proudly Mauro shows on his smartphone some pictures and explains the characteristics of the different rooms.

This kind of collaborative research invites them to talk and relate with each other differently. It unfolds small shifts in either images, beliefs or actions of one another that create new foundations for different ways of relating to each other (Vermeire, 2020).

Is there anything you already discovered that is helpful or makes the question marks smaller? Are there special shared moments that can be an antidote to the question marks?

New ways of mutual understanding can also open possibilities for more collective agency while new relational dances can emerge.

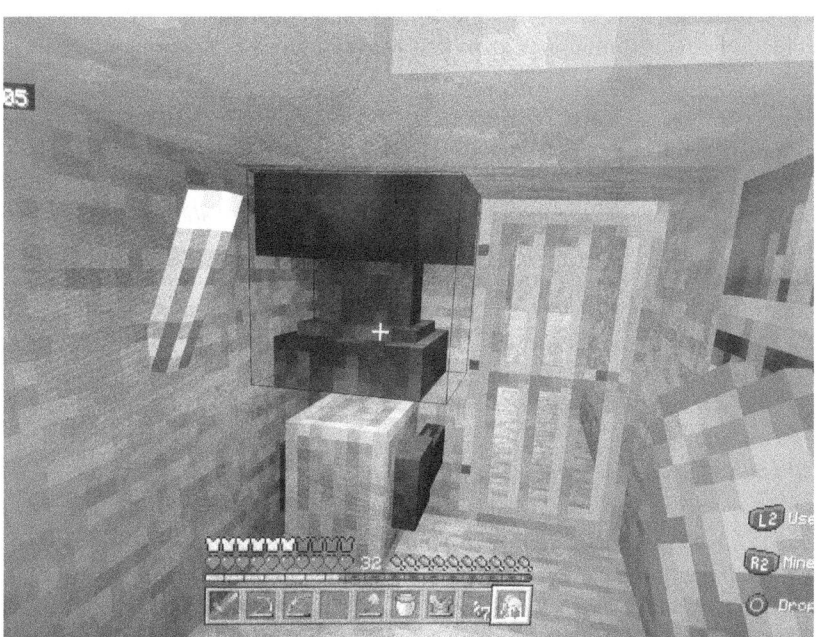

Figure 5.3 Minecraft house. Photograph by the author.

As we find out that playing Minecraft and his hiding place are all about 'find-ing rest', mainly 'rest in his head', grandfather asks if he can help improve his hiding place in Minecraft. Mauro seems very pleased with this proposal and together we think a bit further about what else could bring some calmness and rest. Grandmother replies that in moments they were jointly making apple pie the question marks seemed to disappear to the background and that she earlier really enjoyed having Mauro around in the kitchen.

Small sparkles of how to make more constructive contributions to one's life become visible. Having a sense of relational agency means that a person has a feeling and an awareness of making a difference in the relationship (De Mol et al., 2018). That one as an agent can add something that is meaningful for the other, for oneself and for the relationship (Bertrando & Arcelloni, 2014; De Mol & Buysse, 2008).

From immobilising verbs towards new actions

Children, families, communities, cultures have taken-for-granted customs or ideas on how to deal with problems, difficult (negative) emotions, stagnant thoughts or painful questions. One way to scrutinise such actions is to have a closer look at the verbs people use in relation to these problems. The Dutch word for 'verb' is 'werk-woord' which could be literally translated as 'work-word'. This suggests that we can conceive of verbs as being at work. Unaware they could take us in a certain direction. So we can try to find out what kind of work they are doing, and what kind of effects (limitations as well as possibilities) they are bringing about.

S: Mauro, when you are in your house in Minecraft what do you try to do with these question marks? Or what is your ambition with this house and the ques-tion marks?

M: I try to hide from the question marks. In my secret room I stick my tongue out at them because they can't bother me any longer.

S: Hiding and sticking your tongue out, can you demonstrate this to all of us, how does this look like?

   Mauro jumps under the table in the corner of the therapy room and sticks out his tongue while saying 'Blargh'.

S: Do you have any idea how grandmother and grandfather try to deal with pain-ful question marks?

M (still sitting under the table): She tries to knit them away.

Grandma has to laugh and again I ask if he can demonstrate to us how grandma is knitting the question marks away. He enthusiastically sits on a chair pretending to knit and constantly shakes his head, muttering to himself.

GM: 'Yes, this is exactly what happens'.

Together we explore how grandfather deals with difficult question marks. 'I try to kick them out. *No one should interfere with our life'.*

...

S: *Besides hiding, knitting away, kicking them ... what are we supposed to do*
  normally with questions and queries? In the classroom, for example?
M: *Raise your finger and give the right answer!*

Together, we discover that answering correctly is rewarded but that the questions everyone struggles with do not have correct answers. On the contrary. They all agree that each one of them is struggling on their own and that their responses sometimes are helpful for a while but not in the long term. I wonder aloud what would happen if we would 'share the question marks' (as we are already doing ☺). A bit later we also try to find out what 'searching for answers', 'puzzling answers' or maybe even more 'knitting answers' would look like. Or are there some verbs that feel more appropriate?

  Before we know it Mauro makes a new drawing on the flip chart.

In our therapeutic work we conceive of language as deeply metaphorical. Metaphors can make themselves felt physically as they are rooted in physical experiences (Lakoff & Johnson, 1999; Rucińska et al., 2021). Words can give us something to hold on to, but at the same time they can push or lure us in certain directions. Language and communication is an activity. Verbs in combination with problem names can be seen as actions that open up a space, but sometimes also close off certain routes and can make us feel trapped (Vermeire & Van

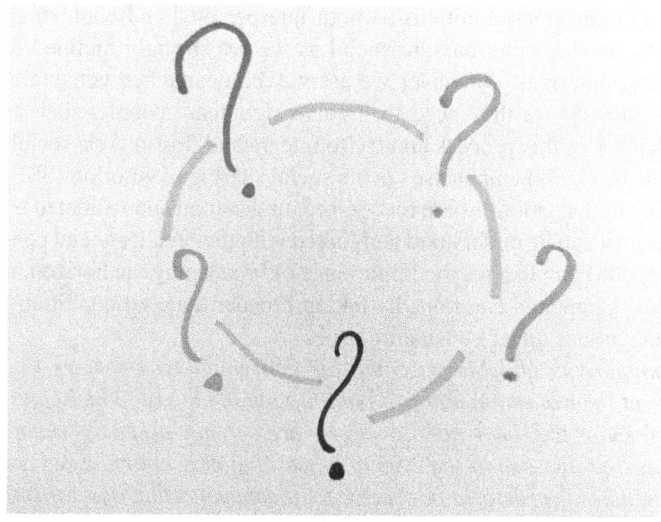

Figure 5.4 Five questions in a circle. Photograph by the author.

den Berge, 2021). It can even become 'fun' but also meaningful in doing these verbs together as embodied actions, like I asked Mauro to demonstrate grandma knitting.

The verbs associated with problems offer a gateway to approach experiences differently and provoke new embodied experiences. Instead of seeing metaphors as linguistic 'comparisons' in which the meaning of the metaphor is sought or found in the comparison itself, we embrace an embodied and enactive perspective that holds that the meaning of metaphors is always situated in unique interactions and contexts (cf. Rucińska & Reijmers, 2014; Rucińska et al., 2021). Metaphors arise where people are connected and can be seen as tools that people use in their interactions and communication with each other. They can become invitations for 'language in action' (Wilson, 2005) and 'pretend play' (Holzman, 2009). We create a context in which the child, the (grand)parents and the carers can explore, experiment, share and find new perspectives or try out new possibilities for action and connection, strengthening a sense of relational agency. Talking and acting together around and from these metaphors is a form of participatory sense-making (De Jaegher & Di Paolo, 2007) that lets them experience that they matter.

Question marks do not fall out of the sky

Sometimes the questions, worries, emotions and thoughts run in circles. They are constantly racing through their bodies and heads and infiltrate their relationships (De Mol & Rimé, 2017). Children (and families) can no longer contextualise their emotions and bodily (re)actions. The instruction often becomes that they have to regulate their emotions. In a predominant sense this boils down to the idea of controlling emotions. We prefer to look at emotion regulation as relational and social and we try to understand emotions as both interpersonal and contextual. Rimé (2009) points out that emotions are social as we are strongly inclined to share our stories, our emotions, whenever we are moved or touched personally by events. Therapeutically we thus need to involve significant people, such as (grand)parents or carers in this process and try to understand this in their social-cultural contexts. Rimé (2009) emphasises in his social sharing of emotion (SSE) theory it isn't sufficient that emotions are recognised, understood and validated by others but also that they can be understood and linked with the broader social context. Denborough (2008) emphasises the importance of broadening the horizon of the origins of the problems and emotions by taking broader material conditions, discourses and social issues under consideration.

Next time, grandparents and Mauro come for conversations I remark that probably each one of their question marks do not fall out of the sky. Which questions that trouble them or they have no answers for are actually asked by whom? Are there questions that they see in the eyes of others, but may not be asked out loud? Do they sometimes get remarks or receive tacit comments that upset them?

Almost immediately Mauro tells us he hates 'Mother's Day'. In school every child is expected to make a present and to share stories of how their mother cares for them. He always freezes in his seat, anxiously waiting for the teacher to ask him this question. He adds: 'I just want an ordinary family. I want to be normal'.

Children and young people very quickly feel that theirs is an exceptional family. Any statement or question, implicit or explicit, about families, about their family or about a particular family member can be heard as a statement about themselves.

S: Could we collect some more of these questions or remarks that are bothering you and maybe are good food for the feeling of not being normal?

On the table we put all the people who are part of these dialogues. We write the questions on post-its and stick them next to them. They can be questions from classmates, or children from the neighbourhood, or from involved adults. Some questions are actually asked of them, others might just not be asked of them. (Where has your brother gone? Why don't you live with your parents? Is your father a real criminal? Did he have guns? Why isn't your mum coming to your birthday party? ...).

People are constantly preoccupied with who they are to each other and constantly make statements about each other, often unintentionally and without being aware of it. Laing et al. (1966) referred to this as interpersonal perceptions. Children and their family constantly receive impressions of who they are in the eyes of others, their family and their community. Their self-perception is a temporary synthesis of their view of themselves with the view others and society have of them, which arises in an ongoing social dialogue in which they participate in active and meaningful ways (Gergen, 2009; Faes, 2005; Vermeire & van Hennik, 2017). Children and families in such contexts often reach conclusions about themselves and their families as failing, abnormal or wrong.

GF (pointing to what appears on the table): That's why I try to kick the question marks out. I want to protect Mauro from all these questions and painful remarks. I, too, have a hard time accepting that his father is in prison. I am still furious about what he did to our daughter. I wish he could disappear from this globe. How could it go so wrong? What have we done wrong? I agree with Mauro: I wished we were a 'normal family'. Sometimes I really get angry when the neighbour shows off holiday pictures of her grandchildren at some exotic travel destination.

As several family therapists (De Mol & Rimé 2017; Walsh, 2006) emphasise, it can be useful to explore with children, parents, carers the complexities of their social relationships not only inside the family but also outside the family and ask if there is someone in that context who can recognise something of these complexities (De Mol & Rimé 2017; Walsh, 2006). By exploring together with the family the relational complexities that exist for each family member, the family is approached as a resource and not as the problem, which facilitates processes of recognition and responsiveness.

While doing so we are contextualising the question marks and feelings of the child and the parents or carers within the many relationships, social representations and broader social discourses. Just like 'pushing and pulling' beliefs and norms about 'good families', 'family relationships', 'motherhood', 'fatherhood', 'being a good son or daughter', etc. become more and more visible. Together they can reflect on alternative positioning or new ways of relating and even rehearse alternative responses.

Re-membering the body

Not only can feelings become contextualised but also bodily (re)actions not understood like bedwetting, tics, panic attacks, etc., can be collectively explored. Not as an ultimate explanation but more as part of our participatory sense-making process and becoming a solid team.

I ask grandparents and Mauro if they sometimes notice a connection between the many annoying questions, the feelings of not being 'normal' and the tics and grimaces. Are there moments the grimaces are definitely present and don't let themselves be controlled?

Together we find out that class moments when he has to perform or present something, but also moments on the school bus or unknown visitors at grandparents place are ideal contexts for the tics and grimaces to appear. Grandfather remarks that he noticed that when Mauro fears that the subject of his mum or dad will come up, this is also a good breeding ground. Grandmother continues: 'And for sure, the weeks and days before we are going to visit his mum in hospital'.

Children's felt connection with their bodies can be under pressure or lost altogether after radical or traumatic experiences or in contexts of distress. The body starts reacting uninvitedly and seems to go its own way completely autonomously. They experience the various body reactions as uncontrollable and incomprehensible while they often get understood by others as 'residual symptoms' of the trauma or typical aspects of diagnoses (Fisher, 2005). The idea that they can control their bodies if they really want to and try hard enough sometimes puts extra pressure on children in these contexts. Here, not only alienation from the people around them, but also from their bodies may arise.

Mauro tells us he hates the moments classmates ask why he is blinking his eyes or making these strange faces. That's the moment it becomes even worse although he does his best to stop it. Also, grandmother sometimes gets nervous of the grimaces and makes unhelpful remarks while asking him to stop. Step by step they realise they get in similar entanglements as with the question marks.

These children sometimes start to 'mistrust' and even 'hate' their own bodies. Their body becomes like an enemy. A sense of failure or worthlessness comes to the fore. Engaging everyone in a collective exploration of the bodily (re)actions in contexts and relations can open opportunities to reconnect children with their bodies. Tom Andersen (in Shotter, 2010) invites family members to question the body as a valuable partner in our conversations and asks, 'What is the body saying if it could speak?' We are not searching for 'underlying emotions' or 'the right deeper meaning' since we cannot know from the outside what the body is saying. We rather hope to unfold new felt perspectives.

After inventorying the bodily reactions, I ask if we could listen very carefully what the body maybe would report about the situation Mauro is in at that moment.

M: *Watch out! Danger!*
GM: *Does it warn of the annoying questions?*
GF: *Maybe it is more that you don't know what is going to come?*
S: *At such moments are you listening to your body or just getting into a fight with it?*
M: *Don't know??? I just try to stop it! I only wish I could disappear!*

Listening carefully and 'understanding' what the body might say is an active process between the child, the therapist and many people involved in which new meanings can arise that are different from the original meanings of the child and loved ones. In doing so, we become a mutually supportive team.

Scientific research found that children in war zones hiding in bomb shelters often make all kinds of movements while adults cramp up and make themselves small. Children who make these movements seem to have less post-traumatic stress and move on quicker with daily living (Berceli, 2008).

Inspired by this research I ask if these bodily reactions can have the ambition to blow away the tension in order to keep going on. In saying this I ask grandmother what her body does when pressure comes in and what her bodily ways of responding are. It seems she used to bite her lip, sometimes to the point of bleeding, but now she sometimes picks at her fingers in an unconscious way.

...

I tell them that I have a colleague who sometimes asks people to move their bodies as 'a double duvet flapping in the wind' when distress comes in (thanks to Renild for this wonderful idea). Or would the idea of another colleague, Els, be more helpful as she asks to do 'The shake your body'? I wonder how this would look for them? How can they collaborate in this with each other and their body?

I am the only one on this planet ...

Children and youngsters feel isolated and alienated from the circles they live in and the conviction that nobody can understand what they feel, think or do, can get deeply nestled inside them (Vermeire, 2017). They often feel questioning eyes poking in their direction or are actually asked all sorts of questions about their situation, to which they are unable to give an answer. Although these children themselves have questions about what happened to them in their lives, mostly they don't ask these questions freely, or they even stop asking questions out of fear of receiving answers that may be too painful (Vermeire, 2020). Sometimes they became quite sure of their own negative conclusions.

Mauro can't believe that there are other children struggling with all these family complexities and not knowing how to deal with these questions. He is surprised and looks at me unbelievingly when I tell him that I know several other children living away from home and struggling with 'family difficulties'. I ask if he is interested in questioning these children or youngsters. He immediately replies: 'Do you also know children whose parents stay in prison or in hospital?' We prepare a questionnaire based on what occupies his mind and what we already explored and discussed together with his grandparents. We come up with the following questions: Do you sometimes have other people asking annoying questions or looking in your direction in a strange way? Do you sometimes have question marks that make you worry? Do you know good tricks to stop this worrying? Do you sometimes do weird things when the question marks are around? Do you miss you mum or dad? Or your siblings? Do you sometimes think it's all your fault? The moment grandparents get to know we are preparing a questionnaire, they are happy to add some questions that concern them. Are your carers sometimes worried and how do they express these worries? Do you know what helps to feel okay with your carers or the people you stay with?

Over the years, I have compiled a list of possible interviewees for such surveys. At the end of each therapeutic process I ask children or families if I can contact them later on to interview them about their experiences in order to help other children. They often feel honoured when they are actually invited for such an interview. The way they want to contribute is thoroughly negotiated. Sometimes I also ask trainees of mine to anonymously interview children they meet and bring back the answers to such questions.

Mauro and I interview several children and youngsters 'live' as well as by video call and e-mail. Mauro is impressed to learn that a lot of children live in comparable situations. Discovering that other children and young people are prepared to answer his questions surprises him even more. He finds recognition for the worries and suffering, reassurance for not being 'too abnormal' and inspiration in the actions of several children that help them to persist (Vermeire, 2020).

I meet Rayan (17) via video calling. The conversation is recorded so that I can watch it later with Mauro. Rayan's mother works as a prostitute (his word) and lives on the other side of the country. He has not met her for years. He says he is often nervous when his mother is mentioned. Especially when a Facebook post of hers appears. Recently, he saw a picture of her in a restaurant together with his stepbrothers. This felt like a dagger through his heart. His foster parents feel like his 'real parents' to him, even though there was a period in which he did 'crazy things' like cutting up his clothes and distributing absurd photos. This made things very difficult between them. Rayan has been writing rap songs for a year now. This helps him a lot to sort out his thoughts and share his anger. His friends now know that he sometimes has hard times. They give him a pat on the back and that helps.

Through the other children's stories, local knowledges and life-acquired skills, Mauro's experiences become recognised and acknowledged. One of the aims of such work is that Mauro can feel a sense of belonging with important peer groups and the broader community. This aligns with the ideas of Reynolds (2012, p. 23) to create a 'community of solidarity' so people become 'allies'.

Two weeks later Mauro receives a special rap song written and recorded by Rayan. He cherishes the text and listens several times a day to the recorded version. Together, we will explore what resonates most with him and what gives him something to hold on to.

Lisa (19) says in response to the questionnaire that there was a time when she was constantly in a kind of struggle with her foster parents. As soon as they started to trust each other a bit more and she felt she had 'some breathing space', they settled down a bit. She remembers how things really changed when her foster parents stopped warning her not to become like her mother, and they started to appreciate some aspects of her mother.

Lisa's stories and inspirations help Mauro's grandma to talk differently. She asks new, more connecting questions about his father. 'What does having a dad in prison really mean to him? Can he still handle the situation in his mind?'

These 'research projects and interviews' not only help people to develop new or alternative perspectives on the difficulties and their responses but it also enhances, in multiple ways, a sense of connectedness and a sense of belonging. The position of 'investigator', 'interviewer' or 'videographer' offers the child and its family a safe place in which to stand and ask the questions that occupy their mind. At the same time this position opens up the possibility of hearing different or even new stories. Other children may prefer to construct a questionnaire for a glossy magazine and do the interviews from the position of a reporter. It is important to let at least three voices speak and be heard to prevent the given answers from becoming truths. Inviting different people brings in multiple realities and perspectives. This creates freedom of choice and activates reflection (Fredman, 2014). Knowledge is always situated. We can bring in different kinds of knowledge to produce a many-voiced, polyphonic conversation (Gergen, 1999; Vermeire, 2017). Expert knowledge as well as local knowledge can be voiced.

We need to discuss thoroughly whose voice and knowledge we want to invite into the room. We will ask the child (and family members) whose ideas they're most interested in, or whose voices they would love to hear. Each voice has a different weight, a different value and a different meaning for the child. We can listen to real or imaginary voices. We can invite them 'live' in the therapy room, we can go out on the street, or we can make questionnaires and send them around through the internet. We can question persons closely involved (family, friends) or complete strangers; peers or buddies, cuddly toys or idols, or people in specific positions such as police, judges or psychiatrists (Vermeire, 2017).

- *Xander (Chapter 1) had a lot of questions about 'borderline', the medicines that his mum had to take and if there were some tricks not to get borderline yourself. He didn't want to question his mum's doctor because he didn't trust her. She would give answers just to reassure him. Together we interviewed a psychologist, a psychiatrist, and the sister of a person diagnosed with borderline. We discovered through the responses that he knew already a lot of tricks to stay on track.*

- *Lisa was struggling with diabetes (Vermeire & Van den Berge, 2021) and together we interviewed some people about diabetes, the fear of needles, how to co-operate with your body and how parents or carers respond to such medical issues in some helpful but also unhelpful ways.*
- *John whose father stepped out of life, interviewed people about all kinds of emotions in these contexts and how to save memories of someone who died. As one of his aims was to become a policeman, we even interviewed two policemen on these subjects. It helped him to develop a new kind of emotion theory.* (https://www.youtube.com/watch?v=S-EgBNofpu0, Vermeire, 2017)
- *...*

Ever widening circles

By collecting all these ideas, listening to them and thinking about them, new actions become conceivable and can be undertaken.

A few weeks later, Mauro surprises us all by telling he wrote a letter to his two best school mates (inspired by what Rayan had said). He explained to them why he hates birthday parties or talking about family holidays and how his body sometimes is protesting to 'family talk'. Although it makes him sad he doesn't want them to stop sharing stories about their mum and dad because then he would feel even more pitiful.

At the end of his letter, he asked: Do you want to stay my friend forever?

Yes   No

Please, cross out what is not correct!

As soon as new ways of relating start to appear and relational meanings are expanded we invite Mauro and his grandparents to widen the circles of important others who get to know about their worries, challenges. As such we encourage them to regain even more relational and collective agency.

Grandfather and Mauro have a conversation with the football coach about how he can feel more part of the team. Mauro explains to the coach how difficult it is to hear all those other fathers encouraging their child from the side line on Saturday morning matches. Together they agree on a secret code language as special support during the match. They also agree that the coach will inform Mauro's father in prison about his progress in football.

By letting the stories and ideas circulate amongst other people involved it then becomes a performance of meaning (Freeman et al., 1997).

Mauro leaves a message in the therapy room for other children and young-sters. On the board he writes in big letters 'Never give up! When you are sad, tell a friend'. He also adds that anyone can contact him when they have questions.

At this stage Mauro is no longer positioned as a child in need but as someone who can make valuable contributions to the lives of other children or families. He has knowledge to share that can be helpful to others. This is also in line with the ideas of Myerhoff (2007): the suffering wasn't for nothing; it can be meaningful to others. This holds true for grandparents too who re-found a sense of mattering. Together, step by step, they create a network of resilience.

Back to start?

Therapeutic journeys are not motorways that lead directly to solutions, certainly not in contexts of multi-stressed families and developmental trauma. These journeys are rather characterised by setbacks and losing one's way. Sometimes it seems as if one is back to square one. In their daily lives and intimate relationships, they encounter many obstacles, pitfalls, etc., and before they know it, they get caught up in unhelpful reactions and dances again.

One Monday morning I get a phone call from grandma. Mauro had a major temper tantrum last weekend. He was with her in the park and after a while he went to play with friends at a forbidden place. When she found him she became quite angry, he called her names and said he hated her. Grandma grabbed him by the collar and pulled him home. In the evening he pooped in his trousers. On the phone she asks if I can talk with him about the incident. She has had enough of it. Our conversations seem to make no difference.

Before we know it the child and their parents or carers lose their sense of agency again. They face each other again as opponents or get stuck in feelings of hopelessness.

Mauro and his grandfather come in a few days after the incident. Grandmother could not be present. When I ask him what happened he indignantly yells: 'grandma does everything to bully me! A real mother would never do such a thing!'

The incident has trapped them back into single, reduced, old familiar stories and solidified perspectives of themselves and each other. They lose sight of each other's relational commitment, hopes and wishes and the possibility of a variety of understandings. Luckily, once their worries and frustrations have been noticed and shared in this very moment, it becomes easier to reflect on what happened. The whole incident is reduced to a few sentences so together with Mauro I try to situate the incident in broader, multiple landscapes of events and actions.

I ask Mauro to re-enact with the Russian dolls on the table the whole Sunday afternoon, not just the incident. He chooses the tallest doll for grandma and the smallest one for himself. Grandfather watches the performance from a distance. We stage everything carefully. What happened before the incident? (He was

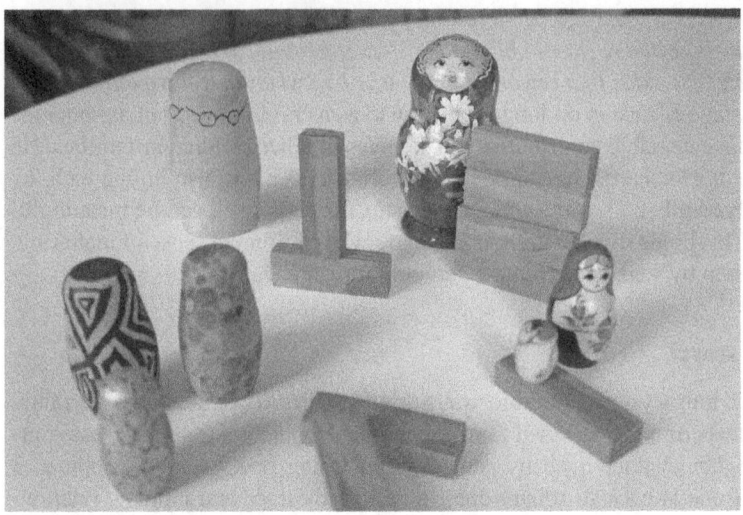

Figure 5.5 Russian dolls and wooden blocks. Photograph by the author.

already lying for hours on the couch refusing to do anything). Who was in the park, who stood where and who said what exactly? (He met two boys from a previous school he hadn't seen for ages) ...

I want to take Mauro step by step from an insider's perspective to an outsider's perspective so that he can look at, and reflect on, what happened from a kind of platform. I hope that in this process we all get a richer understanding of what bothers him and that perhaps new sides to the story will become visible. As we zoom in, we simultaneously zoom out and connect the events to many influencing contexts.

During the play, I ask him what the different people probably thought, felt, perhaps did not show, ... I ask for instance what grandma might have thought when she discovered that he had disappeared from the park. He shrugs his shoulders at many of these questions. They remain unanswered. Several times he repeats that a real mother would never get so angry, would certainly not hit him (as grandma patted him on the arm on the way home) or refuse to talk about it afterwards.

I clearly hear that he feels so wronged. It seems that the disadvantage during the incident has landed on a huge mountain of disadvantages, pain and sorrow. How can we acknowledge this almost existential pain, bring it back to the here and now and bring some differentiation and relief to these painful experiences?

Mauro, I have a small suspicion about this whole Sunday afternoon, but I don't know if I can say it out loud. I don't want to drag all the frustrations and pain into this room ...

M: Go ahead. Give it a try ...

S: Is it possible that this whole Sunday afternoon also has something to do with 'Missing a real mum', 'Wishing to be with your real mum' and maybe at the same time 'Just being bored and being excited meeting these old friends?'

M (with a soft voice): Maybe ...

S: Would you be interested in knowing how real mums feel, think or act in such a situation?

As he curiously looks up, I propose to invite my colleague next door who is a mum, present her the enactment and ask all the questions we have about 'a real mum' in such a situation. Mauro and grandfather use the camera to film this enactment with the Russian dolls and record 'the real mum's responses', which allows us to share it afterwards with grandma.

In such situations it requires some effort by myself to sit on my hands and not to start to 'explain' that probably 'real mums' would also be worried, would be irritated and frustrated. This would put me in an expert position with the risk of convincing him and becoming the 'norm giver'. It is much more powerful when children are enabled to discover things for themselves or measure their experiences and thinking up against a third person's perspective in which they are really interested. It keeps the door open for our collaboration to reflect together later on what is being introduced by the thinking, feeling and acting of this third person. A more triadic questioning and reflecting becomes possible.

I ask this colleague-mum to go through the Sunday afternoon scene together and put into words what she would think, feel and do during the incident. In this way, we find out that this mum would become very scared noticing her son disappeared. She would not tolerate the reproaches he made, but at the same time would not want to ridicule her son in front of his friends so she would be in doubt how to go on. During the enactment her son is even told that he might get a tap as well, but mainly in an attempt to calm him down and not make things worse, in no way to hurt him.

This drama technique and interview are reminiscent of Minuchin's enactments (Minuchin, 1974), but differ in crucial respects. They are not based on observations of interactions and I do not instruct the child or family how to do things differently. This enactment brings about change in the thinking and actions of each family member. Perspectives of others are brought in so that they can be heard. They start to see events with new eyes and begin to notice multiple worries, involvements, intentions, hopes, beliefs, values, etc. in the actions of the other.

When grandma watches the recorded session she remarks that the whole incident maybe wasn't that much about Mauro hating her. She also guesses it has something to do with missing a 'real mum', whatever that may mean and combined with the complexity of meeting his old friends. She really feels pity they lose each other in such moments.

Russian dolls unveiling unsuspected intentions

Children and youngsters in contexts where intimate relationships were hurt and attachment figures as parents or siblings were not perceived as reliable may come to regard all kinds of other relationships as equally unreliable. Intimate relationships can become experienced as contexts of insecurity and each communication or interaction gets experienced as personal, negative, intentional and controlled. What the other person says, does or thinks is interpreted as 'That other person wants to hurt me deliberately and is fully aware of what he is doing'.

Katinka (see Chapter 4) is convinced that her mum and the child care workers at the children's home are all the same. They only want one thing: to ruin her life. You can't trust them. After an argument with slamming doors with her mentor, Justine, she refused to talk to her for a fortnight.

Children and youngsters don't present their understandings as interpretations but rather as indubitable truths about the other, their relationship and themselves. When people interact, they can experience pleasant as well as unpleasant feelings. Philosopher De Botton (2000) remarked that in the latter case, they then typically attribute negative intentions to the other participant (even when this is a non-human actor, e.g., a computer). We often notice that this attributing of negative intentions gets associated with generalisations, and with decontextualisation. 'The other person is always and everywhere only trying to abuse or disadvantage us, wilfully and on purpose'. Often both (or more) participants in the process become trapped in this kind of generalising and decontextualising of what is happening, without being aware of it. The other gets easily totalised (Freedman & Combs, 2002). This becomes part of an ongoing recursive process. That's why it is important (once more) to find playful ways to contextualise events, to introduce doubt and relief concerning the other person's 'inside'. After all, such 'misunderstandings' or unchecked interpretations of each other's 'inside' can easily lead to estrangement and alienation from each other, therefore it is necessary to develop richer descriptions and to look for more connecting interpretations.

I take the Russian dolls from my desk and ask Katinka some questions about moments lately when she really thought Justine was out to 'get' her. I invite Katinka to describe the 'outside' of her mentor, Justine. She gives an example from a few weeks ago. She came back with some notes from school and had to stay after school. The group was very busy. Everyone was coming in and out. There was already some tension because the day before she already had a quarrel with Justine. Pointing to the outside of the Russian doll representing her mentor I ask: 'How did Justine respond to these notes? What gestures did she make? With what kind of voice was she speaking?' Katinka tries to recall this moment and says that Justine opened her eyes wide when she saw the notes, turned a little red and, with great indignation in her voice, had asked: 'Are you going to ruin it at school too?' Katinka put her fingers in her ears and screamed. Justine urged her to go to her room. Since that moment she refuses to speak with Justine although Justine each day knocks at her bedroom door.

While I open the outer doll and look at the first doll inside, I question Katinka about what aspects of the 'outside' of Justine, like her actions, words, gestures, ... make her conclude about the possible (invisible) 'inside' namely her relational involvements, intentions, beliefs, hopes or wishes?

K: *She loves to reprimand me. She is always disappointed in me.*

S *(while I take the next doll out of the previous one and put her next to the others): Do you think that opening her eyes wide and turning a little bit red just means she loves to reprimand or could it also mean that she is worried and cares for your school career? Are some of her hopes for you under pressure?*

K: *Yeah, she really wants me to get a diploma! She sometimes speaks French with me as a kind of rehearsal because I struggle with French at school and I don't get good marks.*

S *(taking the next doll out and showing Katinka): Sometimes speaking French with you, ..., wanting you to get a diploma, ... What is this about? What kind of possibilities for you is she noticing or hoping for?*

K: *She once said, 'Please, be wiser than some people in your family'. I think she believes I can make something out of my life.*

Step by step I put the other smaller dolls next to each other and together we look for other, alternative perspectives in relation to Katinka so that a more nuanced and multi-layered image of Justine and her actions emerge, taking into account different contexts. Their relational involvement gradually becomes visible. When

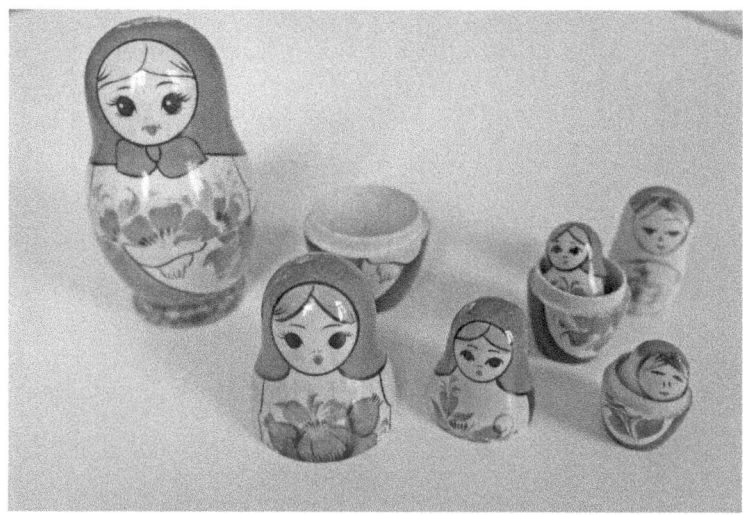

Figure 5.6 Russian dolls with opened Russian doll. Photograph by the author.

*the smallest doll appears and we are reflecting on the 'knocking at her door',
Katinka says, 'I think she doesn't want to lose me'.*

By describing in detail what a person does or says in a specific situation, we get
a richly developed picture of the person. By unravelling their relational involvement, some of their intentions or hopes, their beliefs or values and even some of
their goals can become visible and accessible to themselves. They can find new
actions, new ways to talk and reflect with each other.

*This small conversation with Katinka aided her to ask Justine if she really
cares about her. Justine had to give a number from one to ten for how much she
was convinced she wouldn't just disappear out of Katinka's life. Eight was given
which felt as a reassuring number to Katinka.*

Chapter 6

Injured relationships and 'broken homes'

As noted already in this book, adversities in families also evoke relational pain, suffering and relational traumas. These radical events break apart the 'usual, daily and obvious', and pierce social and cultural conventions about families and family relationships, beliefs, expectations and dreams. Intimate or attachment relationships, structural positions and roles come under pressure, their bounds are sometimes broken or wounded. In this chapter we will focus on seeking new ways of relating or finding a 'home'. We will address more directly the issue of injured relationships, including tendencies of things to become worse due to paralysing feelings of shame and the sometimes emerging tendency towards revenge.

Mauro's mum is in a secure unit in a hospital. She can no longer fulfil her motherly duties, even an 'ordinary' parent-child conversation isn't possible. His father is in prison, is described as 'a criminal' and 'the one who caused all the troubles'. Mauro constantly gets the message his father is a 'bad' person. He is often warned not to become just like his dad. As he lives with his grandparents in foster care, his grandparents can no longer just be 'grandparents' but have to be educators, parents and attachment figures. In relation to their own adult daughter they have to re-position themselves and find a liveable stance.

Ambivalence and complexity

When children's intimate relationships are wounded, they often struggle with a number of ambivalences, confusions and dilemmas. From the perspective of the child a mixture of feelings can become present in relation to parents, siblings, grandparents, offending and non-offending family members, etc. Although children often get caught up in the complexities of these relationships, many of them aren't eager to talk about them. Conversations about their mum, dad, important family members, offending as well as non-offending, can appear to be a no-go area. Many factors influence the way these children try to deal with injured relationships. There is shame, hesitation, not being able to make sense of things, the wish to avoid further disappointment, the wish not to cause others discomfort let alone harm them, the lacking of words or remaining stuck in solidified negative conclusions, all of which can contribute to the experience of not knowing how to

DOI: 10.4324/9781003167860-7

go on. Bird (2004) makes a call to expect and accept ambivalence and explore clients' experience of 'moving between multiple positions'.

Missing 'a mum' but even more 'his old mum' as he calls it and listening to the stories of his friends going home and being cuddled by their mums feels hard to Mauro. At the same time he doesn't know how to behave when visiting his mum in hospital. This mum feels so strange and different from the mum he loved although he feels guilty about refusing to visit her. Sometimes he is so angry with her because of the drugs she took. When he notices in every fibre of his grand-parents' body the anger towards his father and the sadness and pity towards his mother, he becomes silent and wishes to disappear. He does not understand himself, because he often longs for her and explodes inside when someone asks a question about his mum.

Missing his father is also painful because he remembers the many jokes and playful moments they had together. He does not dare to express or share this lack and desire to see his father. He is not even sure if he is allowed to have these feelings and thoughts. Does this also make him a bad person? Should he reject his father and be angry for what he did to his mother, just like his grandfather? Or does the fact that he dreams about his father prove that he is becoming just the same person as his father?

Even more, Mauro isn't just interwoven with his parents or attached to one emotional bond: he misses most of all his older brother, Rico, as he could always count on him when there were troubles at home. His grandparents are afraid that Rico will have a bad influence on him when they have contact. As long as Rico doesn't apologise and shows he can behave properly, he is no longer welcome. Moreover, Mauro thinks that he should be grateful that his grandparents want to take care of him and that he should punish himself whenever he does stupid things and disappoints them.

There is not one simple categorisation that fits the multifaceted identities, roles and tasks that does justice to parents or family members who were harmful. The meaningful family member is not to be known from one fossilised context. Yet children and young people, and also the people around them, sometimes adopt a radical position in relation to their parents or family members, often in the hope of reducing this complexity. In the stories they tell others, some praise their parents as if they were some kind of God, while others reject them as if they were the devil, but many others also remain silent as if they do not care and their parents do not concern them. Not talking about them seems to help them get on with their lives and keep the all too confusing complexity at a manageable distance.

Children and youngsters can get stuck in the complex amalgam of different and often contradictory circling ideas and stories about their parents. These can reach them in a direct or an indirect way. They originate from all kinds of people involved, with different positions and different interests. Sometimes they come from anonymous communities, i.e., from what 'they', for example in the neighbourhood, consider to be decent behaviour, or good parenting. When they measure their parents against dominant social representations and discourses on parenthood, they are quickly labelled 'deviant, abnormal or wrong'. This also raises the question: 'What does this say about me?' bearing in mind the expression 'the apple doesn't fall far from the tree'.

The multi-stress contexts in which their parents or family members lived and often still live and the effects on their lives mean that some parents remain unavailable. Some are in prison, others stay in a psychiatric ward, still others simply seem to have disappeared from the face of the earth. Offending family members sometimes deny all the pain and suffering and decline any responsibility, while other parents or family members try in all kinds of ways to restore what went wrong or to make up where they believe they failed, often driven by all kinds of worries and feelings of guilt. This can all contribute to the children's confusion.

Confused feelings and radical choices regarding family members are easily evoked by circumstances that are not always immediately clear to outsiders. So we need to maintain a broad take that accounts for multiple contexts. It can be helpful if children experience a degree of commonality, i.e., feel that certain aspects of what they are going through are known to others, that the way they suffer from certain experiences is common to other children and families who have dealt with traumatic experiences, abuse or violence (Sheinberg & Fraenkel, 2001).

Similar responses or circumstances should not mislead us: how children as well as family members or carers make sense of what happens to them is always idiosyncratic, and demands a continuous stance of respectful curiosity. Just like keeping in mind that each new event, each new developmental stage or new context that comes to the foreground can bring shifts in meaning and ways of relating.

Some preliminary thoughts on violence

Before we proceed, I would like to consider briefly our being confronted with violence, abuse or neglect. Addressing injured relationships can be quite challenging for everyone involved. As far as I'm concerned, as a systemic and narrative worker, I feel the need for a vision that allows for accountability as well as contextualisation. On such a view, on the one hand, an offending family member can be seen as the one who has acted, who has crossed physical, legal and ethical thresholds, and as such must be held accountable. Sheinberg and Fraenkel (2001) for instance take the stance that the offending family member must always take 100 per cent responsibility for the abuse. This links with a feminist perspective that whatever understanding we might construct of family dynamics or the impact of social-cultural-gender discourses that facilitated abuse, including systemic circular explanations of interactional patterns to which more than one family member contributes and for which more than one member holds responsibility, acts of violence, intimidation and abuse must be understood from 'a linear perspective in which one person enacts power over others and hold complete responsibility for these actions' (Goldner, 1998). On the other hand, there are always experiences or contexts that make it partly understandable (not acceptable) that someone has acted in that way. Holding on to this 'double vision' helps me, as a therapist, to respond to stories of abusive and violent actions, for instance by bringing both perspectives into conversation when possible and appropriate while taking a clear, moral position that violence, abuse and inequality are intolerable in any form.

In fact, all those involved, professionals and non-professionals alike, can always find themselves balancing somewhere in between the two viewpoints. Different people involved may find themselves in different positions at the same time. Children have to deal with the fact that sometimes they have a milder view of their father or family member and will find people who agree with their point of view. At other times they may be shocked to learn that their 'father is a psychopath', or that 'their mother should have taken care of them, instead of just doing what she liked'. We are interested in the dilemmas and contradictions for parents and children as they address the difficult questions to which parents who were offending can be held accountable. The relationship between blame and responsibility is also influenced by the position taken by others, which in turns affects the narratives available to children (Daniel & Wren, 2005).

Opening conversations about troubled relationships

Charlotte (13) and her mum come for conversations about the painful experiences in the past and the endless quarrels that got nestled into their relationship. Domestic violence went on for years in the family. Four years ago Charlotte's father left the house and formed a new family. There is no contact although they heard lately a half-sister has been born. One of the stories circulating in the family is that her father married her mother in order to obtain a residence permit as he comes from Ghana. Six months ago, Charlotte disclosed sexual abuse by her older brother (16). He was sent by juvenile court to an institution for delinquent young people. Her mum tries to visit him each weekend. Charlotte accompanied her mum once at her mum's request. Both of them didn't say a word, not even looked at each other. Charlotte went to a psychotherapist shortly after the disclosure but after a few sessions she refused to go on.

Often the ongoing confusion, dilemmas and misunderstandings in the context of family relations form obstacles in the lives of these children. We learned that it is therapeutically important to put these complexities on the table. We invite children and family members to collaboratively explore the multiple meanings in significantly different ways from how they usually address them. Sheinberg and Fraenkel (2001) highlight that change in relational struggles can begin at the level of meaning, providing direction for change at the level of action. Likewise, change sometimes needs to proceed at the level of action before meanings can shift: families may need to try something new, adopting an attitude of experimentation and creativity in the face of the unknown and see how this affects their feelings and beliefs.

Charlotte, her mum and I already had two conversations in which we explored their concerns together, while creating a safe base and engaging a team of support and solidarity. They agreed to talk together, and as such to engage in new forms of action, because they both wanted things to improve between them. The moment they came in, mother started to cry. 'I am desperate. I have no idea how this is ever going to work out'. Last week, she and Charlotte had a huge row, hurling the most terrible things at each other. At the end of her story, mother says: 'I've lost everything'. Charlotte immediately bites back and yells: 'And me, do you have any idea what I lost? ... Do you want me to disappear? Maybe it is better to kill myself! Would that be helpful?'

Ending up in this quarrel or getting embroiled myself is not an option. So I ask them if we can stop for a while explaining that I don't want them to repeat and relive all the painful reproaches. Then I ask if we can agree on the idea that it is much easier to lose each other than to find and support each other? In doing so, I want to contextualise and make a statement that they, due to all these complexities, are in turbulent waters and get entangled in all kinds of patterns that lead nowhere. Sometimes I bring in my experience with families in similar circumstances, and tell that I have often seen families struggling in crazy ways to stay afloat when the water was lapping at their feet. These families need a therapist or a team of support that can position themselves in these storms. Someone who isn't going to run away, become desperate or gets overwhelmed themselves but instead offers maps to navigate through these relational storms.

So I invite them to talk in a different way, to listen and to think about what is bothering them relationally. We make room for what they miss(ed) from one another, even maybe how they feel abandoned by each other and what they blame each other for. But also for what they still hope and wish for in relation to one another, or the often invisible or unnoticed efforts made by each one of them. As such we hope to be able to step into new, more helpful ways of sharing, understanding and relating.

Family constellations on the table

Personal, relational and family identity conclusions are a complex fabric made up of many 'strands' of meaning. We need to explore collaboratively how children and family members made sense of the different painful experiences, how this also infected their relational experiences and relational meaning-making process. The shifting of beliefs often create problems and restrict possibilities (Sheinberg, 2001). When the child's relational pain or fear is barely noticed or expressed, I often first invite them to share their experiences.

As Charlotte yelled 'Don't you know what I have lost', I take a box with blocks and wooden family figures out of the cabinet. I ask Charlotte if she could pick for each family member a wooden puppet or maybe, if she prefers, a block. Can she put them on the table in a way that feels appropriate to her and show how she feels they are relationally (dis)connected? I ask her mother to listen carefully and try to grasp what touches her, what surprises her or what is new in what she hears or sees.

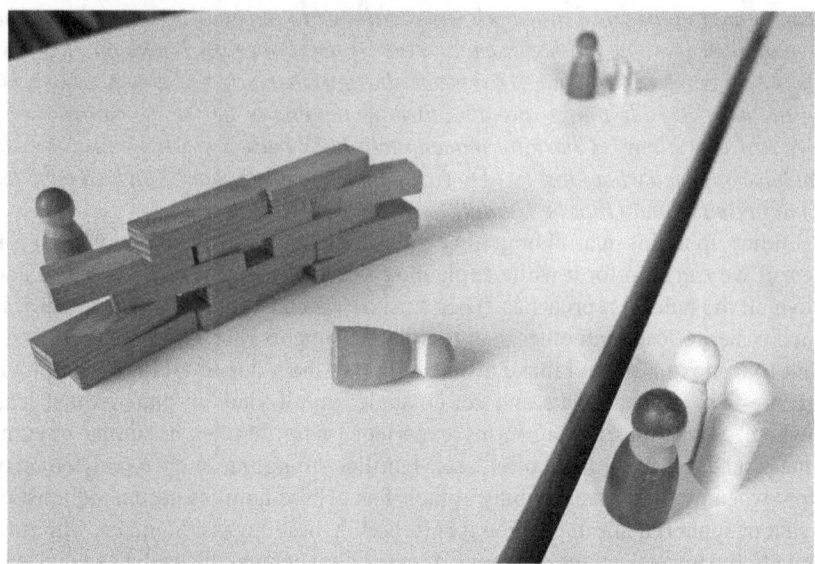

Figure 6.1 Wooden puppets with wooden wall and green puppet laying down. Photograph
    by the author.

*Charlotte takes a figure for each of them. She puts her father (the darkest
brown figure), together with his new family at the end of the table. He has his
back turned to them. Her brother gets situated at the other end of the table and
she asks if she can put a wall in front of him. Hesitantly she puts down the figure
of her mother, also with her back turned to her own figure, faced towards the one
representing her brother. While doing so, it seems as if she doesn't dare to look
at her mother. Her maternal grandparents' figures she places just behind herself.*

By making visible this family constellation from Charlotte's perspective, I
hope she gets the opportunity to express and share some of her relational struggles. As I (and her mother) don't know what these different ways of positioning
particularly mean to her, I ask questions to help her articulate, name and explore
what is on the table. This visualisation or kind of sculpting opens opportunities for
a more participatory meaning-making process. At the same time, I hope that this
will prevent her mother from getting stuck in single, often negative and unverified
interpretations.

S: *Charlotte, can I ask you something? Did I notice correctly that you were hesi-
    tating before you laid the puppet of your mother down? How do we have to
    understand this?*
C *(before speaking she takes a deep breath): Since my father left, mum was
    depressed but after I told what Brian (her brother) did she hardly gets out
    of bed during the week. She constantly asks if I am all right or if things are*

already better. I don't know why she asks this as she is all the time trying to arrange things for Brian. Lately she even asked if it is okay that she is visiting Brian. I think she is angry at me because of what happened. I stand in the way.

...

I ask Charlotte to add to the constellation on the table the obstacles and problems, from her point of view, that brought them to this point.

She chooses a small monster for the fights between her dad and mum and a big one for 'the things that Brian did' because she fears this will tear the family apart completely. Even her grandparents and auntie Babs are angry with her mother and Brian. Lately she heard grandma yelling on the phone at mum. On the one hand Charlotte is glad that her grandparents support her but on the other hand it is really confusing to be with grandma and her mum together in one room. She has no idea how to behave. It reminds her of the fights between her mum and dad.

After some more clarifications, I ask mother if she also has questions about what Charlotte has put on the table (before I further inquire about what struck her and what resonates). In doing so, I engage mother in our explorations. I hope she has already got an idea of what kind of curious questioning I am proposing. It is certainly not about 'finding the truth'. We hope to develop a 'both-and' thinking about the different family members and relationships instead of one single description or 'truth'. In this way we hope it becomes possible to hold the tension of these, often contradictory, mixed feelings so that one does not have to deny one set of feelings (Sheinberg & True, 2008; Sheinberg, 2014).

Mum: Why did you build a wall in front of Brian with some holes in it?
C: Because I hope he doesn't disappear from our lives, just like dad did. I am really angry at him but I didn't want him to be locked up. I think he will be missing us but I have no idea if I can still be together with him. When there were the fights between you and dad, he was always there to comfort me. He helped to keep the monster small and now he became a kind of monster himself. I don't know what to think.

By allowing the mother to respond in an engaged and relationally involved way, the events and relational complexities are given a right to exist in their relational and social world. It may be the first step towards some recognition of the relational pain Charlotte experiences and expresses.

Mum says how she was moved by Charlotte who laid her puppet down with her back towards Charlotte and looking in the direction of Brian. Instead of being turned away from Charlotte she would love to be present for Charlotte for the full 100 per cent. Her constant questioning of Charlotte is her way of checking and trying to stay connected. Mum recognises the constant struggle about Brian and what to do. She tries to explain she is struggling with how she can stay a mum for both of them. From her side the thing she least wants is that Charlotte would think that she is angry with her. She had already wished a thousand times she could turn back the clock. Sometimes she just wants to shake Brian and yell 'Why? How could you do this?'.

By adding mother's perspective a multi-perspectival view is developed. They are both on this journey, not having had the same experiences, not having been affected in the same way, not positioned in the same way, etc. but together now in the activity of sharing and exploring. In doing so they investigate how they can be supportive and meaningful towards each other again so that a sense of mattering and relational agency can be restored.

Going back to Charlotte, I ask her if she has a notion about how she would like her mum to be positioned and connected with her? Can she guide us in the family constellation on the table?

Charlotte picks up the wooden figure that represents mum and puts it upright. She places her into a kind of triangle where she can see both Brian and Charlotte. She takes another figure out of the box. Smiling, she says: 'I'm going to de-double Mum'. She makes one of the mum-figures look at Brian and the other at her and puts them back-to-back. She brings her own figure very close to the mum figure that looks in her direction and adds: 'I wish we could be together again like long ago'.

While repositioning the figures as a kind of 'embodied enactment', the child or youngster can try out some 'options', taste how things possibly feel or could be. At the same time some intentions, hopes and wishes become visible. We can also notice this repositioning as an invitation to mum or other family members.

Together we try to figure out what 'de-doubling' mum could look like in daily life and what intentions go along with this. She doesn't want her mum to choose

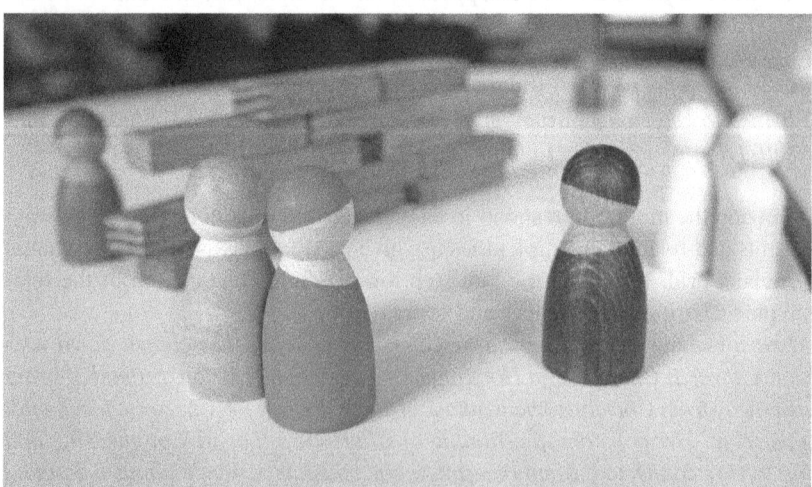

Figure 6.2 Three wooden figures green, red, blue in front. Photograph by the author.

between her and her brother. She just wants her to put no pressure on her in relation to Brian. She wants to feel her mum believes in her. It would make a difference when she is nearby in doing, not talking. This makes us reflect on how their relationship and emotional bond used to be. As it seems difficult to grasp I ask Charlotte if she can do this family constellation again, but then with a view to a time before all the problems were present in the family.

When children, youngsters and families can't recall answers in the here and now, it can be helpful to explore moments, areas or times not yet affected by the painful experiences.

Charlotte goes back to the time when she was six. She decides to put her father, mother, her brother and herself close to each other. They are in a circle looking at each other. She remembers mostly the holidays and weekends together at the seaside camping. It felt as if they were 'on the same side', everyone was playing with one another. She adds also her maternal grandparents because they came a lot to visit and each Sunday afternoon there was freshly baked cake or cookies. I ask what kind of valuable stories she remembers in relation to her mum, dad and brother.

...

Watching the two family constellations on the table, I ask Charlotte what got lost or what she is missing most in relation to her mum that could already make a small difference in the here and now?

C: *Baking cookies together would not work now. I think we would kill each other in the kitchen, but do you remember the lullaby you used to sing? You used to come and sit on my bed at night ... Now and then just sitting next to me would be nice.*

M: *I can sit next to you on the sofa while you watch your favourite series? ... And am I allowed to bake some cookies alone for you?*

As we walk around in their relational lives, little by little they get reconnected. They start to notice that they can still be meaningful to each other. Small inspirations for actions appear. Also mother can discover some ways of again being supportive to Charlotte and how to 'do mother' again.

Although some alternative relational pathways and stories are opened, it is an illusion to believe that all relational struggles can be explored and unravelled at once, or once and for all. While they are speaking and talking about relational dilemmas or relational pain they can hurt each other again. In order to avoid such ongoing painful exchanges, they often try to spare each other and keep silent (see also Chapter 3). Reassuring them that not everything has to be told or shared with each other can be a relief. It can also be helpful to invite a parent/family member for an individual conversation to make room for their specific relational disadvantages, pain or sorrow. So we can avoid competing hierarchies of pain and create space to acknowledge everyone's pain, while keeping in mind that everyone's context is very different.

Since mum continues to struggle with the question of how to be a mother to both her children and it is currently too complicated and painful to talk about Brian together, we all agree that I will have some conversations with mum alone (see Chapter 7). Charlotte also wants some individual conversations to talk about the painful experiences and to think about Brian and what happened.

Which acts and utterances will be seen as relationally supportive and what kind of relational narratives will develop further between Charlotte and her mum, is not exclusively negotiated between the two of them. This happens in ongoing dialogues with many other people and communities involved.

A few weeks later Charlotte comes in confused and sad. Grandma furiously told Charlotte that her mum has to choose radically for her instead of 'secretly' visiting Brian each weekend.

At different points in the process, children can become upset in the many interpersonal and social perspectives that surround them. Their positioning or the way of relating that was temporarily found can come into question again when confronted with statements about the events, or certain explanations and especially the viewpoints of their parents and important family members. Statements by important people can also bring them into all kinds of conflicts of loyalty, making them unsure how to carry on.

Articulating the unarticulated

When intimate relationships are injured, questions about what parents and other family members mean to the child may haunt their minds. Children often desperately search for a sign that they matter to their parents or other significant family members. In what follows we try to create momentum so questions that haunt children in silence can become articulated, and presented to the person. Doing this opens the way to unravelling associated and never questioned convictions.

Charlotte keeps on worrying that her mum somehow blames her for the situation they are in. The conviction 'it would be a relief to my mum if I just disappeared' keeps popping up. Each time again she loses sight of what she may mean to her mother.

We first collect the questions on the child's mind and then invite the family member to respond to the questions by way of an interview. When asked aloud in this interview setting, children often get more nuanced and multi-layered answers to their questions than they would have expected. By first collecting the questions individually with the child, they can taste in this safe context how these questions sound when asked aloud, some thoughts and feelings linked to the questions can be clarified and we can wonder together how their parent or family member will respond.

The first question Charlotte has for her mother is: 'Did you want me to be born? Or would it have been better if I was never born?'

When I ask her how long this question has been bothering her, she answers resolutely: 'Since my father left. My mum yelled once that he just made some kids with her, had his pleasure and then left her with the shit'.

Other questions follow:

- *Do you blame me for what happened?*
- *Did the depression come because of what dad did or because we were too difficult to handle?*
- *Do you believe that it is all hopeless? Do you think it will be all right?*

Suddenly she says there is one final question she really doesn't dare to ask because she fears it will make her mother furious. 'Do you think contact with my father will ever be possible? Would you ever allow it?'

We agree that we keep this question until the end of the interview at which point she can decide whether the question should be asked or not.

After collecting the questions we negotiate who will do the interview, and how these questions will be asked. Some younger children like the puppets to ask the questions as they can 'hide' behind them (see Chapter 4). Some prefer that I ask the questions and they just listen from a 'safe' place. As the prepared questions are often of great importance to the child, almost of existential value, such an interview has to be well prepared and can evoke some stress or feelings of insecurity. Just as we can't predict the responses of the parent or family member, we have to take into account that these responses can be hard to hear and can initiate unhelpful dances. In choosing how we are going to set up this interview we need to talk about the child's ways of responding to stressful, fearful situations and what could be helpful when 'stress levels' are becoming too 'high'. How will I be able to notice this? Will they signal it? Will they leave the room for a while? Do they want me to stop the interview? This listening from a safe distance can be done by letting them take a 'distanced' position as for instance behind the camera, or allowing them not to be present, or by letting them sit in a chair at a certain distance and so on.

Only if all this is settled can we invite the parent or relative. We explain the set-up, the importance of the questions for the child but even more the importance of serious, honest and respectful responses. My experience is that parents or family members quickly grasp the importance, at the same time become very curious, nervous and often feel excited. They hope to make a meaningful contribution, to make a relational difference, that makes a difference. It is also good to take into account that this method is used in the context where there have already been quite some therapeutic steps taken. Child and parent need to be on speaking terms and there still has to be some degree of mutual commitment, even when it is no longer noticed by everyone involved.

In search for sparkling lights

Charlotte and her mum come in for the interview. Charlotte has chosen to film this interview and she positions herself safely behind the camera. First of all I thank mother for coming and for her willingness to be interviewed.

Charlotte's mum is completely surprised by the question 'Did you want me to be born?' She says with conviction that she would not have wanted to miss Charlotte for the world in her life. When Charlotte was born, difficulties were already simmering between her and her father. She was especially worried about how she was going to cope. She didn't want to talk about it with anyone because the family had already said so many times that father was a wrong choice. It is true that she was not planned and yes, she had been angry for a while when she found out she was pregnant but this did not mean that she was not welcome. Her concerns were mainly about whether this was a good place for Charlotte to grow up.

I ask her if she can tell a bit more about the first months after Charlotte was born and if she remembers some 'sparkling' moments (Freedman & Combs, 1996).

The interview setting, including the preparation, generates a conversational context, in which existential misunderstandings can become noticed and unravelled. Acts that got a solidified meaning, leading to negative conclusions about the other's identity and intentions, can be revisited, can become re-contextualised. In my experience this often has very connecting effects on the participants.

After unfolding many different aspects of stories, I check with Charlotte whether I may ask the final question about her father. From behind the camera, she nods. 'Do you think contact with my father will ever be possible? Would you ever allow it?' Mum starts to cry. After a while she says that it would be okay if she was sure that it was helpful for Charlotte and that her father would not hurt her. Unfortunately, she doesn't have this peace of mind. I ask if she was okay with Charlotte having and asking this question. Mother replies: 'Yes, of course, I can understand she has this longing and that this is difficult for her, even though I would like nothing more than to never have to think about him again'.

After the interview I sometimes ask the child, when it is present, to join the conversation and to share with us some of their reflections. Within a safe and structured framework, the child could listen to the responses. Charlotte saw and heard that her mum still cares, and that she matters to her mother. She also discovered that mum can understand some of the things that are on her mind. Her struggles and questions were given a right to exist. Although this interview offers an *indirect* way of conversation between them, it definitely has very direct effects and often brings change at the level of meaning and relations. Again, these are not absolute, perpetual shifts as the outside world and important others co-speak, but changes that bring hope and make new relational narratives possible.

Relatives off stage

In contexts of injured relationships, parents and family members sometimes disappear, cannot be reached, stay in prison or in a hospital or have died. Sometimes they started a new life, founded a new family and broke off all contact with the child. Contact can also be prohibited by the juvenile court, social services or other family members.

- *Mauro misses his brother who has been placed in a children's home and keeps silent about this loss because he does not want to cause any trouble to his grandparents. There is also much hesitation about whether or not to visit his father in prison.*
- *Xander was not allowed to visit his mother during the first months she was in hospital. His mother had to be 'stable' first.*
- *For Charlotte, it is unclear whether her father himself decided not to see her or whether it is rather because her mother has forbidden him to do so, or possibly even because his new wife does not want him to do so …*

When children and youngsters have to deal with these issues it is important not to collude with the ideas that these children are at the mercy of the parent or the decisions taken by other family members, social services, etc. Feeling sorry for them, just explaining to them what makes it difficult for their parents to connect or why decisions were made, puts them in a situation to be pitied. We prefer to think and talk in bidirectional ways about these relationships, and prefer to address the children as active participants and full agents in these relationships to help them to experience a sense of relational agency.

As many parents in contexts of trauma feel judged, blamed or struggle with ongoing feelings of inadequacy and mental distress, it can be hard for them to be reflective about how to contribute to the life of the child that no longer lives with them (Richardson et al., 2016). Instead of 'waiting' until the parent or family member takes action or contacts the child, we can initiate conversations with the child (and their carers) about what they would like to share with their parents or significant family members and what kind of 'connection' might still be possible.

We can reflect on what important events, milestones, significant steps, but also small stories they would like to document and keep track of until they can be shared in some way. Can they imagine what their father or mother, their siblings would like to know about them or their life? Engaging carers in all kinds of ways of collective actions of connection with a parent or sibling can be very valuable. In order to develop a greater sense of agency and even a more constructive and coherent sense of identity, it is important to enable and highlight meaningful relational actions towards other significant persons in the child and carers' network (Vermeire, 2020).

Mauro decorates with grandma a beautiful 'mum box'. Together they fill it with photos, school reports, presents for Mother's Day, a baby tooth, a few shells from a trip to the sea and fragments of our letters I have written after each conversation. Whenever he visits his mother, the box accompanies him. The ingredients give him something to hold on to and keep his mother present in his daily actions. At the same time, he has something to tell and to offer during the visits. While he and his mum take a closer look at the content of the box, they have a pleasant

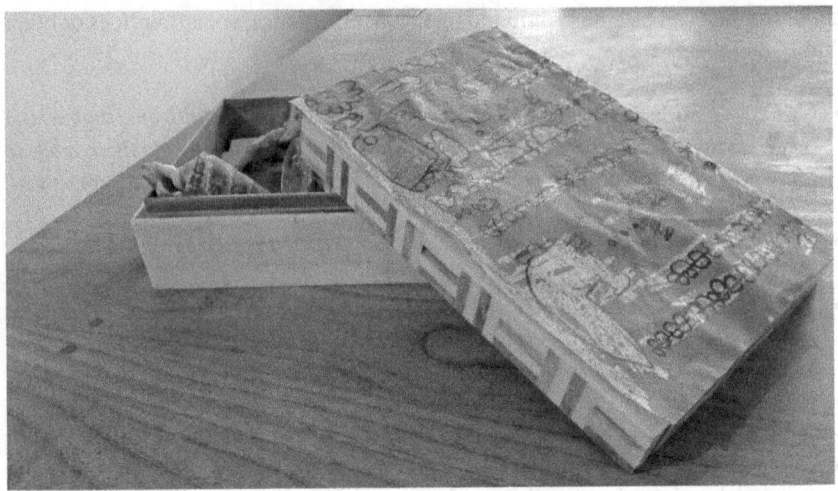

Figure 6.3 Open box with drawing on the cover. Photograph by the author.

moment and he can experience that he is somehow making a small contribution to his mother's life. Keeping the mum box up-to-date also creates nice shared moments between grandmother and Mauro. It gives grandmother the opportunity to tell stories about his mother. In a manageable, delimited way his mum can 'inhabit' his world.

Besides documenting and sharing events and special moments, we can also ask if they want their parent to know about their worries, struggles and mixed feelings.

As his dad is in prison Mauro says he doesn't want to upset grandfather with his questions and stupid feelings. He knows grandfather is angry with his dad but Mauro can't help it, he is still longing for him. Grandfather and Mauro choose a small box out of my collection to put Mauro's mixed feelings in. Different col-oured beads represent the anger, sadness, missing and even for the funny jokes that father made he chooses a bead. When we explore what has to be done with the box, he prefers to keep it in the drawer of his bedside table. 'I don't want to bother my father with these things'. But when grandfather notices how much 'The Missing Bead' hurts Mauro and suggests to write a letter together to the prison social worker, Mauro immediately agrees. Next time, he proudly reads the letter to me before sending it to the prison. The letter also includes the scores of the last football matches.

We engage the adults (professionals and non-professionals) from a position of responsive, collaborative participants. This allows them to notice the relational struggles and to be supportive to the child in finding ways to relate and matter to their parents or significant family members. When things go well, they become a team of solidarity and networks of resilience are woven. We often do not know in advance how these parents or involved family members will react, but even when they do not respond, these children can look back on their actions with some pride. They did not let the whole situation put them off, but they took steps in the hope of making a difference. Often I am surprised by the inventive ways children find to connect with their parents, siblings, etc. and to try to make valuable contributions.

Suddenly, in a meeting with grandparents and Mauro, he confesses he is connected with Rico, his brother, by Facebook, ☺. Grandparents are completely surprised. Together with his two schoolfriends (the ones he wrote the letter to), he made a 'secret' Facebook account, became friends with Rico and now they chat sometimes by Messenger. Once recovered from the shock, grandparents become curious about what they are 'chatting' about. Surprisingly, besides the newest Playstation games, they seem to be reminiscing about when mum was still healthy. Mauro finally adds: 'Grandma, do you know that Rico would love to taste your apple pie? Can you prepare it for him once more, please?'

As Mauro demonstrated, children can not only be active participants in the steps explored and deployed in relation to their parents and important family members but they can even become 'directors' of these networks.

Attachment unlimited

When family relationships are injured, we can take all kinds of directions to allow for some acknowledgement of the pain and to re(dis)cover connections but often it is important to look outside these intimate family relationships to enhance processes of resilience. No child is an island. Children don't live in one, all-important and all-encompassing relationship. For too long there has been an almost exclusive focus on the importance of the mother-child relationship and by extension the parent or primary caregiver–child relationship for the development of attachment and emotional bonds. Byng-Hall (1995) enlarged our view as he claimed that just as a secure attachment between a mother and child enables the child comfortably to explore her or his environment, the notion of a secure family base provides a reliable network of attachment relationships in which all family members of whatever age are able to feel sufficiently secure to explore. In multi-stressed contexts it is important to extend this notion of a secure base to all kinds of relations that can offer emotional attachment and open doors to comforting and exploring. There is also a growing consensus that the damage done to a child as a result of broken relationships is not irreversible (Hoogsteder & de Vriese, 2012) and that a child can enter into multiple attachment relationships. In the meantime we also know that attachment relationships develop into adolescence or even into adulthood (Rutter, 1999; Rimé, 2009). So, especially in contexts of relational or developmental traumas, it is important not to narrow the gaze and to appreciate how generous children can be in attachment (van der Pas, 2004).

In the years I worked with these children, their families and networks, I have become more and more fascinated by their creative and original ways of doing attachment in relations. Traditionally, theorists and researchers have assumed that because this process is innate and evolved, only humans are capable of meeting a person's needs for security. Recent research challenges this assumption by demonstrating that an array of targets, such as places and pets, can also satisfy needs for security, particularly under conditions of threatened or absent connection to other people (Keefer et al., 2014).

Acknowledging the 'safe and comforting relationships' developed with animals, cuddly bears, special objects, a favourite singer, songwriter or football player, a god, a fairy-tale character and so on can open interesting conversations about local knowledges and skills, about relationships, the building of emotional bonds and what is valued in these relationships. As we are widening the scope of attachment, we can discover together what these relationships mean to them. We can not only focus on how they find comfort or a peace of mind with these special attachment figures or places, we can also ask how they care(d) or contribute(d) in reality or in imagination to the 'life' of that person, animal, object or figure.

- Yana (see Introduction) was attached to her cuddly bear 'Little Orange' and she seemed to grow, literally, when we discovered how they already took care of each other for years.
- The Minecraft house that Mauro built together with a friend, is a 'safe place' offering peace of mind during confusing times. Just like the secret place at the end of the camping site kept hope alive for Xander. Acknowledging and exploring the knowledge on how to construct such places and what their important ingredients are proved very helpful.
- The nightly conversations Emma had with Wendy (and the lost boys in Peter Pan) meant she had someone to share her worries with. Wendy was an inspiration to go on when Emma was sad and was overwhelmed by emotions.

While diving into these relationships, we also try to enlighten what their contribution was to these pets or figures. When children notice that they made a difference to them or their life, their sense of mattering enhances as well as their sense of relational agency.

As an illustration I add the letter to Laura, after a conversation with her therapist. On one very dominant account she was a victim of serious child neglect.

Dear Laura (16),

Last time we met you talked about Boy, the puppy that has been living with you for a few months. There was a big smile on your face as you talked about him ☺. You explained to me how special Boy is. He gives you a warm feeling and makes you happy. Playing with Boy is always an experience! He wags his tail enthusiastically and runs in circles of joy. I immediately understood that you are a dog lover and I got the feeling that you can sense what dogs need.

You told me that you actually like all animals. This aroused my interest, because I do not know much about animals myself. Maybe you could teach me something.

When you used to live with your parents, you had many pets: dogs, cats, birds, a mouse, ducks, a pony and even spiders. You had a good relationship with almost all of these animals. They came to cuddle with you, the dog slept in your bed, and you even taught the birds and ducks to enjoy being stroked by you. The bird Frodo put her head on your shoulder to be cuddled. I was amazed! I asked how it was that these animals came to you. You told me that they felt safe with you. I became curious about how you can make them feel safe!

Fascinated by the bird Frodo, I asked what you think you meant to her. You were a second mother to her. You always took care of her when she needed something. Unfortunately, you haven't seen Frodo for a long time now, because she still lives with your parents.

...

(Thanks to Laura and Sophie Geerinckx, her psychotherapist, for sharing this letter.)

In addition to looking at non-human figures of attachment, we need to be alert to people involved, who are often not immediately in the foreground, but who are still figures of support, even if they do not always do so intentionally. We have to open our therapeutic conversation and invite them 'in the flesh' or in imagination. As the children we are talking about here often experience insecurity in their intimate relationships or have to deal with unpredictability, it is important that they can experience a sense of security, comforting and mattering in other relationships. We have to look for relationships that are not yet contaminated by all kinds of complexities. People who are not at all aware of what is going on in their lives or not directly connected with family members can be part of a supportive network, intentionally but also often unintentionally.

The lady of the camping shop was of great importance to Xander. When he stepped out of the school bus, he always hoped she was on the lookout and waved at him warmly. Not knowing what to expect once in the caravan of his parents, the awareness of her presence made a big difference in bearing the burden. Making visible what she meant to him, and what he probably meant to her, made him literally grow in the conversation.

Because the football coach discreetly winked at him at difficult moments, or sometimes put an arm around his shoulder when he scored a goal, Mauro felt like he was receiving a lot of special support, and also as if he was really part of the team.

His dance and rap mates appreciate the efforts and progress Xander makes. He is often asked to correct or 'uplift' the songs they wrote themselves or perform in the YouTube movies they create.

MacLeod (1997) says: the generosity of a neighbour can make them feel reconnected with the idea of 'hope in humanity'. It is important to make these, often unnoticed, social networks visible and to strengthen them by enhancing a sense of mutually mattering. In doing so we weave networks of resilience in ever-widening circles.

Revisiting shame and revenge

Feelings of shame aren't far away when family relationships are injured. Children and youngsters can feel the many judgemental and shaming eyes piercing their backs. They try to 'hide' the situations they are living in, avoid talking about the deviant relationships and sometimes try to 'disappear' themselves. Fear that someone will find out about their family and family member and thus about 'themselves' can have a grip on them. Just like lying or telling grand imaginary stories about their so-called family may be attempts to stand their ground and counteract the shame.

Shame can pop up in all its 'glory' with its tentacles holding everything and everyone in its grip. The different relational experiences, their effects and impact become one large, absolute mass without any differentiation or nuance through time and situations.

Xanders' mum was found dead in an apartment a few days after he became 18 (for the beginning of my journey with Xander: see Chapter 1). A few months later, panic attacks rule his life. Taking public transport, going to school, being out in open spaces with a lot of people becomes a challenge. At the most unexpected moments he starts to shake and tremble, his breathing goes wild and his body screams out in fear. Such a panic attack can sometimes last for two hours. People around Xander have great difficulty calming him down. After such an attack, shame has full grip on him. For Xander this is really proof that he is a failure. And these thoughts make shame grow even bigger. He hasn't been for conversations for a few years but is now urgently knocking at the door.

Xander sits huddled and stammering, he tells me he is ashamed of the panic attacks, of himself, of who he is, of his parents, etc. The latter, being ashamed of his parents in turn makes him ashamed of being ashamed of his parents. 'Surely that's not normal'.

'... Shame is a vicious giant porcupine. The thorns give me all sorts of bad thoughts: "Soon you'll be exposed and everyone will see how worthless you are", "You shouldn't be here!" These thoughts make that I hardly go outside'.

A timeline of shame

When shame has acquired an absolute meaning it can be helpful to make differences and nuances visible in a multitude of contexts. Together we collect the pieces of the puzzle by which the arrival and presence of shame can be related to

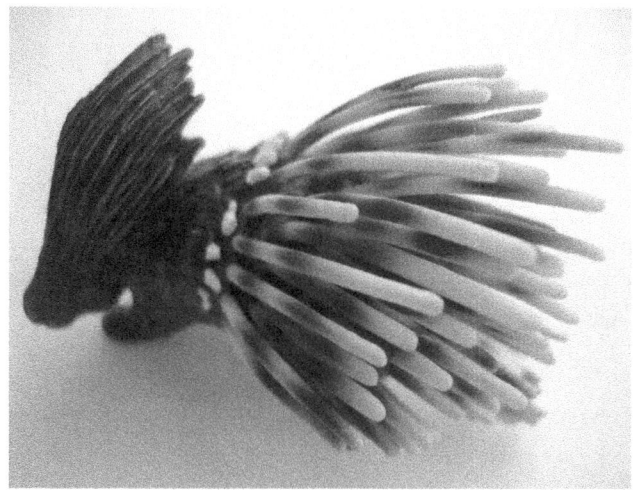

Figure 6.4 Plastic figure of porcupine. Photograph by the author.

different events in a person's life. The toxic side of shame often has long histori-
cal roots both in the personal life and in the family and cultural history of those it
visits (Weingarten, 2003).

*In Xander's life, some roots can be found in the memories of his childhood.
His parents who often were drunk on the bus or tram. His stepfather who used
to swear in the street. His mother who behaved strangely in front of his schoolfriends. At times like that, Xander wanted to be invisible, to disappear under the
seats of the bus. Shame swelled ... and still does. For example, when he is now
sitting on the bus and feels people looking at him, Xander has to get off the bus
as quickly as possible.*

By linking step by step these feelings and bodily responses through time with
more specific moments, the different influencing aspects, the many eyes watching
and voices speaking in these contexts and the social prescriptions about families and family members, these feelings get unravelled and understood in a much
larger, multi-layered landscape of contexts. Constructing a timeline of *Shame* can
widen our understandings.

*Shame popped up for the first time when Xander went to special education.
Little Venomous Shame was connected with his parents being drunk in public and
Toxic Shame was there when his mum was in hospital and finally The Scorpion
Shame came when his mum died.*

Relating them to several contexts of his life, the panic attacks and feelings of
shame get connected with worries and disadvantages. Once we have a broader view,
we do not only focus on the painful, pernicious or toxic aspects of shame. By double
listening (White, 2007) we can also look for intentions, relational involvements,
wishes or dreams. If one regards feelings of shame as relational, value-filled and

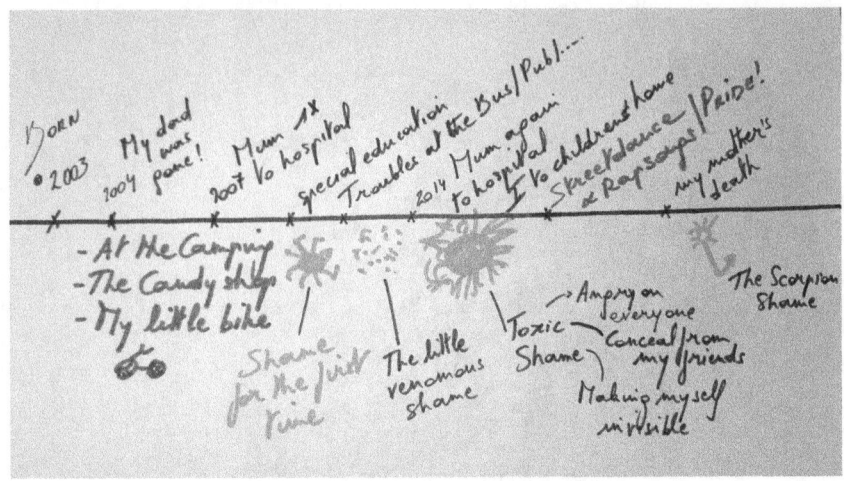

Figure 6.5 Timeline with orange symbols. Photograph by the author.

moral responses from the body to 'specific experiences and what is going on in the child's life', we can ask different questions, such as: what does this feeling of shame or the panic attacks say about what you value? What does this shame say about who or what you want to be? What is shame a testimony to? What or who is so dear to you? Weingarten (2003) states that people can transform the pain caused by feelings of shame into a 'reminder', a testimony to the values they cherish.

One can assume that shame is always in relation to someone or something. One can read 'feeling ashamed' as an expression of relational and social commitment. This brings other questions to the foreground: to which group of people dear to you does the feeling of shame, of being worthless, distance you? To which you have a sense of no longer belonging? And where do you want to belong? With whom do you hope to stay connected? These questions can be helpful because they make visible who is valued by the child and where they want to belong.

Finally, one can think about what social, cultural and political issues shame raises. What dominant social representations and discourses about families or family members make shame grow when they don't reach the standards? What social standards is someone wanting to achieve? What social problems and social expectations of our society interfere with this? This means we can understand shame in some situations as a disagreement with the state of affairs, as struggling or protesting against certain social, cultural or family practices. This means shame also has a political side.

Shame infiltrated Xander's life very early on. In primary school, he was sent to special education. They thought he was stupid because he did not speak Dutch well. He never dared to say this at secondary school. He also never mentioned that he lived in a children's home. He wanted eagerly to be 'normal', just to go home after school and invite friends over. He ended up talking to just a few classmates so children wouldn't ask him any awkward questions. He hoped that carers treated him 'normally' and that they would not try to fit him into the strait-jacket of their institution's rules. Xander thought it was completely unfair that he had to live like this. He didn't deserve this, and yet shame overwhelmed him again each time. He wanted so much to grow up in a normal family.

As an increasingly rich web of meaning unfolds around shame, and the child or family has an increasingly differentiated view of its effects, we can invite children or youngsters to (re)position themselves in relation to shame and the feelings of shame, the impact and the linked discourses. Do you still want shame to direct your life and actions? How big can the impact of shame still be? What place do you want to give shame in your life in the next period?

Xander would like shame to fit into his hands as the porcupine toy, so that he can put it in his pocket. The quills should not disappear completely. They should only be pinpricks. 'I don't want to be locked up in my little room. I just want to belong somewhere, have fun with my friends without constantly having to think about whether I'm worth it. I don't want to feel ashamed all the time. I keep the prickles as they can keep me going. I want to keep trying to fit in and not become a weirdo but at the same time just "be myself"'.

A sense of belonging as an antidote to shame

Children often try to cope with shame on their own, while sharing with others and engaging a support network can be an important and powerful antidote to shame when it becomes toxic. Polyphony can provide further enrichment and, at the same time, connectivity. Others can recognise and understand what someone experiences in their wrestling with shame, and the difficulties or painful histories that are related to it. People never have the same experience 100 per cent, and do not experience oppression or power in the same way but can meet and connect at crossroads (Reynolds, 2012). Once a 'team of support and solidarity' develops, it really can stop shame in its tracks.

In the presence of two witnesses, his social worker and a 'rap' friend, Xander talks about how his girlfriend's mother buys him clothes or gives him pots of food to take to his studio. He feels that she looks at him with eyes full of pity (cfr. What he earlier on called Harry Potter eyes). These are moments when shame swells up in him and he feels his family, his mother and also himself completely failed.

During this telling, Xander shares the toxic influences of shame with others. He is no longer alone.

I ask him if he had met people in recent years who addressed him as 'normal' and appreciated him. A teacher immediately flashed through his mind. This man knew the circumstances in which Xander lived and his life history, but not once did he ask about them or referred to them. On the contrary. He always came to talk about how his street dance was progressing and gave him advice on writing rap songs. I ask what this teacher would whisper in his ear the moment Shame walks in on him. Xander immediately replied: 'Listen to the beat of your favourite rap song' and 'Don't let yourself be pushed around, go your own way!' We decide to write these two sentences on a card and keep them in his wallet.

Kicking against the world

When relationships get injured, revenge requires special attention because it is often at the root of the escalation of non-helpful relational dances, while at the same time it is difficult to deal with therapeutically. The disadvantages and the relational pain, injustice or trauma children or youngsters experienced can take on huge proportions. Their feelings of anger or hate towards the offending people, the family members who abandoned them or society that didn't respond in an appropriate way can be so omnipresent that they become destructive themselves and break the conventions of society. Abusing drugs, fighting, running away, stealing, getting trapped in situations of sexual exploitation, etc. risk becoming dominant in their life. They seem to take a stance of 'Nothing or nobody can hurt me anymore!', 'I don't care about anything or anyone'. Or even 'From now on, they will know how it feels. It's my turn'. They seem to detach from people, places, even the world or get entangled in relationships, peer groups or communities that lead to negative, destructive chain reactions. Everyone seems to lose their grip on them, while the child is also losing their grip on themselves.

Naomi (16) expresses this very clearly by saying: 'Nothing more dangerous than someone who doesn't care any longer about anything. So you better watch out when I come in'.

In contexts of injured relationships it becomes very hard for the people involved who still care about them to connect, because each step they take towards the child might be rejected. Just like for carers and parents, also for counsellors and therapists it can be a daunting task to find points of entry to go on a journey and open conversations with them.

It becomes a real challenge to create a conversational context where parents, carers and their children or youngsters can talk and listen to each other without reproducing violence. Jenkins (2009) put the challenge in a question form: 'How can we invite these youngsters to enlarge their moral potential instead of becoming ourselves a moral knight?' Put slightly differently, we can ask: 'How can we acknowledge the difficulties and injustice they have been through without ignoring their destructive actions in the here and now?'

These youngsters often come in with an attitude of unapproachability while at the same time they can feel lost and powerless. Quickly the conversation can get bogged down in a me-against-them dynamic. The battle against the adult world that doesn't understand them becomes the focus. They claim others have a problem, not themselves.

Farida (16 years) is the youngest in a family with 11 children. Her parents come from Morocco, she was born in Belgium. Until she was 12 everything seemed okay. Since her transition to secondary school, she argues at home and refuses to help in the household. Regularly there are fights at school, with teachers and classmates. Her school results have reached rock bottom and drugs have taken a leading role in her life. Nobody seems to know where and with whom she is hanging out. Her parents feel powerless. Finally she runs away from home. In the meantime her father gets sick and is dying. Farida is placed in a youngsters' home but keeps on kicking against the world.

Often these young people can smell 'therapist's blood' from a distance. I definitely don't want to repeat what has been done so many times before, so I would like to hear different stories in the room and possibly new perspectives on her life and relationships. Moreover, I don't want the stories to be told to me, but rather to the people they concern. That is why I invite her to a meeting with her mother, sister and the social worker.

To first questions she shrugs her shoulders and is dismissive: 'I don't know', 'Why do you want to know this?', 'Mind your own business'. Suddenly she says rather provocatively: 'Nobody gets into me! I've built a solid fence around me'.

For as long as we don't know what is still somewhat worthwhile or important to them, it will remain difficult to talk about the violence. This means we have to make space to listen out for more silent or subjugated stories and make some of their still important values or connections as guidelines for life visible (Vermeire, 2017). In doing so we hope to invite the youngsters to reflect on which direction they still want to go in life instead of telling them what they have to do or how they have to behave.

I ask Farida what is so important about this solid fence around her. What is she trying to protect with this wall that is so precious to her?

F: Me, myself! I don't want people to know who I really am! They always judge you wrong. From the moment they know you are vulnerable, they will try to get you.
S: How would you like people to judge you?
F: For sure, not as stupid or weak.
S: How then?
F: As someone who can achieve something!

This exploration reconnects them to their values and beliefs under pressure (Jenkins, 2009). Questions such as: *'What ideas are being challenged that frustration is all around? Showing all this anger, what are you protesting? What are you refusing to accept that is important to you? What do you want to renounce or set right that has been done to you?'*, can open up other, new perspectives on their actions and let them be seen as young people who find certain things worthwhile or worth fighting for.

Disadvantages then and there

Curiously listening to their intentions and commitments creates a platform to stand on together looking for links that help to understand the difficult, sometimes destructive actions and emotions. We can start to look for and notice disadvantages then and there linked with local and social contexts.

I ask Farida what in her life made it necessary to build a fence around herself.

F: *I was bullied from the first until the fifth year in primary school. I let people walk over me. When pupils asked me to do something, I did it immediately, even the most stupid things. When I refused, they said that they would punch me in the face. I worried a lot and I could no longer study. At home there was no one to talk with. My parents were in a constant fight and I hide in my room.*

S: *What made them bully you?*

F: *It was a school with mostly white children. Most of them came from other neighbourhoods than mine.*

S: *Children you didn't know? Children you didn't felt connected with?*

F: *No, I didn't have friends.*

S: *Any idea why they picked on you?*

F: *At that time I was also very shy. I tried to stay in the background to avoid problems, but it brought even more problems. I didn't fit in their world.*

S: *Did you feel lonely at that time?*

F: *Yes!*

S: *Were there people around you who knew how bad it was?*

F: *No, I didn't talk about this at home. They already had enough worries. Once, I told it to a school counsellor, but they never did anything about it.*

S: *Then that fence appeared?*

F: *In the sixth year of primary school I made a click in my head: 'From now on I will show them who I am. I will decide who is going to get close to me and who isn't'. I put myself at the centre'. I wanted to show them that they couldn't fool around with me any longer.*

Listening to the stories that are prior to the 'problematic behaviour' does not have the intention of looking for an 'excuse' for the present destructive actions, neither is it to neglect the problems the youngster is causing by these actions. It offers the possibility of tuning in to the efforts the child has made to stay on their feet during episodes of relational and social pain. We can address their attempts to resist, the considerations and ethical choices they have made and what they have deemed important in all this (Wade, 1997; Reynolds, 2012).

What about 'revenge'?

Through sharing these stories the youngster is no longer just defined in one single story as 'bad', 'delinquent' or 'violent' and we create some solid ground beneath our feet to stand on and talk about the violence, terror or destructive actions. To begin with we don't try to find out what exactly happened, but together we search for a description of the violence that fits for the youngster, people involved and connects with their experiences without minimalising their actions.

Through an externalising dialogue we create a context in which the youngster can investigate the history of this violence or (self)destructive actions, the impact and effects and of course their relation to 'this violence'. This does not relinquish youngsters from the responsibility to address the problems they caused both intentionally and unintentionally. We hope a range of possibilities can become available to revise this relationship (White, 2007).

Farida talked about how, in school, she changed in a few months 'from being the one bullied to being the bully'. Her main motivation was 'revenge'. We decided to take a close look at 'the revenge'.

S: When did you first notice 'the revenge' nesting itself in your life?
F: When I decided to fight back. After a while I didn't care any longer who or what was harmed.
S: What did the revenge make you do?
F: I started to rant and rave at children, to yell at teachers, to threaten, ...

The revenge had a complete grip on Farida. The injustice that she experienced in primary school and home had to be put right. She started to use drugs and skipped class more and more. On the one hand she no longer dared to face her parents and on the other hand she blamed them for the trouble she was in. In the end she ran away from home.

Often it is a tangle of relational difficulties that youngsters are struggling with. Through mapping the violence, exploring what 'promoted' the revenge and how it infiltrates their relationships and lives, the youngster can start to re-evaluate their relationship with these destructive actions.

Farida explained that the revenge, the drugs and the running away made the relationship between her and her parents explode. She doesn't really understand it herself any longer. She acts wickedly towards the people she actually loves. The revenge has created a real mess. She says she still would like to set things right. At the same time she doesn't want to walk around so filled of rage. She doesn't want to be a burden to her parents any longer but doesn't know how to do it in a different way.

Youngsters always try to respond to radical or difficult experiences and in those responses we can hear what still matters to them. Listening to their efforts to measure up to certain dominant discourses and making them explicit, allows their moral viewpoints and relational choices to be visible (Jenkins, 2009). Together we can find out how they can enlarge them or give further form to them.

Signs of involvement

Youngsters locked up in spirals of violence often have their focus on what is done to them and on the struggle to make the other or the world clear that they no longer care about. But there are also moments when they hesitate, notice that they have hurt someone or that they suffer from being distanced from the people they care about, sometimes even feel guilty. Noticing those moments and making them into the subject of discussion opens the possibility of questioning their strongly held convictions or their chosen directions in life. Also, it allows them to be seen as youngsters who still care about others.

F: *My father, my mother, my sisters ... I tried to avoid them. The drugs made me unpredictable. On the one hand, I wanted to be with them, but on the other, suppose I suddenly craved the drugs ... I hid this from my family for a very long time. I didn't want them to know about it!*
S: *What did you try to spare them by running away?*
F: *They had already suffered a lot with my elder sister. They wouldn't have survived a second bout of misery.*
S: *Although you wanted to spare them this misery what caused the running away and all those quarrels?*
F: *A lot of sadness.*

When we notice their acts of caring and moments of being moved, we can invite them to take a look at the effects of their actions on other people. This means moving process wise: at one moment youngsters can see and talk about the impact and effects of what they do, but at other moments they are absorbed by the revenge and conflicts. The more hesitations or doubt about their own actions and their 'silent' hopes for their relationships gains a prominent position in the conversation, the more we can move on. Making visible how these youngsters want to relate to others, who they want to be as a son or daughter, as brother or sister, as friend ... but also how they want(ed) to be cared for, open possibilities to explore step by step how the youngster still can be meaningful to the important persons in their lives (and vice versa).

Witnessing as small steps to reconnection

When thinking about youngsters kicking around, from the outset, we have to take careful consideration of the setting. In some situations it is important to start by having some conversations with the youngsters and parents separately. When it is possible, and the youngster and their parents or carers agree to it, we invite them as witnesses.

These youngsters often struggle with feelings of being unfairly treated and have a strong feeling or conviction that nobody cared. It is not enough that these richer, multi-layered stories exist in the therapy room and are recognised by the therapist or counsellor. They must especially be heard by and shared with the family members involved and their carers. Stories are not yet stories until they find their audience (White, 2007). As Myerhoff (1982, p. 103) emphasises 'because unless we exist in the eyes of the others, we may come to doubt even our own existence'. Hearing these stories can broaden the view of their parents or carers and meanings can start to shift. Indirectly they can acknowledge the struggles then and there, subscribe to hope for their relationships and collectively develop new small steps to reconnection.

Farida's mother was touched by the 'hiding of the drug stories' and Farida's intention not to hurt them as parents. It made her realise that it is difficult to discuss many things in their culture, even though she would like her own daughters to be able to tell her everything.

Her sister had some interesting thoughts about the bullying and the difficult years at school. She had also experienced hard times at school, but there was a niece in her classroom so she never felt alone. The family counsellor while listening to Farida's story had written the following sentence down 'Once, I told them at school but they never did anything about it'. She was touched by the feelings of injustice and how revenge took a hold on Farida.

These responses bring in hope that maybe there are still new directions in life and relations possible, away from the lure of 'revenge'.

Chapter 7

Engaging with parents, carers and professionals

First of all, I would like to emphasise that discussing the theme of 'engaging with parents and carers' just now does not mean that I believe these conversations to be less important nor that I want to put parents and carers on the side-lines of this process. On the contrary, it is my sincere belief that parents and carers have to be taken into account the whole therapeutic journey. This importance has also been emphasised by research, if we want treatment and care to be effective (Tarren-Sweeney & Vetere, 2014; Tarren-Sweeney, 2021). Those people who know and love these children are best placed working together to support them to move towards emotional and mental health (Lobatto, 2021). I have chosen this order because in daily practice I noticed that the many perspectives 'about' the child are still central in conversations and I wanted to let children speak for themselves as much as possible in this book, also in relation to their parents and carers. In this chapter, I will first focus on conversations with the parents and carers present in the daily life of these children and later focus on the conversations with parents or family members who were offending or injuring and are only partially or remotely present in their lives.

A special bond and position

This said, children, their parents and carers are inseparably connected. What this connection looks like, how it is experienced, its impact and effects on their lives, what names and meanings are given to this connection, is time and time again the ever shifting result of a dynamic, unique interplay of multiple influences. Parents and carers each of them have a social position and role that is coloured by many people, institutions and communities and is constantly being (re-)negotiated. In addition, each of them develop a special, unique emotional bond with the child and have a specific social task. This means we have to consider parents and carers as valuable collaborative partners playing an important part in what and how new steps will be developed. Their perspectives, their worries, their struggles, hopes, wishes and ideas have to be taken seriously and listened to, not only in function of the child but also for their own sake.

In the first conversation with Yusuf and his mother, she tells she is extremely worried about him. She no longer knows how to deal with the nightmares and

DOI: 10.4324/9781003167860-8

his temper tantrums. She became convinced that he is 'damaged' for life by what his dad did to him. Even more, she blames herself for staying so long in a violent relationship with his father. These worries and feelings of guilt immobilise her and make her feel powerless. She no longer notices that she matters to Yusuf. She desperately seeks for reassurance that everything will be all right. She wants 'peace of mind'. We decided to have some conversations about all these worries without Yusuf being present as they concern questions about her parenthood and her past experiences with Yusuf's father. In these conversations her hopes and wishes as a mother, and how she could accomplish them, can be explored as well as how to find a helpful stance towards the feelings of guilt that are haunting her. Yusuf remarks that he is glad that someone is taking care of his mother. It even brings some relief that he no longer needs to keep a constant eye on her.

Mauro's grandparents want some conversations separately from Mauro. They want to talk about their anger towards his father and the grief for their 'lost' daughter, Mauro's mother. Since they have different ideas about how to deal and proceed with this in relation to Mauro, they would like to find out together and no longer burden Mauro with their quarrels. They also want to reflect on how to prevent things going the same way as with his brother, Rico.

Over and over again Charlotte's mother gets stuck in how to be supportive to both her children. As talking about Brian in the presence of Charlotte is too complicated and painful we all agree to have some conversation with her as a mum alone. We want to make room for what is pulling and pushing at her as a mother and how to respond in an appropriate way to Charlotte. We also negotiate how and when things out of these conversations will be given back to Charlotte.

Foster mum Daisy is desperate. Lately, Kimberly (eight years) has bitten and kicked her several times. She regularly hides dirty pants and foster mum recently found poop under her bed. An argument recently got out of hand and Daisy had shaken her. Kimberly's mother has been missing for several months. She ran away from a rehab clinic. In the past, Kimberly was sexually abused by a partner of her mum. Kimberly's father is unknown. After each escalation between foster mother and Kimberly, Kimberly is extremely sweet and begs her to forgive. Foster mum feels incompetent and helpless. She gave everything she could to Kimberly and can't any longer make sense of her actions. Even more, foster mum no longer recognises herself. She thinks it is maybe better to find a new place for Kimberly. Kimberly doesn't want to talk with anyone so we decide to have some conversations with foster mum and the social worker from foster care.

In multi-stress contexts where children experienced trauma, or intimate relationships got injured, or attachment problems are in the foreground, the pressure on the parent or carers living daily with the child can be enormous. Not only children's expressed demons of the past, overwhelming emotions or destructive thoughts, but also their actual struggles and the relational entanglements in the here and now can become an exhausting challenge to the parents or carers. On top of that, a list of social instructions weigh heavily on their shoulders. They often have the feeling they have to make right or repair what went wrong and have to be better educators than the offending parent or family members who failed in the eyes of many. They often have to be able to do trauma-sensitive parenting, be an attachment figure and thus be fully emotionally available. Above all this they also have to find, together with the child, their way in the wasps nest of family relationships and loyalties. With all these complexities and high standards, pressure, doubt, feelings of guilt or a sense of falling short are never far away.

Even more, in these contexts, from a professional stance, the focus is often exclusively on the child and what is believed to be their interest and need, although the interest and the need of the parent or carer also concerns the child. If we are not alert, the parent or carer risks becoming reduced to an important instrument in the upbringing and more specifically in the healing of the child. They often are not approached as a fully-fledged person intertwined and struggling in the interplay. It is a helpful thought to assume that if their child is in need, the parents or carers are in need as well. Based on how things are going with the child, in our society, the parent or carer receives 'a scorebook'. A lot of parents are watching themselves and measuring their doings against the societal standards of 'good instruments' in the upbringing of these children (Ramaekers & Suissa, 2012; Van den Berge, 2013). As children in these contexts often present problems and struggle in many ways and in multiple life areas, parents or carers no longer experience that they have a grip on the child's actions or their relationship. They no longer sense they matter in the life of the child. Even more, some of them start to think and become convinced that instead of being supportive or helpful they are in fact harmful to the child. Sometimes they can't make sense of the child's actions at all and only experience hostility and rejection from the child. Jakob (2011) emphasised that this rejecting behaviour can hinder caring responses in adults. Adult and child increasingly operate with negative conclusions about each other's identity and intentions.

As it is precisely the adults that are often the ones who first knock at our door, it is important to make room for their questions, requests and perspectives. It can even be worthwhile and more effective to talk with them without seeing or talking to the child or to offer them a conversation and reflecting space with a colleague. In this way we respect, honour their position, expand their insider's knowledge and skills and hope to strengthen their relationship with the child and their belief in themselves as parents or carers. At the same time the child isn't burdened with our conversations, maybe less addressed as a problem child but hopefully can be supported in more helpful ways in daily life by their parents and carers. Sometimes children and young people may not wish to access direct therapeutic work, but their key adult networks can support their mental health and wellbeing by working together (Lobatto, 2021). When it is not preferable to work this way, we still have to reflect carefully about how to cooperate with parents and carers as full-fledged partners during the whole journey even from a distance.

We provide moments where they can speak and reflect, as parents or carers, about their position, role, the felt dilemmas and ambivalences, in order to find ways to enhance their sense of agency and mattering. Taking good care of the parents or carers can be understood as taking good care of the child. Just like children can feel isolated, also these parents or carers can get disconnected from important others and communities. This means we have to weave with them networks of support and solidarity.

A parent or carer in need

Taking all these previous aspects into account, we consider the parent or carer from the very first contact as an adult in their own right with their own worries, challenges and specific constraints and obstacles in relation to their parenthood and the upbringing of this particular child. We don't want to reduce them to instruments in an education or healing process of the child but make room for their full range of experiences and stories. The more serious the problems the child presents or the more desperate the parents are, the greater their call for help can be.

We need an eye for the effort and courage it takes to put their concerns on the table so stories about what chafes, makes desperate and even makes losing themselves and feeling ashamed, can be shared. Parents and carers come to see us with a heavy heart. Often, a lot of worrying, well-intentioned advice from others and all kinds of trial and error have preceded. Some in their network have been supportive but others have further eroded their self-esteem with their comments or stares. Making room for what it means to ask for help here and now and having to have this conversation can be an important starting point.

Daisy, Kimberly's foster mother, tells that she could never have imagined ending up in this situation. She is ashamed and at the same time furious with Kimberly's mother. She holds her responsible for the mess they are in. In fact, Kimberly's mother should be sitting on this chair instead of herself. Two years ago when Kimberly came into foster care, Daisy had high hopes for her. She thought she could give her a new future and all the love Kimberly had been missing. The first year seemed like a breath of fresh air as Kimberly blossomed. But then the hassle with her food began. Followed by the comments from school, the bullying of other children and finally the silent protest at home. It all became too much. Talking doesn't help a bit as Kimberly's promises aren't worth a cent. Foster mum finishes her tirade by saying with a big sigh 'It is all lost. I don't think Kimberly is ever going to be okay. What do you think? What did I miss that it went so wrong?'

After such an outburst, it is important to slow down. We need to resist many temptations. We do not immediately answer the questions. We do not focus first on what the child's problem is and neither we put the parent on the examination table. We do not analyse what he or she should have done more or less or differently. Instead, we try to notice what 'pulls and pushes' for this particular parent or carer, what weighs most heavily on their shoulders, what concerns them and which of their beliefs and values are affected (Van den Berge, 2013; Vermeire et al., 2022). Which single stories have a grip on them? Which stories became overshadowed by the problems in the here and now and in the past? We invite them into an exploration of their struggles in the multi-stressed contexts they are living in (Madsen, 2007).

Noticing parental pain and values

For a parent or carer, it can be particularly painful when children seem to reject or even ignore them through their actions. It can become even more painful if they notice the child is harming others or themselves and they can't prevent this nor stop it, although it feels as it is their responsibility. Parents and carers often do everything they can to turn things around. Sometimes the craziest roads are taken. Because all their efforts and expressions of relational commitment seem to make no difference, they no longer notice the hard work they do. Consequently, they tend to define themselves as worthless and failing or to define the child as 'lost' or 'irreparably damaged'. Noticing and acknowledging their disadvantages and their relational efforts often is a necessary step to bring them to a riverbank position, overwhelmed as they are by all the storms and swirls.

Asking what hurts and worries the most and locating these disadvantages in daily life by asking for a recent moment or a situation when the troubles explicitly were present, makes it possible to take the parent and carer seriously in what worries them but also to start to unravel the tangles that pull and push on them. By searching together for some nuance and difference in the painful stories, we create some relief in the landscape of negative experiences that bring at the same time a glimpse of hope. *'It isn't always or completely negative or hopeless'.*

Responding to the question 'What touches you most deeply in all these difficulties?' Daisy replies that it is Kimberly's attitude that seems to mean that she does not care at all. 'On the contrary. It is as if she enjoys hurting me'.

S: *Can you share a moment when this attitude was entirely present?*
D: *Last week. I discovered some pants with poop all the way in the back of her closet. I confronted her with it as soon as she came from school. She denied it completely while her face remained unmoved. She swore they were not her pants and she certainly did not know how they got there. It almost felt as if she was mocking me. She stepped away and ignored me when I called her back. This felt like a knife through my heart!*
S: *What do you think: does she really not care or did she rather get specialised in pretending not to care or ...?*
D: *I cannot find out any more.*
S: *After this confrontation are there some small signals that might indicate that she nevertheless cares about what happened?*
D (thoughtful): *Maybe later that evening, she offered me her favourite spot in front of the TV when otherwise she claims it unconditionally.*
S: *What are your main worries for Kimberly when she acts like this? What values that you want to pass on to her get under pressure?*

When we notice the parent's or carer's disadvantages, we can also read between the lines and notice that what the child does, says or feels does not leave them unmoved and that they actually do still care about the child. This also opens the possibility to explore what they hoped and maybe still hope to achieve in relation to the child. As parents or carers would like their child to find their way in the community and society and to uphold certain values and norms, we can ask what kind of values, beliefs and commitments get hurt or become under pressure in these interactions (Van den Berge, 2013).

Being listened to, being taken seriously in what worries and hurts without a feeling of being blamed and starting to notice some bright spots makes it possible to invite the parent or carer to have a closer look at how and when they still make a difference to the child.

Noticing moments of mattering

As parents or carers lose their sense of agency, the moments and stories in which they do matter can become covered by these negative, sometimes explosive, moments (Beckers et al., 2022). The same applies to the moments when the child matters to them and makes a valuable difference in their lives. It is therefore worthwhile to bring these moments to the foreground, making visible that at certain moments and situations they still make a meaningful mutual contribution to each other's lives.

Asking Daisy some more about the time she was sitting on the couch in front of the TV, Daisy realises that Kimberly slowly got closer to her and even asked her if she would like a drink. So I ask Daisy what this probably would say about the importance of the relationship for Kimberly.

A bit later in the conversation, I ask if she remembers some other moments Kimberly tries to get her attention, asks for her help or tries to make up for things. Suddenly Daisy thinks of a moment when Kimberly came home from school crying, huddled in a corner and finally allowed Daisy to put her arm around her. The whole story of school difficulties, bullying and feeling like a strange creature who doesn't belong anywhere, had come out in fits and starts. For a while, they had even cried together but then they encouraged each other. Again I invite Daisy to reflect about what this might have meant for Kimberly. Hesitatingly she responds 'That I still care for her?'

Strolling through these moments and stories together, there is a growing awareness that the parent or carer still matters to the child and that the child matters to them. Collecting these moments with parents or carers can enhance the awareness that their efforts still make sense. When a parent regains insight into their possibilities for action, hostility decreases and room is made for a focus on the needs of the child (Jakob, 2011, 2013).

Turning the spotlight on the child

Once parents and carers emotionally end up in calmer waters, and are no longer encapsulated by their own struggles, we can invite them to take a closer look at what might bother the child. We turn the spotlight on the child's perspective, their worries, struggles, wishes and hopes. We ask the parents or carers if they can try to look from the child's point of view, and if they can think of difficulties the child is facing at the moment.

S: *Daisy, can I add a chair here in our conversation for Kimberly? (While asking, I already move an empty chair closer). If we had the opportunity to ask Kimberly what is currently bothering her most, what do you think she would answer?*

D: *Probably, several things. The bullying at school, ..., the toilet problem, ..., our quarrels and fights, and maybe not knowing where her mum is?*

S *(addressing the empty chair): Dear Kimberly, how would you call these things your foster mum lists? (I turn back to Daisy) Any idea how she would name this? Any common factor in these?*

D: *'Being a misshapen alien'. After a huge discussion, she once shouted 'I am a failed alien. I can better disappear'.*

S: *Does this mean she has a feeling of not fitting in this world? Or does she no longer have a sense that she matters to others? Does she report that she experiences no grip on the things happening in her life? ... Daisy, what's your guess?*

D: *I think all of this.*

S: *Would it be a good idea to explore this a little bit further?*

The actions of the child are often experienced and understood by parents and carers as negative, personal and deliberate. Sometimes the child's actions take on such incomprehensible proportions or are so bizarre from an outsider's perspective that parents or carers no longer know how to relate. Their responses seem to evoke more of the same. The many influencing relations and contexts in which these actions are embedded disappear from view. By asking the parent to step into the shoes of the child and gain a broader view of the child's world of experience and meaning, we can delve into the possible influencing relationships and contexts that may have been left out of consideration until now. We may be able to gain richer understandings of the child's actions, emotions and beliefs. At the same time we invite them to empathise with these contexts and what this may mean for the child.

Daisy and I explore a bit how things might go at school for Kimberly but also what it might mean to no longer feel in control of your own bowel movements while sitting in school.

What impact and effects does this problem have in the different areas of her life and in the different relationships?

As Daisy gets a better idea of what all this might mean for Kimberly, she exclaims: 'It must be dreadful, how on earth can you not have control of your poop? Is this all a consequence of what happened in the past? Is there still any way I can be helpful to her?'

I propose to try to find answers to one question at a time and ask if we can make a list of all the things in the present, the past and even the future in relation to which Kimberly probably no longer experiences a sense of (relational) agency.

Unlocking shared opportunities

Together with the parent or carers we are not looking for an unambiguous and correct explanation of what is happening in the here and now nor a 100 percent correct analysis of the child's troublesome actions and problems. We try not to step into simplified linear causal explanations. We are looking for ways of understanding that are therapeutically helpful, that do justice to the complexity and that open new ways of relating. Problems and problem stories are woven into a web of constantly mutually influencing relationships and contexts. After having disentangled this web to some extent, together with the parent or carer, and after having identified significant contexts, we can begin appreciate the complexity of the problems, get a richer notion of the problem stories and at the same time discover some new points of entry in relation to the child.

While unravelling all kinds of influencing contexts, Daisy notices that the difficulties became worse and worse when Kimberly's mother disappeared from the clinic. 'It seemed as if Kimberly blames me for what her mother has done. Since she can't kick her mother, she seems to be kicking me more and more. I think she feels abandoned by her mother for the umpteenth time'.

Focusing on communicative processes runs counter to the conceptual insulation of the child and opens therapeutic possibilities to make visible the child's relational involvements as well as what is valuable to them. In this exploration we can invite or engage the professional and parental network (Carr, 2012). The purpose is to help them, in a collaborative way, to find their own helpful responses to the child's utterances. As such we start weaving networks of care (Vermeire, 2020) and become ourselves part of networks of resilience.

S: *What might Kimberly be hoping for or trying to make clear? Could it be that she is inviting us to notice some particular things? Any idea how she would like us to respond?*

D: *Maybe she is convinced that I also shall disappear out of her life? Maybe she is looking in a crazy way for reassurance? Now, she only gets confirmation of her conviction of 'being an alien' and that no one wants her. It is she against the world.*

As soon as the parent or carer can see that the child also no longer has a sense of agency or mattering, we can try to find out how they can help the child re-experience a sense of agency.

D: *Maybe I have to talk with Kimberly about this painful missing of her mum and not knowing how to deal with this; I don't want to replace her mum but maybe we can find a way to give some more room for her mum in our house.*

S: As you know Kimberly best, what would be a good moment or way to have such
*   a conversation?*
*   ...*
S: Where does this conversation bring us in relation to the 'poo-problems'?
D: I want to find a way to be more supportive in this because now it is tearing us
*   apart.*

Step by step we can collect ideas and develop concrete actions in which parents
or carers acquire an active role and (re-)discover what possibly works in relation
to the child and the problems.

While telling these stories, parents or carers present moments they experienced
themselves as skilled parents or carers who still make a difference in their child's
life. Although this doesn't mean all the problems are resolved nor have disappeared, they both obtain a sense of 'being on track again'.

A village of parents and carers

A frequent challenge for parents or carers is that they can get stuck between educational obligations on the one hand and acknowledging the painful experiences
or ongoing adversities of the child on the other. It is for instance not because
parents or carers call their child to order, or ask them to do something boring or
tell them to tidy up their room, that the bond between them disappears, although
it can be felt that way by the child. So making this distinction between these tasks
of raising the child and the ongoing process of being emotionally and relationally
involved can be helpful for the parents and carers as well as for the child. Noticing
that other parents or carers are struggling with comparable dilemmas and facing
similar obstacles can be a relief and offer new insights.

As they easily can have the feeling of standing alone in these enormous challenges, it is important to weave communities of solidarity. We have to create
spaces where parents and carers can share with each other their experiences and
stories, their worries and dilemmas as well as their small, or less small, actions.
Their hard-won skills and knowledge until now can contain valuable ideas for
other parents or carers in similar contexts. They can become an (anonymous)
learning community and the reciprocal nature of a peer helping process offers a
sense of belonging and a sense of hope.

Coincidently, in the therapy room there was a drawing in the Kamishibai
(Japanese storytelling theatre) of a ten-year-old girl also struggling with 'toilet
problems'. Her adoptive parents were at a loss as to what to do about the poop
problems. In the conversations with these parents we reflected on how this girl
frenetically tried to please everyone by being the perfect girl. She seemed to be
convinced that a princess doesn't go to the toilet, just like mermaids don't pro-
duce poop. Through the process the girl made a drawing in which she showed
how mermaids poop. The drawing was left in the therapy room because the
girl, together with her parents, wanted to inform other children and parents

about 'poop problems' and resist some simplified ideas about how to solve problems.

I draw Daisy's attention to the drawing and she immediately becomes interested in the experiences of these parents and how they managed to survive in these difficulties. As I had permission of these parents, I share some stories and invite Daisy to collect some questions she would like to ask these parents (see Chapter 5).

In weaving these communities we try to create polyphonic webs of solidarity. Parents and carers in these contexts can also become disconnected from the many adult bystanders, professionals as well as non-professionals. Even worse, they can have the feeling they are called to account or held responsible for the child's actions and wellbeing by the schoolteacher, the neighbour, the baker, the case manager, parents on the side-lines of the football field, and so on. Often they are actually called to account. They come up against each other or get trapped in problematic dynamics instead of forming a cooperative team and facing the challenges together. Often the bystanders also have lost a sense of agency and no longer know how to go on or how to relate to the child or the parent or carer.

This means it is important to take these bystanders and their viewpoints and actions into account. In conversations with these parents and carers we look at how they move in this community tangle, how they still experience some connection or how they can relate to specific people in their community. We invite

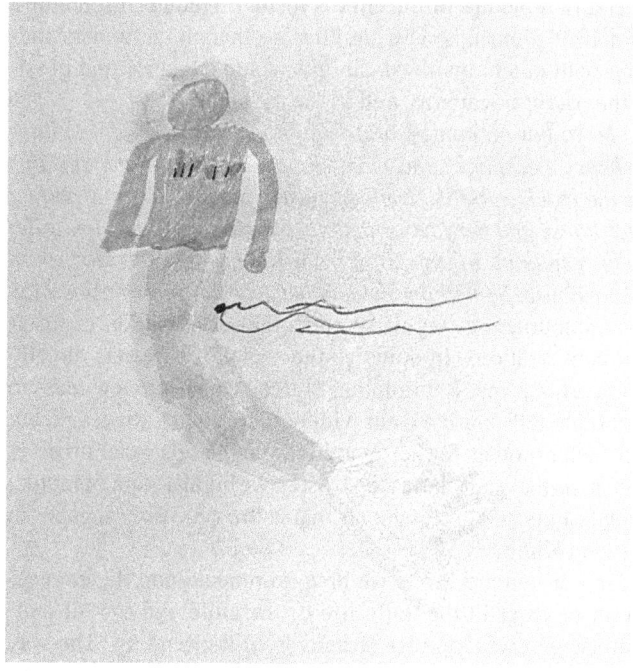

Figure 7.1 Drawing of a mermaid. Photograph by the author.

them to (re)engage with significant bystanders, share experiences but also skills and knowledge of what can make a difference to the child. Lobatto (2021) refers to a foundational position within systemic practice, which involves attempting to appreciate the position of all those present and not present in the room. This position does not mean being uniformly congratulatory or positive; rather it denotes a practice of seeking to transform problematic dynamics, bringing to life the shared intention of adults to care for and nurture these hurt children.

Daisy and I reflect a long time on how to talk with the school about all these difficulties. There are a lot of irritations on how school deals with the 'toilet problems' and Daisy has the impression that they rather want to get rid of Kimberly as she is causing too much trouble. Who would be best placed to have what kind of conversation? What has to be said? What are we hoping for? What kind of information and stories about Kimberly and her life have to be shared with the schoolteacher so she gets a richer understanding and in telling so maybe regain a sense of agency in relation to Kimberly and her actions? How can we involve and engage Kimberly into this conversation?

In this reflecting together we find words and provisional broader descriptions of what is going on and how we ended up here. Outcome research points out the importance of psycho-education for foster parents in helping them to understand where children come from and why they act as they act (Tarren-Sweeney, 2021; Herring, 2021). Elaborating these ideas, it can be helpful when parents and carers can co-construct a rich picture of the child's history, feelings, difficulties, strengths, challenges and relationships with significant others in an understandable language. Sharing with others involved can give some guidance and possibilities for action for the parent or carer as well as the bystanders.

Finally Daisy decides to have a conversation with the schoolteacher explaining Kimberly has a 'heavy backpack' and a sense of alienation. Later on, this conversation inspires the teacher to take Kimberly aside during playtime and let her tell about her foster house and her favourite dolls but also about the new toilet seat. This unexpectedly results in an invitation from Kimberly to the teacher to come and visit her foster house. Something the teacher was happy to respond to.

During our therapeutic journey we regularly invite the social worker of foster care as witness of our conversations. In doing so the social worker gets directly informed of the ongoing process that is unfolding. She can connect as a witness to the stories that foster mother tells, enrich them with her ideas and knowledge, but also indirectly honour foster mother for her many efforts, the relational involvements and the different steps that she takes. Step by step we build a team of mutual support with the parents, carers and professionals that at the same time engages in new relational dances with Kimberly.

Last but not least, in our conversations we have to reflect upon the connection between the parent or carer in the daily life of the child and the 'absent' parent or family member who was, and sometimes is, still offending. The way this parent or carer speaks, thinks of and positions themselves in relation to the offending or injuring parent or family member and the different meanings given to this, will influence the child, their relationship with the child and the child's actions. We cannot pretend that these are two separate worlds. Just like we should not ignore this parent or family member although sometimes the child itself tries to close this door to make the complexity somewhat manageable and liveable.

In the beginning Daisy avoided talking about Kimberly's mum with Kimberly. She thought it would hurt her too much. She was afraid that in speaking about Kimberly's mum her anger would echo in her words. She didn't want to burden Kimberly with her anger. She was convinced this was not okay. Certainly, as the case manager had given Daisy the instruction not to speak badly about her mum.

By making room in our conversations with parents or carers for sharing emotions about painful actions of family members and about the child's hurt relationships, we bring these experiences and stories into the social and relational world. Rather than operating under the skin or having unnoticed effects of all kinds, they become visible, discussible and we can start to reflect upon them. We can try to figure out what is a helpful, valuable and response-able positioning for the parent or carer towards this offending person also bearing the child in mind.

Once Daisy, in our meetings, begins to express her anger towards Kimberly's mother, we discover it is mainly anger about 'abandoning Kimberly each time again'. I invite Daisy to imagine Kimberly and all the emotions probably connected with her mum. Would it be just sadness about missing that Kimberly experiences, or possibly also disillusionment and disappointment? Is it thinkable that there are also some moments of anger? Would Kimberly allow these moments to exist? What would it mean to Kimberly to know that Daisy is also angry sometimes about the abandonment by her mum?

These questions don't have the intention to direct the parent or carer towards certain actions but rather want to nibble away at some beliefs or dominant social instructions that may have a hold on them, such as 'you must not speak ill of the parent'. These social representations, often containing valuable viewpoints, may prevent them from doing or saying certain things, but may also remove them from each other and keep things unspoken. Making these ideas and emotions visible allows us to unravel them and find a way to relate to them with Kimberly in our minds and their possible effects.

While talking about the anger in relation to Kimberly's mum, we try to find out what would be helpful or supportive in this. It makes us also reflect on how to relate to Kimberly's mum the moment she will reappear and what Kimberly would hope for.

For Kimberly it seems to be a relief to know that Daisy also is sometimes a bit angry because of 'her mum's abandoning' but that this doesn't mean that her mum is no longer welcome or, even worse, that she is a 'bad mum'.

Parents (or family members) falling short

Parents or family members sometimes hurt children, cause terrible harm, fall short or are absent at moments they should be present in the life of the child. They have intentionally or unintentionally disadvantaged, in one way or another, the child or youngster and sometimes they continue to disadvantage the child. This means that society and many people involved will look at them as failures or even as wicked. They are considered not to be okay for the child, sometimes not even to deserve the title 'parent'. They must be kept at a distance from their child, sometimes punished or they must admit guilt, apologise and rectify what went wrong. Often these parents have internalised these perspectives on themselves. In their struggle about who they still are or can be in relation to the child, they respond in many different ways. As their parenthood is called into question, they can become elusive and even their parenthood can become elusive to themselves.

All this can urge parents to 'disappear' out of their child's life, while others will do everything to try to convince the child and everyone around it wasn't their intention or their fault. Some of them will do everything to prove they are a better parent and will try hard to put right what went wrong. At the same time the child will respond in many different ways. The connection between the parent and child can be coloured by uncertainty, doubt, ambivalence, suspicion but also sometimes by mutual reproaches, lies or silence and solidified ideas about each other and about what has happened.

In conversations with these parents it will be important to take these complexities into account as it will inform our working alliance. Just like the constant palace of mirrors as to who this parent is or is not, can interfere in our conversations. Several studies have described the interactions between parents and child protection care as challenging after parents lose their children to public care. In a study from the U.S., Sykes (2011) showed how mothers developed strategies to avoid being labelled as bad parents. These strategies led to little productive collaboration, with caseworkers being frustrated that parents took little responsibility for what they believed parents had inflicted on their children, with parents spending energy on defending themselves (Syrstad & Ness, 2021). How can we have conversations in which we invite them as parents, reflect with them on what happened, (maybe still happens) and the impact and effects on themselves, their parenthood and the child without ignoring the responses of the social world? Can we question how they still want to be, or can be, a parent in relation to their child and at the same time take into account the many interfering contradictory perspectives?

So, also in these contexts it can be helpful to remain true to the idea 'the problem is the problem, not the parent' (White, 2007) and invite them to explore the obstacles, constraints and concerns in raising their child, their relationship with their child and of course what in the broader picture of their life and community is good food for these problems. This doesn't mean we want to disconnect them from their part in the violence, harming actions or acts of neglect. On the contrary, we want to create a way of talking and reflecting in which we don't have to become 'moral knights' ourselves but can invite them to start to enlarge their moral potentials as parents (see Chapter 6) or reconnect them with their hopes and wishes as a parent. We don't want to put them on the investigation table but we would rather find manageable ways to name the struggles and disadvantages and put these on the table. We need to create a space that feels safe enough and allows them to be aware of what happened and happens in their lives and to think about themselves and their child.

Solange (32) is desperate. Her daughter, Grace (15), is back on the run. Grace has already been placed several times in a closed facility after being removed from situations of sexual exploitation. Until she was 11 years old, Grace lived with her mother and alternate partners. There was frequent domestic violence and Grace also shared in the blows. Solange was in that period heavily alcohol-dependent. Reports on Grace refer to emotional and psychological abuse and an attachment disorder. For two years Solange has been trying to get her life back on track and attends weekly AA-meetings.

She was referred for therapy by the institution where Grace was placed. This referral was accompanied by a warning: 'Consider it as a try-out and don't take it too personally if she doesn't show up more than she does'. The first period they were right. For Solange it wasn't clear what she could get out of these conversations or how these conversations could be helpful. 'It was her daughter that was in need and had to be helped'. She was even doubting if she had the right of sitting in this chair and spoiling my time. While she just as much felt some pressing instructions on her shoulders from the professionals around her: 'You have to come to certain insights and work on yourself'.

Parents in these contexts are very sensitive to the ways people look at them. It can be very confusing for them and for ourselves to get entangled in these often shifting perspectives. One moment they are expected to do something for or with their child, and on other occasions they are not allowed to take care of them, to be a parent. We prefer to put these complexities on the table. We address them radically as parents. In doing so we take a clear political stance ourselves. This opens the possibility to ask them what preoccupies them here and now from that position and role and how past events and histories contributed to these worries. We invite them explicitly into their parental position and encourage them to think and speak from that position.

S: *Solange, can I ask you,* as the mother of *Grace, here and now what is your biggest struggle being a mother or what do you worry about most?*
Sol: *That Grace will end up in horrible situations where they will do all sorts of things to her. That something irreversible is going to happen.*
S: *Have you talked to her or anyone else about this?*
Sol: *I have tried to make clear to her countless times how dangerous it is ... but it always ends in an argument and mutual recriminations. She says I have nothing to teach her ... I am powerless. There are periods she refuses to see me.*

S: What is it that you keep trying to make clear to her?

Sol: I don't want others to hurt her. I want so much for her to have a good life, different from mine.

S: Is it an idea to explore together what in the past or in the different areas of life she is embedded maybe contribute in the here and now to closing her ears to your warnings and constantly tumbling over in reproaches?

Sol: This is clear: she is angry because I was not there when I should have been. I was in a bad place and she has had very hard times. Often I think this will never be right again. I'll always stay a bad mother.

The history of the problems is often so long, the negative experiences so over-whelming and the isolation such a heavy burden that these parents lost a sense of hope and no longer see a conjoint future for their child and themselves. Many parents who acted in deficient or abusive ways know that they crossed lines and failed in the eyes of many. This means it isn't our primary job to make them clear they were wrong or did wrong; it is much more interesting to explore how they understand how this could happen and what constraints and obstacles came along. These constraints and obstacles can be personal but also interpersonal and social, all entangled in one nested knot. Existentially, they have often lost the ground under their feet, no longer understanding themselves in what they have done and so who they are. Negative, simplified identity conclusions become central. We have to detect local and broader contexts so that what they have done begins to make sense to themselves although what they have done isn't acceptable (also to themselves).

I ask Solange to tell me a bit about the first period of her motherhood. She was just 17 and Grace's father denied he was the father. Although she was not surrounded by supportive family, she decided to keep the baby and quit school. Together with her friends at that time partying and drinking cocktails was almost a daily habit. Once Grace was born, the parties were mainly at her apartment as she wouldn't leave the baby alone. Men often stayed over for the night. She fell in love with one of them, Arvid. In the beginning he was really gentle to Grace. She thought he would be a good father to Grace but pretty soon the humiliation and the violence came in. Drinking helped her to bear the difficulties. In the meantime she was also financially dependent on him ...

While making all kinds of influencing relations and contexts visible, including the parent's doings, we try to listen for small actions of caring for the child, small actions revealing they were still worried for the child, or tried to protect them from worse or took decisions for change, etc.

Sol: Once I brought Grace, at the age of five, to my mum. I begged her to take care of her although this request was a giant step for me. I no longer wanted Grace living in such a devastating environment. It was clear she was better off without me.

Understanding their actions and themselves in a much richer, nuanced and multi-perspective field of relationships and contexts can help them to see themselves as parents who failed, but also as parents who tried their best and to whom their child mattered and often still matters. They have to get out of their own some-times traumatised position so it becomes emotionally doable to focus on the needs of the child. We help them recognise and mitigate their own responses so that they regain some strength to approach their child in a slightly different way and not to allow themselves to be thrown off balance by the rejectionist, dismissive responses of the child (Jakob, 2011). Step by step we can invite them to try to figure out what the child experienced in the past and what this means to the child. How did their child respond? How did they try to stay on their feet? What did they miss? What did they worry about? And so on. We invite them to move from a rather self-centred view towards an other-centred view (Jenkins et al., 2003). Parents often didn't notice the child's efforts to make a difference nor their acts of relational involvement. This also means that there never came any recognition for the child's pain, hard work nor ambivalences and contradicting emotions.

Sol: I remember once she ran to the neighbours to call the police. My partner was beating me almost to death. Once the police left I was furious at her. Instead of appreciating her help, I pushed her further away. ... It is only recently, I can consider that she must have been scared too and not just wanted to betray us.

> *...*

S: Can you imagine how scared she must have been? Would it have needed cour-age to run to the neighbours? And what would she been hoping for? Or rather prevent, maybe protect?

These conversations may also reveal what they blame themselves for, what the child blames them for or even more the significant people around them. Just like it brings a richer understanding of the painful or unhelpful dances in which they got involved through time.

Suddenly, I receive a call that Grace has returned to the institution but that Solange may have been hiding Grace those last days. When Solange, a few days later, comes for conversations, I tell her about the phone call. She starts to cry. 'I didn't know what to do ... I was so angry that she had disappeared for so long. At the same time I couldn't refuse her to stay with me when she, last week, was on my doorstep. At least, I knew where she was. And of course, after a few days, the quarrels started again'.

S: How would you call the struggles you get trapped in together?
Sol: Not being able to live without, but also with, each other. We always end up in mutual blaming.
S: What is good food for this mutual blaming?
Sol: My many failures in the past. I wish I could undo it.
S: How have you tried to undo this so far?

Once parents are able to take the child's perspective and start to see what they have done, feelings of remorse, guilt and shame tend to become omnipresent and even toxic (Weingarten, 2003; Vermeire et al., 2022). This can appear in all kinds of ways like making themselves invisible, trying to make things up, begging for forgiveness, etc. This often makes their relationship with the child tumble in even more complex dances. Just like for the child or youngster the relational obstacles, questions, hesitations, concerns and accusations can grow over the years. Which means that every attempt at contact, an outstretched hand, a parent's apology often falls on a ground strewn with these complex histories leading to further rejection, distrust but also sometimes to new sparkles of hope and yearning.

Guilt and reconciliation

Notions as apologies, atonement, reconciliation can easily be experienced as big words or felt as hollow phrases. Just like they easily can become a path that the parent supposedly must take and where the counsellor should lead the parent to. Jenkins warns against simplifying such concepts by reducing them to single actions. Popular notions of atonement, just like notions about forgiveness, generally relate to notions of acknowledgement of abusive behaviour, restitution to the abused person and resolution or moving on (Jenkins et al., 2003, p. 41). The relational and contextual embeddedness of these concepts is in danger of disappearing altogether here, as does the process character whose end point is not fixed. It makes a difference when they become mandatory obligations or rather are possibilities, choices and 'directions of travelling'. Can we unravel these concepts and ideas and draw distinctions as informing respectful choices?

Jenkins suggests that a person can develop a 'journey of atonement', which may involve acceptance of responsibility and restitution for their actions. This often means moving from a self-centred thinking towards an other-centred perspective. By investing in processes and practices of realising that the child and their feelings have been hurt, a commitment to take responsibility can be enhanced.

By not only focusing on the feelings of guilt and experiences of 'failing as a mother' but also inviting Solange to try to get a more full understanding of what these past histories meant and still mean to Grace, she can start to acknowledge the effects without trying to 'solve' them or 'erase' what happened.

The actions of the parent stay interdependent of the responses of the child, as their relationship is interdependent, just like they are influenced by the many voices involved. The parent who was offensive is often not in a position to demand forgiveness, let alone enforce it. If this were to happen, we then repeat what has already happened, namely abuse of power relations. We, as therapists, can be supportive in helping the parent to endure and carry feelings of guilt, shame and even remorse in these contexts.

Sol: The day they took Grace away from me and brought her to the children's home, will be etched in my memory forever. I cannot, must not and will not forget how wrong I was.

S: Etching this day in your memory, what is this all about? What does this say about what you want to keep in mind for Grace as a mother?

Sol: I want to remember what I have done and keep in mind that I want to go about things differently now.

We can reflect together on what kind of acknowledgements the child would hope for and in which ways some restitution could be possible and meaningful to the child, again without any pressure, expectations or condition towards the child.

Throughout our conversations, Solange notices more and more what it meant to Grace to feel abandoned by her as a mother. Grace must have felt very lonely, maybe even still is. She suspects that Grace is still looking for someone who loves her unconditionally. Realising that she can't ease this longing, feels very painful. Just like all her 'good advice' and 'ways of trying to help' are waved away. However painful it may be, Solange no longer wants to hide her shortcoming and accept for this very moment that maybe things will be irreparable. Together we think about what Grace would appreciate for Solange to notice and take seriously. What would Grace possibly want recognition for and what would that look like?

Solange remarks that Grace never had the chance to tell quietly what it all meant to her and how hard she worked. Grace often screamed: 'You do not understand anything. You have never listened'. Solange thinks it has a lot to do with not having noticed her worries and concerns, let alone her hard work.

It requires a careful process of attunement, to find out together with the parent what they can do that would make a difference for their child, that would be useful for their child's life. Gradually, we gain an understanding of what is still possible or desirable from the child's perspective. Reflecting together on how the parent can still be valuable and meaningful, even if the answer will be 'by being absent or keeping a distance', can be an important step in opening new conversations and relational positioning for both the parent and the child. Also, the way in which the envisaged possibilities can be checked, needs to be carefully examined as we don't want to force or convince the child in some obvious direction nor want to be intrusive. The child must have the opportunity to develop their own thoughts and ideas and must be able to set their own limits. They should be able to draw a line when they feel the need to.

A few weeks later, Solange asks Grace if it would be helpful if Grace somehow could share what it meant to her in the past and the efforts she made. Grace replies immediately: 'Yes, of course, but only when you could keep your mouth shut!' and she adds: 'And I don't believe you can do this!'

We suggest that she and her mentor from the institution carefully explore what she wants to share and how, but also what she hopes for and what would be a valuable outcome for her in this sharing. In the meantime, I further explore with Solange how she can position herself and respond to Grace's expectations.

Finally, we organise a life review interview with Grace. Solange is present as witness. She is asked to remain silent for almost one hour and to listen very carefully to the stories told before responding (see Chapter 8).

Involving parents from the start

When it becomes clear there is a situation of abuse or neglect, the focus is mainly on the child and on creating safety for the child. In these actions for security, harming parents can easily disappear out of sight as possible valuable and resourceful partners in creating safe grounds. However, it can be important and helpful to the whole journey to take the parent into account from the first moment. The precious story of Isabel, Ilya and Kevin shows what important steps can be taken from the very start.

Isabel is brought in crisis to a psychiatric unit after a psychotic episode. The father of both children returned to Syria a few months ago (as an ISIS fighter). Kevin, their eight-month-old baby, and Ilya (four) are brought to a foster family. The juvenile court initially prohibits all contact between Isabel on one side and the foster family, her children and others involved on the other side.

Luckily the foster care worker, hearing how both children cry a lot these first days, not really knowing what is happening, asks juvenile court special permission to contact Isabel or a nurse in the hospital. Once authorised, she asks the foster parents to write a small letter to Isabel about how they received her children. They write about what is remarkable in a pleasant way about the children such as baby Kevin's beautiful dark eyes and Ilya's fantastic curls. They also emphasise how polite Ilya is to the other children staying with them. In a few sentences, foster parents introduce themselves and ask Isabel, as a mother, a few questions. They literally ask for her advice and help.

> *... Dear Isabel, we assume that you know best how we should go about some things, so we would be pleased if you could help us a little. Does baby Kevin have a special sleeping ritual? Is there anything we can do to make it easier for him to fall asleep? Also, while giving Kevin the bottle, we were wondering if there is anything we can do to make it more comfortable for him? Ilya's curls are beautiful, but they get tangled easily. Do you wash them with special shampoo?*
>
> *Finally, if there are things that you think are important for your children and that you would like us to take into account, please let us know. We cannot promise that we can do everything, but we will do our best.*
>
> *...*

One of Isabel's responses, although she was in the beginning still very mentally confused, was a children's song she asked to sing to her children. It was a Spanish lullaby that she sang every night beside their bed. It could be found on the internet and was easy to learn.

This letter was the beginning of a valuable collaboration and of weaving networks of resilience from the very start.

Chapter 8

Laying down a path in walking

In this chapter we make room for the many ever-recurring questions that children who experienced painful life histories and those involved ask themselves, e.g., *'How could this happen? What does this say about me and my family? Is it all my fault? Will it ever be okay?'*

Despite many efforts, some of their concerns, obstacles and difficulties do not get 'solved' and it is an ongoing quest to find a way to relate to them. Children often have incoherent and confusing stories about their history, their family, themselves and their relationships. Together with the child and important others I show through the co-construction of timelines of the past as well as timelines of the future and through 'life review' interviews how we can collect all kinds of jigsaw pieces to enhance step by step a sense of coherence and continuity.

In this final chapter, I also want to challenge some ideas about 'processing trauma and painful histories' and discuss what can be considered good outcomes of our conversations and process. I do not assume that the problems and traumatic experiences can be simply solved, restored or repaired but instead I search for liveable pathways and places to stand that fit with the values and hopes of the child itself, the important people and their community in order to enhance their sense of belonging. We conceive of 'outcome' as a never-ending process of becoming in continuous dialogues with many others and society. Which stories will be told and what ways of being will be performed in which contexts?

A sense of coherence and continuity

Carter and McGoldrick (2004) noticed that children and family members after radical or traumatic events can feel as if they are frozen in time. Many live only in the present moment, without a sense of past connection or future direction. Others are locked up in stories of the past or future.

In my home town now and then I cross a young man that I knew years ago as a little kid. He was placed in the children's home where I worked. Each time we meet on the street, we have a nice little chat but the stories told always go the same direction. In big words he tries to convince me: 'Tomorrow, it's going

DOI: 10.4324/9781003167860-9

*to happen: I will have a job ...', 'Tomorrow, I will find the love of my life ...',
'Tomorrow, I am going to move to a wonderful flat in town ...'*

Children that are labelled as insecurely attached often have shredded, reduced or unfinished stories about their history, their family, themselves and their relationships (Byng-Hall, 1995; Walsh, 2006, White, 2007). Stern, et al. (1999) distinguish two types of stories that people tell about their difficult life path. There are stories of restitution where the experience of various life events are transformed into meaningful phenomena, and acquire a place in the life of the person. However, there are also chaotic and 'frozen' stories in which experiences remain a series of separate events. Many young people with difficult and stressful life histories tell fragmented, chaotic stories with barely a sense of control or influence. Initially the answers to questions about the past can be limited to: 'I do not know', 'No idea ...' or shoulders are shrugged.

Richardson et al. (2016) emphasise the vital importance for young people in care to have a developmental story of one's life, but the immediate network of family to provide a reservoir of memories is often lacking. Sometimes the stories of the past are too painful to share, to discuss or to question and there is a tacit agreement in the family that one should not talk about them. The many people involved may also have too different, contradictory perspectives on what happened, so that every talk ends up in a truth struggle.

After a long history of domestic violence and traumatic experiences, Ismael's dad ended his life when Ismael was eight years old. He seems to have no memories and stories about his dad nor about what happened, apart from fragments of fights, of crying and being locked in his room. Aged 12 now, he never mentions the past at home, being loyal to the family and out of concern for his mother. Together we find out that there is, what he calls, a 'deafening silence' in the family. But the efforts to 'silence' his father seem to make his father even more omnipresent in the house.

I put two questions to Ismael:

- *If you had questions about the many events of the past or about your father, who do you think are best informed and could provide the most interesting or compelling answers?*
- *If you actually wanted to ask these questions, which person would you think of?*

Together we draw a kind of genogram in which he colours those persons who have the most inside knowledge red and those persons to whom he might ask a question yellow.

This drawing illuminated interesting ideas for next steps. For instance, his father himself, his mum and paternal grandparents know, according to him, the most but he wouldn't ask them any questions. We discussed with whom we could share this drawing and to what purpose. We also tried to grasp who possibly had what kind of information and what kind of stories he was longing for. He himself

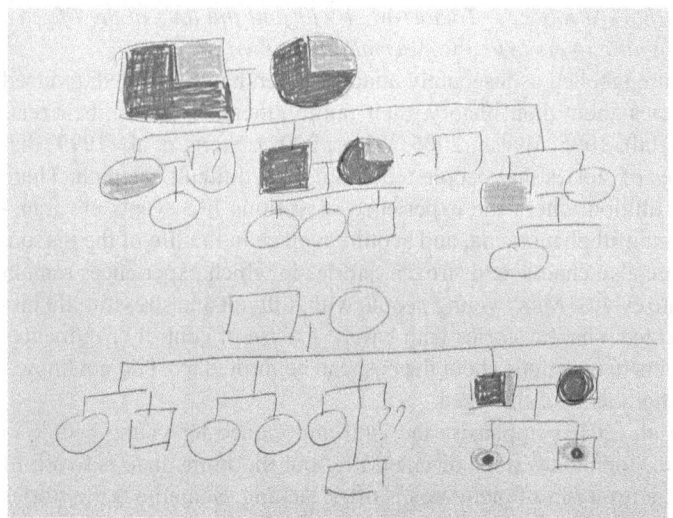

Figure 8.1 Genogram drawing, red and yellow. Photograph by the author.

decided to start a quest about his father. The first person he interviewed was an old school mate of his father still living in the neighbourhood.

Children develop and construct their stories in relationship with others, including their families and communities, and may draw on many other contexts to guide their meaning and actions. Dallos (2005) suggests to create, together with the child, family members and significant people, a secure base from which they can develop narrative skills, explore narratives and invite alternative understandings of experiences and stories. The aim is to co-construct new and more coherent narratives and enhance a sense of coherence. In doing so we don't want to make the children disloyal to their family. We can search for 'subordinate storylines', connect the child with stories of being valued and cared for, and people who have cared about them: wider family, carers, friends and teachers (White, 2007; Richardson, et al. 2016). In what follows I illustrate the possibilities of working with timelines and life review interviews as more straightforward approaches to create a sense of coherence.

Timelines of the past

As children and families can get stuck in single stories in time, it can be helpful to situate these painful experiences from the past made visible within a broader field of experiences, events and encounters throughout time. Each point or period in time is always situated in a zeitgeist, a place in the world and wider social-cultural discourses.

Ismael had come to the conclusion that his dad had to be a monster by nature. His death was the climax of all the disasters which had happened in their life and now the family is in ruins. As he regularly has temper tantrums at home and in school and his auntie already remarked he really looks like his dad, he is convinced he will be a hopeless case just like his dad.

When I pull out a long roll of wallpaper and suggest that we draw the path of his life so far, he immediately jumps up and is into this quest. With a marker, I draw a thick line through the centre of the roll and ask how long our timeline should be. He shrugs his shoulders, his enthusiasm ebbs away and with his head down he mumbles: 'Short... there are only disasters anyway'.

I don't let myself be thrown off balance and ask if it is okay to take about 30 centimetres for every year of life.

S: *What's your date of birth?*
  While he responds I write this date on the line but leave enough space on the line before this date.
S: *Do you have any idea: Was it a sunny day? Are you born during day or at night?*
I *(with a smile, his interest is back): How can I know that?*
S: *Did no one ever tell you any small story about these first days? Was your dad present? Who came to visit you and your mum first?*
I: *My mother once showed me an amulet she wore during pregnancy and I know my father said the obligatory prayers. I think Uncle Eli was definitely present during the circumcision. This should be done soon after birth.*
S: *Shall we write or draw the amulet and the prayers around your day of birth? Should we also indicate circumcision on the timeline and the people present?*

Ismael takes the pencils and draws a multi-coloured amulet before his birth date. He adds his mum, dad (saying prayers) and some important family members.

S: *What does this amulet possibly stand for? What might your mum have hoped for?*
I: *It is to protect me! I think she wished me all the luck in the world!*
S: *Shall we add these words in a special colour?*
I: *Let's take green. That's my favourite one!*
S: *What should we call this moment? And what would your mum, dad, other family members call this moment? Are there still pictures of you as a baby?*

... Above the circumcision he draws a Jewish star as a symbol for his religious connection.

As these children and families got stuck around the painful experiences, it can be interesting to choose a starting point that goes back to long enough before the problems came in. This can open, from the very beginning, some new perspectives as some children and youngsters can't imagine that there was a period when the problems were less, even maybe absent. Just like they never took into consideration that their parents maybe once were in love with each other or were happy with their presence, or even proud of them. I sometimes ask if they know where their parents first met or if they know where they first kissed and who took the initiative. These questions re-activate their curiosity so our co-creation of a timeline can become a vivid journey into stories of the past.

We can re-activate forgotten, buried memories and look for possible fillings of gaps, unknowns in the story. Just like we can actively indicate people who disappeared out of sight on the timeline to re-populate their worlds and lives. At the same time, we do not merely try to gather 'knowledge' or 'information' on the time axis, but try to unveil a rich palette of meanings, actions and gained knowledge.

As we move forward in time, we collect all sorts of small and big moments and encounters, such as learning to ride his tricycle with his father, a trip to the seaside with his aunt, the birth of his little sister, etc. Each time, we look for a naming and what meaning it has for himself and those involved. He chooses in what colour, what form or with what word we put this on the timeline.

In doing so, more and more moments to cherish unfold in which it becomes visible that there was still care for the child and they were meaningful to loved ones. Together we can look upon the timeline from an emotionally manageable distance.

Moving in time, step by step we are approaching the difficulties. When did Ismael begin to notice that things were difficult? Ismael first wants the quarrels and fighting as miniature dots on the timeline, but soon they become larger and

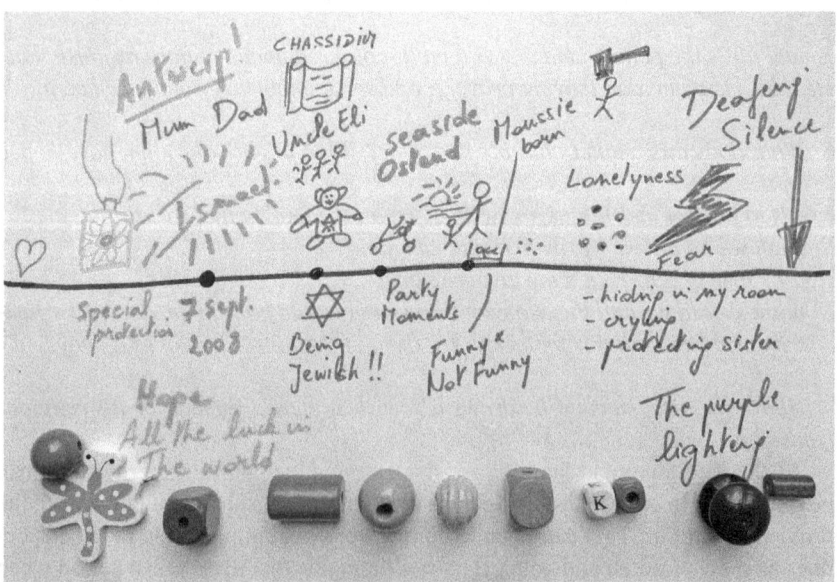

Figure 8.2 Timeline with beads below. Photograph by the author.

larger lightning bolts. As I know he came to some conclusions about his dad as a monster by nature and also linked his temper tantrums with the actions of his father, I decide to ask some more questions that can enlarge our sight on this period and hopefully develop some richer narratives. What was going on in the life of your dad or what perhaps happened before things got out of hand and can be important to write on this timeline? He remembers that since going to primary school his dad lost his job, was at home every day and even stopped going to the synagogue. He could suddenly burst out. There seemed to be no story about his father losing his job and we wondered who could help us in understanding this. We also reflected on what 'losing your job' could mean in their Jewish community.

By situating them on a co-constructed timeline the adversities get situated in a storyline over time. These experiences and stories are given a right to exist, but they also become connected to the stories that precede, succeed or occur at the same time. Based on research evidence, Bruner (1990) shows that people are naturally predisposed to construct narratives that make sense of the unusual and unexpected, and that 'children produce and comprehend stories, are comforted and alarmed by them' long before they are able to express simple logic with language. He argues that logical claims are most easily understood by the child when they are embedded in an ongoing story (Fredman & Fuggle, 2000). Stories are not formed in isolation but in relationship with others, including their families and communities, and may draw on many contexts to guide their meanings and actions, for example, their relationships, cultures, gender and religions (Pearce, 1989; Fredman & Fuggle, 2000, p. 219). This means that our discoveries and possible new links will also have to stand the test of their family stories and their world over and over again.

In between conversations, Ismael tries to fill in the 'gaps' in our timeline. Apparently his uncle Eli is a valuable source of stories and family knowledge. This is how he finds out that the loss of father's job was a 'hard blow'. He got fired because he made a grave mistake. Ismael decides to draw a big hammer above father's head in the timeline. In the meantime, we also add the information he gathered from father's former schoolfriend. The latter described him as a rather timid boy but with surprisingly bright remarks and he recounted a funny incident in class that Ismael symbolically drew on the timeline, remarking 'Maybe my father wasn't a monster after all'.

While children and youngsters get engaged in these 'research projects' they can also get involved in valuable conversations with other significant people. They can even discover that their questions open possibilities of connecting. His father's schoolfriend even thanked him for helping remembering some nice moments.

While Ismael is drawing the red points and lightnings, I ask what they evoked in the house and in his life. He writes the words 'Loneliness and later also Fear' in purple and calls it the colour of The Evil. While co-creating descriptions for the pain and impact, I also ask for his responses to these difficulties. We write down 'hiding in my room', 'crying', 'protecting my little sister', ...

As our timeline isn't an 'objective depiction of reality and history' but a kaleidoscopic web of stories and meaning in which a number of common threads emerge, we can look for responses, skills and knowledges from the past that bring in ideas for the future (Epston & White, 1992). As it is a piece of material, we can literally look at it from a certain distance or even reflect on it from a different time perspective or through the eyes of other people involved. We can even invite them to witness or collaborate in the co-construction of these lines. We may also choose to let the timeline rest for a while, to forget it for some time, and come back to it on a later occasion.

Children, youngsters and family members can also start to think again about how they want to relate to the events and what place they want to give them in their lives in the here and now or in the future. We can gather what they want to take with them or would like to hold on to in the future. What could be an important next step for tomorrow?

As our timeline on the wallpaper gets filled in, I invite Ismael to take a step back, have a look at it and walk to the 'next week' on the line. Looking from this point, what would he like to embrace about his dad and take with him? What are some actions of the past that can be helpful in the future?

While talking, telling and searching, but also reflecting with the child and important others, step by step, we collect new, alternative and more nuanced stories, with new connections and where problems and histories are an important aspect of their lives alongside many other aspects. We listen for the cracks, gaps, ambiguities, historising dilemmas and problems, so we can shine light in a different way (Daniel, 2018) and discover new traces. This journey can also be seen as 'doing hope together'. Still, we have to keep in mind that each timeline is just a temporary result in the ongoing process of becoming and each new stage in life, each new jigsaw piece or simple remark of a friend can form a context that possibly shakes these narratives up again.

Timelines of the future

For some children and young people, a direct exploration of the past is too threatening, too confrontational or too painful and therefore not an option. Every question in that direction is turned down. Although they seem locked up in the here and now, and the future seems empty, exploring a possible image of the future can offer ideas to know how to go on in the present. A trip to the future can be an interesting, alternative route while the past is still implicitly addressed. It may be a much more hopeful route (McAdam & Lang, 2003).

Cindy (16) was abused for several years by her mother's brother and went through a period of drug abuse during which all contact with the family was broken off. Talking about the past years only increases the stress. I ask her what she would like her life to be like in five years' time.

Questions like: *Where do you want to live? How will you arrange your living space? What place will your parents or significant people take in your thoughts, in your daily actions? What do you hope to carry with you (personal belongings as well as ideas, habits, ...)? What kind of values will you cherish?*, will not only evoke a lively picture but also enhance a connection with her hopes and dreams.

All the ingredients that Cindy lists and that she thinks will be important come to the 21-year mark on the timeline. The first thing Cindy says is: 'Then I am grad-uated! I will be living in my own little flat in the city. I have a TV, a PlayStation and music boxes with a microphone to rehearse my songs. I have a job so there will be a Vespa in front of the building ;-)'. We search a picture of a red Vespa on the internet, print it and stick it on the timeline paper.

We unravel step by step what her life will look like at that moment. Besides the material, practical and organisational aspects, we also discuss the various relationships she will be involved in. With certainty, Cindy says that when she turns 21, she will have a tattoo of a rose. Her mother's name is Rosemary, so she will always have her mum close to herself. She hopes that this can make up for the loss of these last years. She wants to invite her mum to her flat and hopes she can be proud of her. She doesn't want to think about her uncle anymore and she doesn't want to waste any more words on 'the events'. The thought: 'What's done is done. That's the end of it. Full stop' will give her something to hold on to. With great care, she draws a detailed rose on the sheet and writes a big 'full stop'. I ask what is so important to her in this 'full stop'. What does this say about her hopes for her life?

We take the child or adolescent's ideas and dreams seriously and do not give in to the temptation to categorise them as 'not realistic' or 'not achievable'. We try to illuminate what is meaningful and valuable to the young person in these longings and choices. From this co-created picture in the future, it can become possible to reflect upon 'how much space they want the previous painful experi-ences to take in their life'. Once the ideas and expectations have been worked out in detail, we can take a step back in time. The more tangibly worked out, the more foundation is created for further work.

If you want all these things realised when you are 21, what should you be doing when you are 19?

Here, too, we try to paint a picture of the child's world at that age but this time in relation with their already expressed hopes and dreams.

I will hang out a lot in the city and probably work in the bakery because I will need money for the flat. I don't want to have money problems like my mum and my family. At that point, I will have had some serious conversations with my mum and not, as I have done so far, with recurring recriminations. This is about 'cleaning up the past'.

Step by step, we bring the child or adolescent's life closer to 'the here and now' (within two years, within a year, ...). Once we arrive in the present on the timeline, it often becomes clearer which steps need to be taken now in order to achieve something of the dreams within five years, especially in accordance with what and who is important to them. At the same time, they sometimes for the first time, get the feeling that there is hope and that they may be able to position themselves in the face of traumatic events, and believe that their lives don't have to be ruined forever.

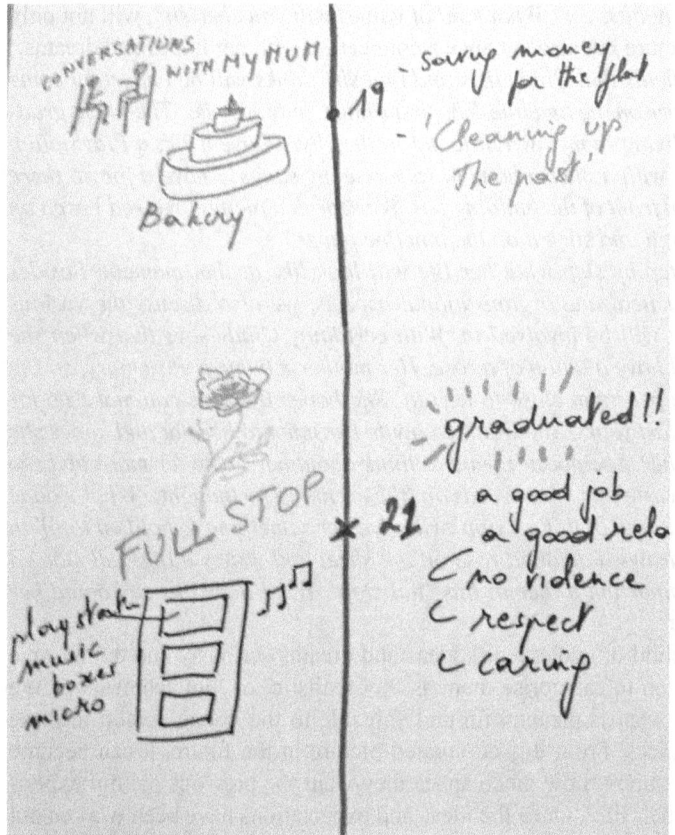

Figure 8.3 Timeline with flower and 'full stop'. Photograph by the author.

Beads to hold on to

While remembering and sharing stories, drawing and writing on the timeline, I also put boxes with various beads next to Ismael. I ask him to choose a bead for each important moment, experience or persons popping up in the co-creation of the timeline. He also searches carefully matching beads for important actions, responses and meanings linked with these experiences and encounters. For instance, Ismael choses a little smiling sun for his day of birth but first he puts a bead signifying the amulet his mum was wearing during pregnancy on the string. He takes a large green ball, as the bead of 'special protection'.

This beading helps children to better hold on to their choices, (re)position-ings in relation to events or injustices, and to keep in sight what they value. The inspiration of working with beads came during a trip through Borneo. I became fascinated by the beautiful bead necklaces, beaded masks and other objects made by the various Iban people in Sarawak. At a local exhibition on the occasion of an international congress on the rich, multiple meanings of the use of beads, there was shown how beads or bead combinations symbolise experiences, radical events, certain knowledge and skills. A new world opened up. Making the beads in clay, glass, wood or even animal bones, then colouring and carefully selecting the beads is an intensive and meaningful activity. Bringing the different beads together in a bead necklace or mask documents lives or certain periods in life. Some bead necklaces function as amulets and offer protection when crossing dangerous territory. Others are made during initiation or transition rituals such as 'becoming a man or a woman', marriage ceremonies or the death of a loved one. The bead necklaces are also attributed with medicinal power to cure a serious illness or injury. The important ornaments or jewels are passed on from generation to generation, with a new piece of beadwork added each time. The Iban wear these necklaces, masks, etc., with great pride (Sarawak Museum, 2010).

Around the same time, I met Sara Portnoy at a conference in London. She presented a workshop on the 'Beads of life' approach (Portnoy et al., 2015) inspired by 'The Tree of life' and 'The Team of life' (Ncube, 2006; Denborough, 2008). It became a cordial, inspiring exchange that continues to this day. Sara works in London at University College Hospital with children, young people and families dealing with profound illnesses. Talking directly about emotions with these children, young people or families is often difficult. This prompted her to look for ways to express painful, sometimes traumatic experiences and to document meaningful moments together, without offending the child or adolescent's feelings. Children and young people are encouraged to tell a multitude of stories rather than being trapped in one story of trauma or loss and to include this wealth of stories into beads.

Aisha (16 years), a Somalian girl, had been placed in a closed facility by the juvenile court after ending up in situations of sexual exploitation. She was given the opportunity by the judge to work and stay with a farmer's family in Croatia for two months as an alternative project, instead of staying at the closed unit. After these difficult but successful months at the farm, she came for an interview in order to reflect on her life and sort things out about the past, present and future. We took a close look at the work project as a value-filled choice and initiative. She chose a bead for each significant meeting, action, thought, etc.

The night before her departure to Croatia, she could not sleep. The doubt crept in again. Two conflicting voices kept her awake. One tried to persuade her to stay in the institution, saying it was a 'stupid' idea to leave. The other voice promised that everything would be better after the work project! This 'hesitation' became the start of our special bead string. She chose a black and white bead to indicate the swinging back and forth. By morning she had said to herself, 'Come on, grow up!' She had got up and taken her backpack. This special moment was captured in a large, red, polygonal bead. It was given the name 'on the road to a better future'. When I asked how things had gone at the airport and on the plane, Aisha told a story about a little girl at the airport gate who reminded her of her sister. The girl had been scared when boarding and had cried. Aisha had smiled at her

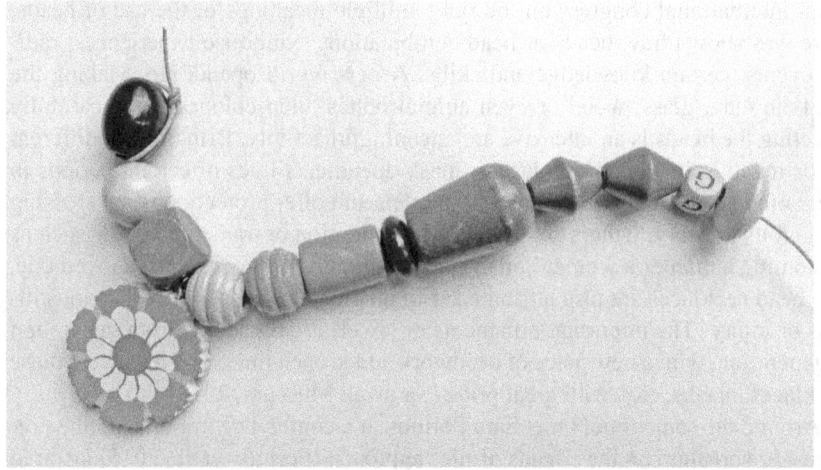

Figure 8.4 String of beads with blue-white flower. Photograph by the author.

and made funny faces like she used to do in the past with her own sister when her mum did crazy things. The skill of 'comforting others' became a flower pearl. Step by step, difficult as well as precious moments and encounters got collected and strung on the beaded strand. This now hangs on her rucksack as an amulet that she can reach back to and hold on to at any time.

Stringing beads is a creative way of expressing, acknowledging and documenting hurt and commitment. It helps to differentiate events, actions and feelings and to place them in a time dimension. This approach allows a sharing with people involved (parents, family members, social workers, teachers, friends) something about their experiences but also about their responses. It can be a testimony of efforts, relational involvement skills, strengths and commitment (Vermeire & van Hennik, 2017). By locating the different stories and their meanings in beads and threading these beads on a strand, we get a materialised novel with a wealth of events, encounters, difficulties, unexpected twists and unique outcomes (Portnoy, Girling & Fredman, 2015). If we want to give complexity a place, we must also make room in the stringing of beads for the variety and multiplicity of clients' stories. In the process, just as working with timelines we are not trying to make a correct, complete chain but try to weave more coherent narratives which also enhance a sense of coherence (Vermeire & van Hennik, 2017). As Bruner (1990) refers to a good novel, which also does not give away everything but leaves space and a certain indeterminacy for the reader, so that people can enter into a dialogue with the many facets whereby new meanings can be created again and again.

In a similar way, documenting with beads can bundle stories temporarily and locally and at the same time be a tangible testimony of experiences, without fixing everything. This local and temporary capturing is important to be able to hold on to what has unfolded in our conversations. It offers a counterbalance to the limited tenability of interpretations after the conversation has ended, as well as a symbolic network to turn to when the difficulties return to the foreground (Sermijn, 2020).

Involving the audience in life review interviews

Through our therapeutic journey with children, families and their network, we reflect on painful events, unravel and process difficulties while gathering new and forgotten pieces and new perspectives unfold. After a while, it is good to collect these different aspects and biographical meanings and bring them together in a more coherent way and connecting our discoveries with significant people. Inviting children or youngsters for a life review interview provides a powerful way to weave several threads so that more coherent narratives emerge.

We take stock together while walking through their lives and do this in the presence of an audience. By engaging witnesses, we hope that what is developed in the therapy room and in conversations will also be noticed and given a right to exist by significant others, and will come more to live in their world, even evoke change in their networks. This 'life review' interview and process can create openings to acknowledge the sufferings and to take steps towards reconnection or reconciliation. Sharing these processed experiences and developed narratives with an increasingly wider audience, brings what happened in their lives and social world back into the community. This process can consolidate, sustain and extend the steps already taken.

I will first focus on the possibilities and context of a 'life review interview' and second on the importance of re-connecting with significant others and a community.

We consider a life review interview as a reflective, recursive conversation about the different processes in one's life. These processes are related to their current situation and their future projects and expectations. We draw on Mary Catherine Bateson's idea that 'composing a life involves a continual re-imaging of the future and reinterpretation of the past to give meaning to the present' (1989, pp. 29–30).

By gathering together for a life review interview, we reposition ourselves as interviewers, the child or youngster becomes the interviewee and the significant people invited become an audience. We open the full stage for them as Taiwo Afuape (2011) says we have to listen to the people who were most oppressed. The children are invited as experts of their lives by experience and the audience can contribute to the further developments of their life. These interviews are also informed by what White (2007) called definitional ceremonies, referring to the work of Myerhoff (1982, 2007). These ceremonies are rituals that can acknowledge and 'regrade' people's lives. They provide people with the option of telling or performing the stories of their lives before an audience of carefully chosen witnesses (White, 2007, p.165).

Denborough (2005) developed an interesting framework for receiving and documenting these kinds of testimonies. Starting from articulating and sharing hopes in giving testimonies, he suggests to explore the values and commitments linked with these hopes and to historicise them. Based on these ideas we invite the child or young person to reflect carefully with whom they want to share their life stories and who they would love to be present as witnesses. Besides questioning what they hope by their testimonies we also ask what they hope the significant people will notice and what kind of acknowledgement they are longing for. In articulating and making visible their hopes and wishes for their lives, relationships and even their communities, we don't accept that their history is a definition of their lives or that they are a hostage of their history (Mukamana, 2021).

Grace (age 16, see Chapter 5) agrees after several conversations with her mentor to come for a 'life review interview'. She wants her mum, Solange, to be present but with the clear instruction that she has to 'keep silent' during the interview. Grace hopes that her mum finally notices and understands what things meant to her in the past and how she missed her mum. Secretly she hopes that her mother can be a little bit proud of her and that all her efforts have not been 'for nothing'. Her mentor from the children's home and her best friend are also invited. To them, she hopes to make it clear that her sometimes awkward, difficult or unpredictable actions are not meant personally. On the contrary. As the interview will be recorded, she hopes some other youngsters can benefit from the stories she will share. Maybe it even can help them not to fall into the same traps and feel less lonely. Finally, she would like to offer some advice to the carers and psychologists.

In the interview we first collect small safe islands to stand on and identify 'teams of mutual support and solidarity' so we can make room for the experiences and testimonies of disadvantage, adversity and injustice. We ask for their responses, their ways to endure and hold on to what and who are precious to them. We have to keep our ears open to particular moments and small actions that often haven't been taken into account as meaningful, valuable responses, invitations or utterances of relational involvement neither by the child nor the audience. These entry points can be stepping stones to reveal alternative understandings and can open new, wider perspectives in everyone present.

We try to spot:

- Moments of 'doing emotions' like crying, shouting, making themselves invisible.
- Moments of 'body (re)actions' or actions in relation to their body.
- Moments of worrying, fretting, hesitating, doubt, suspicion, (dis)trust.
- Moments of making choices, taking a decision, standing up for oneself or others.
- Moments of ambivalence, contrasts, conflict and confrontations.
- Moments of shame, guilt, self-contempt.
- …

Or

We try to spot small acts of living (Wade, 1997; White, 2006; Yuen, 2009).

- Small acts to cherish or hold on to what and who was/is important.
- Small acts of preserving or preventing from getting lost.
- Small acts to stay involved, connected or loyal to certain people, groups, communities.
- Small acts to invite people into their lives.
- Small acts to resist the intrusive effects of the adversity:
  - Small actions not to let the adversity or painful experiences take over and have a total grip on you, your loved ones and your daily life.
  - Small acts of 'keep on going', 'remain standing', 'protect themselves or others', 'try to stay safe', acts of incantation, …
  - Small acts of consolation, calming oneself, asking help, …
- Small acts to keep running daily life.
- Small acts of others that were supportive, offered a stance to go on, …
- Small new, surprising actions, initiatives or discoveries.
- …

During the interview, Grace says she often tried to intervene in the arguments at home. She was always alert to possible signs that the quarrels might flare up. To this day she immediately intervenes in all kinds of discussions in the hope of avoiding quarrels. She explains how she learned to put on a poker face, at first so as not to show how scared she was, but later it helped her not to feel any pain. At first, she was terribly worried about her mother. That something terrible would happen to her was an unbearable thought. The poker face also seemed to be about not wanting to show how much she missed her mother, an attempt not to feel the longing for her love any longer. When talking about the placement in children's homes and her running away, I asked not only what she was trying to run away from but also what she was looking for. Her answer, 'real love', opened the possibility of exploring what she meant by 'real love', where and how she had tasted real love and with whom she had experienced it.

The interview format offers a context in which the child chooses which questions they want to respond to. At the same time, it allows us to ask difficult, abrasive questions. The child can share stories that have not been told before, sometimes 'unfinished', sometimes unflattering, still ambiguous and contradictory (Wasserman & Fisher-Yoshida, 2017). We have to be aware that stories can evoke discomfort and feelings of shame. As an interviewer we keep the audience in mind all the time, as we want them to hear and relate to what is important and of value in the child's life.

As Grace ended up in contexts of sexual exploitation, I ask her what kind of love she found in these places.

G: *I told myself it was true love. In the beginning, D. gave me everything I had ever longed for. I was stupid and naïve but at the same time maybe tomorrow*

I go back to him. I think I became just like my mother. I am stuck: 'Love is blind'.

S: *What does this 'blind love' try to convince you of? What ideas about love are linked with 'blind love'? The moments you are trapped in those painful situations, how do you keep yourself going? What made you keep going in previous periods?*

...

A bit later I ask if she has lost her faith in 'true love' or if there is still a glimmer of hope. Are there any beliefs she kept defending? What kind of values and principles about love has she managed to protect?

Step by step we link all these moments, periods, small actions and valuable encounters into threads that can be woven into the larger fabric of their lives. Throughout the interview and dialogues the youngsters can begin to understand themselves through more coherent narratives and regain a sense of continuity. We hope this also happens to the listeners. These enriched and more coherent (self-) understandings are considered an important component of resilience (Focht-Birkerts & Beardslee, 2000) that does not exist in a vacuum or only within the therapist–child dyad. Furthermore, it is necessary that the child can re-appear as active participants in their lives and relationships, not only to themselves but also to the significant people. We hope the audience becomes moved and connects with the stories in new ways. By listening from a position of an audience they can hear and discover painful as well as alternative stories and new meanings. This allows the audience to respond in novel ways, which can create space for acknowledging the youngster's experiences.

Networks of acknowledgement and care

Weingarten (2003) emphasises that our job as caring individuals is to acknowledge losses, to support mourning and grief, to humanise the enemy, and to witness individual and collective pain with as much heartfelt compassion as we can muster. Life review interviews form powerful contexts where acknowledgement and forgiveness, to a certain extent, can be accomplished. I often notice that children and youngsters are eager to participate because they long to be seen and to experience recognition of their sufferings in the past. This 'life review storytelling' is a collaborative, social performance (Denborough, 2008). It is a joint action that leads to shared understandings and as such to the (re)linking of lives. In the life review sessions we can invite and engage different types of compassionate witnesses (Weingarten, 2003). They can be persons involved in the child's life, or persons that are unknown to the child/youngster, or they can even be an anonymous audience.

After the interview, we ask Solange, Grace's mother, to respond as a witness to these stories being recounted, but also as a mother who is a part of these stories. She is moved by all the painful things that happened and also by Grace's ideas of love. She recognises the many struggles and she says she feels responsible for how things turned out. She would so desperately like to undo her mistakes for the sake of Grace. Unfortunately, she cannot turn back the clock. She wants to try to accept that Grace may have doubts about her for a long time to come. Although she is so eager to help her daughter, she says she understands that she cannot impose this help on her. She hopes that Grace will find a way to deal with all these confusing emotions. Her witnessing ends by making explicit what she is proud of in listening to Grace. She finds Grace incredibly brave and is so glad she keeps going on, and that she is not giving up 'her belief in true love'. She is touched by how Grace managed to cherish a lot of important things. She wishes her enough people around her to support her in the future and if she can, she certainly wants to contribute to that.

A conversational structure that offers family members, parents, carers who hurt the child or failed to empathise more accurately with children's distress, enables them to respond more appropriately and more sensitively to their experiences and nestled stories. The willingness to repair what has been rent in relationships is one of the most precious gifts we can give to others and ourselves (Weingarten, 2003). Hurt creates an opportunity to repair and make stronger what has been torn by harm. Failure to do so can create a second injury. This means the work of repairing relationships extends forward in time, affecting generations of the future. However, it is important not to be too 'idealistic' in these situations. We must not push children or young people and the family members involved in a 'mandatory' direction.

Forgiveness and repairing is best conceived of as complex realms and journeys (Mukamana, 2020). In pursuing them we need to be very sensitive and resist the urge to erase the complexity. Our goal isn't a simple 'moving forward and re-unification of a happy family'. On the contrary, we have to be aware of the political context of obligation and nature of, or motivation for, pardoning. We need to try to introduce the notion of choice (Jenkins et al., 2003) and to create opportunities.

Grace is relieved by her mother's witnessing. She is glad her mum noticed her hard work and didn't try to ease all the pain (like she used to do before). She thinks that there is still a lot that connects them but she feels that there is also a lot that she wants to let seep in and think about. She expresses the wish to have a next conversation with her mum about 'real love'.

At a certain point forgiveness may be important in finding ways to go on. But some people have done such terrible things that from their perspective 'asking for forgiveness' would be considered highly inappropriate. In having conversations with several Rwandan people who survived genocide, I was also inspired by some ideas of the Ibuko team (Mukamana, 2020):

Forgiveness doesn't make the other person who did harm 'clean' but sometimes it makes it possible to 'live' without carrying that weight of trauma. When a person can forgive, it can sometimes mean a step forward living in peace with themselves. It can offer 'a peace of mind' as it stops occupying their mind. This act can also mean letting go of fear and suspicion to some extent.

A few weeks later, Grace writes a letter to her mum in which she says she no longer wants to blame her mother for everything that happened. At the same time, she doesn't want to forget it because she wants to keep in mind what she missed so badly. She hopes that one day they might get closer again. For the time being, she wants to concentrate on 'still making something out of her life'.

A theatre play as compassionate witnessing

The importance of compassionate witnessing does not only concern the important people in the child's life. It makes a real difference whether the child can look at themselves and their history with compassion and kindness. Witnessing oneself, one's injuries, relationships and lives as the ability to reflect on one's experience is found to be a key capacity that fosters resilience (Fonagy & Target, 1997). It allows one to witness the multiplicity of self and to witness others. Without this ability we are much more likely to repeat the past. This capacity to witness can be compromised at any point in our lives, as well as nurtured (Weingarten, 2003).

Aisha, just like Grace, was 'imprisoned' by relationships of sexual exploitation. In conversations about her life until now, some horrible stories about traumatic experiences came in bits and pieces. The ways in which she hurt herself and often still hurts herself were also painful to notice and hear, for instance cutting herself and burning the wounds with hairspray. She herself seemed almost impassive, resigned, still concluding that she was hopeless and worthless despite the many efforts and worthwhile involvements we noticed.

At that time we were engaged in a project 'Voices from the margins' in the context of the 5th European Narrative Conference (Antwerp, Belgium, July 2019). Girls in situations of sexual exploitation are often seen and understood as stupid, naïve girls and as victims of abusive men. Neither professionals nor their environment get a grip on their situation. During our project, we interviewed several girls with adverse childhood experiences and in the grip of sexual exploitation. Together we went on a therapeutic journey and asked them to help us to discover what could still make a difference in their lives.

We asked Aisha if we could bring all the shared bits and pieces of her story together in a text and so into more coherent narratives. Until then, Aisha didn't really 'witness' her own life story during the interviews and conversations but remained locked in the same mantras and final conclusions. We asked a theatre actress to read and perform the text to her. Danny Keuppens, her family counsellor with whom she collected and wove these story pieces into a theatre monologue and I were present as 'witnesses'.

As Aisha listened to and looked at a 'performance of her life' presented by the actress, she was able for the first time to look at herself in a kind of mirror. Tears rolled down her cheeks. She could connect emotionally with the stories and the girl in the stories performed. She noticed that maybe she wasn't as naïve and stupid as said. This girl had still done something, trying to protect her sister and at the same time holding on to some important values. With eager eyes she waited for our witnessing. We offered her a box with beads symbolising what touched us and what she gave us by this sharing. After this 'performance' she asked if we could do this performance once more but this time in the presence of her sister, mother and carers.

Some children and youngsters have lost their capacity to witness themselves. They can benefit from meeting others who are dedicated to restoring the capacity to witness even to those who have endured unimaginable suffering. The knowledge that some people are willing to provide compassionate witnessing reactivates the capacity to witness oneself (Weingarten, 2003).

As music and singing helped Aisha to keep going in hard times and also was linked with her culture and family, we offered her the possibility to record her favourite songs with a well-known Flemish musician. We weaved the Somalian lullaby that her mother used to sing to her as a child but also her recorded songs 'What is love?' (Haddaway) and 'Take a bow' (Rihanna) through the theatre play. The last song she sang together with her sister. This theatre play was also weaved with stories, actions and knowledge of girls in similar situations and became finally called 'What is love?' We started to reflect on the possibilities of a performance for a larger audience that could bring some further recognition, new understandings and reconnection.

Some horrible, all-consuming experiences can be difficult to put into words, while bringing them out into the open can prove very helpful. A few years ago I had the occasion to visit an exhibition of Ai Weiwei in London. He made an artwork, 'Straight', after an earthquake in China that caused school buildings to collapse. The buildings turned out to be very badly constructed, with concrete of inferior quality. Five thousand schoolchildren died as a result. With his team he collected the twisted rebars and straightened them. With the straightened rebars, a kind of memorial was erected in a room that had the names of all the deceased children displayed on the walls.

By incorporating children's sufferings and ways to go on into a work of art, a play, a book, etc., the experiences are transformed, 'delimited' but also given a 'place'. They are situated in a location and in a period in time, but can still be 'visited', 'remembered' and 'witnessed'.

Robby (13 years) made in clay a small 'Gollum' referring to the things his sister did to him. He decided to put this Gollum in a large Chinese vase at his grandmother's. He considered her as the best guardian of these painful stories. It means that they are not always with him but not completely erased either.

The Belgian philosopher Visker referred to 'The Truth and Reconciliation Report' as meant to be an actual report but also as a book of 'monumental recognition'. A monument exists in the public sphere, where people can see it, can walk by it, can ignore it, or become interested. Visker stressed that at a certain point, it is no longer possible to get personal recognition, and then one requires 'monumental recognition', and part of that monumental recognition is that you bring it out into the open (quoted in van den Berge, 2017).

We asked Aisha what it would mean to her if the actress performed the 'theatre play' and so parts of her 'edited' life story at the European Narrative Conference for therapists and social workers and later also in the City Hall for whoever could be interested.

In this way, stories, which were private until then, are processed and carefully made public and visible. They enter the social arena where they are heard and seen by a large, anonymous audience. With works as 'Straight' Ai Weiwei renders social issues visible as a form of political protest. In the same vein we address societal problems while taking the children's voices out of the margins.

At the end of the first public performance of 'What is love?' we invited the audience to witness and write on a piece of paper to Aisha what they took away for themselves, their work, their life and what small actions this could possibly lead to.

A few weeks later I stand at the front door of the building where Aisha lives. At the entrance I have to ask some guys, clearly under the influence of drugs, to let me through. It is a neighbourhood where a small flat is just affordable for a 17-year-old girl without financial support from her family or friends, but where you would not want your own daughter to stay.

Her room is a mess and it is suffocating hot. She is really excited and dressed herself specially for this visit. She asks me to read the letters to her as she is too nervous to read them herself. She says she is even a bit afraid of what people will say about her or think of her story. After reading the first ones, she asks if I want to read some more of them.

'People say such nice things!', 'Do you think they mean it?' I take four more sheets of paper out of the box and start to read. 'Can you read a bit slower?', 'Yes! They noticed very well that my sister is really important and supportive to me'. 'I think people have listened very careful!' 'Maybe they are right: I have worked very hard for my friends and family. There are times I tried to resist and tried to be a good friend'. After reading some more of those messages, she asks if I want to go on … It's true I never stopped believing in love. I still hope for a good relationship! With a big smile on her face, she asks if I would mind to read all the letters and messages … More than 80 personal reflections of what touched or resonated in her story and of what people took with them. Finally, I ask her what name she would give to this moment. She answers: 'Filling my heart with warmth'.

Sometimes we have the opportunity to re-link stories and lives in even wider circles and engage people in unexpected forms of compassionate witnessing. It also enhances a community support system where people feel collective accountability to take care of each other.

A few months later, I did a training in Rwanda and four Somalian social workers and psychologists participated. I showed some parts of the recorded theatre play and they recognised the lullaby Aisha's mum used to sing. These four sang the whole song especially for her and added some messages. We recorded and sent it by WhatsApp video. As Aisha left Somalia when she was two years old, this felt as 'a double heart-warming cultural connection and acknowledgement'.

Re-linking lives as social action

All our meetings and journeys have the potential to become contributions to larger purposes. Convinced as we are of the connectedness of many of these children's problems and struggles with broader socio-economic challenges, we believe it to be our responsibility to consider ways of re-linking the personal with the political. In moving away from singular pathologising and psychologising the child and their family, we make visible the social and political roots of problems.

Girls like Aisha and Grace in the grip of 'sexual exploitation', but also youngsters like Steff, Farida or Ahmed who became violent themselves, are often seen as 'a threat' to themselves, to others and to society. They must, therefore, be protected from themselves and others. They are taken to 'safety' (closed units) and much effort is made to bring them back on the 'right path'. Public opinion but also the view of professionals is often narrowed in the sense that a sensitivity for the social concerns and the idea of collective care and responsibility get lost.

By making their stories public, for example by having Aisha's play performed, we can promote a richer and broader social understanding and hopefully create some ripples in stubborn beliefs of society and communities. Through providing forums for the hardship of youngsters and their families and the many stories linked with this hardship, there can grow a new, shared concern. As Denborough (2008, p. 192) said: the person is not the problem, the problem is the problem and the solution is not only personal, but rather opportunities have to be created for collective contribution and for people to contribute to 'social movement'. Denborough has no grand social actions in mind, but rather local, meaningful, resonant, sustainable, social actions or social contributions.

Contributions to the lives of future generations and those whose lives are affected by these social issues can be done by sharing their struggles, relational involvements and efforts, just like their local initiatives, skills and knowledge with youngsters in similar situations but even more by sharing it with youngsters more widely, people of their community, carers, professionals and policy makers. In doing so we hope to foster collective care and resilience. Just like Reynolds emphasises that our collective care, and our collective sustainability is reciprocal, communal and inextricably linked with spirited practices of solidarity (Reynolds, 2012).

A documentary, 'Zone(n) 050', has been made by Danny Keuppens, the family counsellor of the theatre project. Boys in our hometown, mainly from immigrant families, hanging around at 'problematic places and parks' and who were

referred to by the police as 'hopeless criminals' have been narratively inter-
viewed. They were invited to present their world to us and asked what and who
makes or made a valuable contribution to their life until now. Most of them had
been placed in youth prison in the previous years. The documentary was shown
to the police, the mayor and to social workers of our hometown, Ghent. After
the performance these boys debated with them about their wishes and hopes for
their neighbourhood. This evoked some important ripples in how the government
positions and acts in relation to these areas and children living there. http://www
.zonen050.com/en/front-page-english/.

In these projects the personal, social and political get interweaved and can
cause small ripples of social change. These local, social actions contribute to a
sense of belonging and solidarity.

Ongoing conversations of documents and testimonies

The harvest of our conversations and quests can easily be overshadowed by the
daily rush, interpersonal hassles and dominant social perspectives and discourses.

> Conversation is, by its very nature, ephemeral. After a particularly meaning-
> ful session, a client walks away aglow with provocative new thoughts, but a
> few blocks away, the exact words that had struck home as so profound may
> already be hard to recall.
>
> (Freeman, Epston & Lobovitz, 1997, p. 112)

Letters, written parts of our conversations just like documented images or created objects mirror the words found, emotions shared and developed thoughts of
the child, carers and therapist and give them something tangible to hold on to. In
these specific contexts these documents can have the effect of acknowledgement.
They provide existence to the sufferings and the work done by the child or persons
involved.

Selin (17) came for more than 30 conversations to talk about traumatic experi-
ences in the past. After each meeting I wrote her a letter in her words about what
we discussed, what we discovered, how she wanted to relate to these things and
new meanings found. I sent the letters by email attachment. She never read the
letters, kept them in a digital map on her laptop. Each time I asked if she still
wanted to receive a letter, she nodded convincingly 'yes'. It became a kind of
testimonies of what had been done to her and, above all, of her continued efforts
not to be overwhelmed by it or letting her life be dominated by it. At the end of our
therapeutic journey, she brought a special box to put the USB stick in.

When children or youngsters read the letters afterwards, they may experience
acknowledgement both to the sufferings and to the steps forward or steps in new
directions. They may feel heard and supported by the coherence provided by the
written text. In the process of talking, writing and reading, one takes up different

positions each time again. The letters or any form of recording allow for an ongoing conversation in which, on re-reading, re-watching, re-taking, one can reposition oneself or new reflections and ideas can emerge.

It can also help to enhance connection between family members, the environment and the professional network (Wilson, 1998).

After each session I send Toby (age six) and his foster mother a letter about what Toby and I did together, talked about and discovered. The foster mother reads these letters to Toby in between the sessions.

These letters contribute to the continuity and consolidation of the newly found stories regarding aspects of the relationships and the person. They are a kind of 'travel document' that sustain a sense of coherence. The letters weave threads between the different conversations, the different stories, and at the same time they document and strengthen the collaboration between Toby and foster mother. They can also share these letters with others and receive new reflections.

Parts of the letters were sent to the case-manager. When Toby's mother was located after having disappeared for months and brought back to the rehab centre, he handed her some of the letters (Vermeire, 2020).

During this process we document a kaleidoscopic palette of these children's and their families' lives. These travel documents can be seen as testimonies of our therapeutic journey and their migration of meanings and identities. They may facilitate transitions, in the sense of 'rites of passage' (van Gennep, 1960; Fox, 2003). They can contribute to capturing and integrating new identities (Madsen, 2007, p. 237).

Each time, we can carefully reflect on using creative ways that connect with their world and fit into the circles in which they live. Denborough (2012, 2018) refers to the use of locally resonant songs and folk cultural treasures that sustain people in hard times.

Xander (see Chapter 1) at the age of 14 became increasingly interested in hip hop, street dance and rap songs. We thought together about what was occupying his mind could be put into rap songs and how this was connected with other rappers in Belgium and the world. Especially when his mother left life and two years later his father, writing rap songs and finding the most fitting beats became an important source of support and help. Through words, images and music, he created a whole vocabulary and language linked with this rap culture. By sharing the lyrics and songs with his friends and the community of rappers, he felt understood, supported and connected in the circles and language of this culture. Once the rap songs were put on a streaming platform, more and more other youngsters joined and shared their songs. He was even invited to share his stories on a Facebook page, 'ScarsBe' (LittekensBe). On this page young people share their 'survival ways' of adverse childhood experiences.

Making these works of art, plays, books, rap songs public can offer recognition or comfort to others in similar situations. A collective archive that children, youngsters but also adults can consult and in which they can be part of building is a valuable aspect of enhancing collective agency and resilience processes. Their suffering has not been for nothing (Newman, 2021).

A rap song Xander wrote after his mother died

Mama (Mommy in Dutch)
My mother didn't bother,
Looking for answers on the bottom of a bottle.
Falling like autumn leaves.
But never left me.
She sometimes smelled like paralyses
But never wavered giving me a kiss
With open or closed wrists
She would embrace in bliss.
Never dismissed from the fact that I miss.
Mommy you know I try to resist resistance.
Our distance is another plane of existence I would like to visit,
But people still need my assistance
I hate my persistence in this system
Mommy do you read what I have written?
Mommy the snake of your absence has bitten.
The poison has driven me insane
And this time I can't put the blame
So I am not able to frame and give my pity a name,
I feel so ashamed
That I couldn't tame the sadness
I need your experience in my creative madness,
I levitate but I can't find your spiritual address
I access states that relaxes me
But actually I'd rather be with you
But I have something to do, a dream that I have to pursue,
And a nightmare that I have to go through that is ...
Living life without you.

These and other kinds of creative 'documents', like the bead strands, are ways of symbolically giving experiences and their meanings a place. At the same time they become testimonies as you can keep them close or even 'hold on to them' when required. Art works, rap songs, just like tattoos can have symbolic meaning and contain important values they want to cherish.

Guluzar survived many painful adversities as a child. People became unreliable and still feel completely insecure. Only animals keep her here in this life. She speaks their language as no one else. Seventeen dogs, a horse and a bear sanctuary are her daily concern. Every significant animal in her life so far is tattooed on her body. It also symbolises who she was in this life until now and wants to be. It reminds her of what it means to 'care' and 'be loved'.

Letting go

Resilience does not mean bouncing back unscathed, but rather struggling well, effectively working through and attempting to integrate one's experiences into the fabric of one's life (Higgings, 1994). The fact that children and their families regain a sense of agency, mattering, belonging and coherence doesn't mean that things are 'solved' or 'processed' once and for all. Significant journeys are rarely linear experiences, simply moving in one direction, ramping up continuously while life improves measurably with each day that passes (Duvall & Béres, 2011). One's 'life story work' is a never-ending puzzle as each new puzzle piece can become an invitation to reinterpretation. Each new experience or story told, each new developmental stage and so each new context can reshuffle the puzzle pieces and bring back old memories that threaten the hard-won sense of coherence. Just like new and old obstacles, constraints or problems can lurk around the corner.

Special family events such as Mother's Day or Father's Day, as well as special family moments such as becoming a mother or father oneself or the death of an abusive parent, can be moments that bring certain intrusive questions to the foreground or reopen certain wounds. Just as these children or family members regularly have to weigh up who they can tell about their life stories and when. *When do you tell your new boyfriend that your father abused you, or is it better to keep quiet about it?* They can be confronted like in each person's life with new and old contexts of unsafety or uncertainty and so the risk of getting entangled again in unhelpful dances is ever present. Transitions, tilting moments or pivotal moments ensure that they have to relate again and again and take a position with regard to the events.

A few years ago, Flora came on regular basis for conversations to talk about the abuse by her grandfather. Now, she is a grown up woman, happily married and recently she gave birth to a lovely baby girl. In panic, she calls me and asks for an urgent appointment. Since the baby was born, she can't sleep and can't leave the baby alone. She has to check each five minutes if the baby is still breathing. Together trying to get a notion of what is going on and what is having a grip on her, she says she promised herself and her child to protect her fully 100 per cent. She doesn't want her to go through what she went through. She is already 'falling' in her own eyes as she can't protect her totally. Together we try to understand, in a broader picture, what is happening, reflecting on the different reciprocal influencing relations and contexts and recall all the ideas, skills and knowledge collected previously.

Rutten (1999) and other researchers found that responding well to adversity is a resilience factor in itself. Our attitudes to ourselves and our confidence in our ability to deal effectively with life challenges are likely to be influenced by how we coped with stress and challenges in the past.

Once the child, their family and networks can go on without the therapist or counsellor, it is important to let them develop their own tracks. The ultimate meaning of their experiences cannot be pinned down in a story and is always evolving.

Weaving threads of care, hope and agency is an ongoing collective process. So every now and then it may be necessary to 'refuel', in the same way that the need to constantly find unique, creative ways of moving forward never disappears.

Xander is now a youth worker in a music and dance studio where disadvantaged children and youngsters living in a tough neighbourhood, can record their own created music. A few months ago, life became increasingly hopeless for Lewis, a young man in foster care. Skating and writing rap songs were a few things that kept him going. We asked Lewis if he would be interested in meeting 'Xander' and recording one of his rap songs. He immediately said 'Yes'! That evening they met, together with his foster care counsellor, I witnessed two young men speaking the same miraculous language: a hand gesture, a head nod, 'rap-music-slang', English terms whose meaning escapes me. Above all it was a shared language of painful histories, anger and sadness but also resilience, going on and not giving up. A team of resilience emerging in front of our eyes.

In contexts of adverse childhood experiences, doing hope means an ongoing weaving of networks of resilience and resilience processes. In the book '*The boy, the mole, the fox and the horse*', the boy asks: '*What do we do when our heart hurts?*' The horse replies: '*Then we wrap it in friendship-shared tears and time, until it wakes up happy and full of hope*' (Mackesy, 2019). Although we often cannot cure a child's heart, we can try to wrap it up in a joint and persistent search for ways to a liveable future.

References

Afuape, T. (2011). *Power, resistance and liberation in therapy with survivors of trauma.* New York: Routledge.

Alon, N., & Omer, H. (2006). *The psychology of demonization.* Taylor and Francis Ltd.

Anderson, A., & Gehart, D. (2007). *Collaborative therapy. Relationships and conversations that make a difference.* New York/London: Routledge.

Anderson, H., & Goolishian, H. (1988). Human systems as linguistic systems: Preliminary and evolving ideas about the implications for clinical theory. *Family Process, 27* (4), 371–393.

Antonovsky, A (1987). *Unraveling the mystery of health.* San Francisco: Jossey-Bass.

Arao, B., & Clemens, K. (2013). From safe spaces to brave spaces. A new way to frame dialogue around diversity and social justice. In L. Landreman (Ed.), *From the art of effective facilitation* (pp. 135–150). Stylus Publishing LL.

Audet, C., & Paré, D. (Eds.) (2018). *Social justice and counseling. Discourse in practice.* New York: Routledge.

Barrat, S., & Lobatto, W. (Eds.) (2016). *Surviving and thriving in care and beyond. Personal and professional perspectives.* London: Karnac Books Ltd.

Barrett, P.M., Rapee, R.M., Dadds, M.M., & Ryan, S.M. (1996). Family enhancement of cognitive style in anxious and aggressive children. *Journal of Abnormal Child Psychology, 24,* 187–203.

Bateson, G. (1979). *Mind and nature: A necessary unity (advances in systems theory, complexity, and the human sciences).* New York: Hampton Press.

Bateson, M.C. (1989). *Composing a life.* New York: Atlantic Monthly Press.

Beckers, W. (2016). Netwerkversterking als antigif voor strijd voor hoogconflicten na echtscheiding. *Systemisch Bulletin, 34,* 277–293.

Beckers, W., Jakob, P., & Schreiter, M. (2022). Mattering and parental presence in systemic therapy using nonviolent resistance: The utilization of imaginary methods. *Family Process, 61,* 507–519.4.

Berceli, D. (2008). *The revolutionary trauma release process: Transcend your toughest times.* Vancoucer: Namaste Publishing Inc.

Bertrando, & Arcelonni (2014). Emotions in the practice of systemic therapy. *Australian & New Zealand Journal of Family Therapy, 35,* 123–135.

Bird, J. (2004). *Talk that sings.* New Zealand: Edge Press.

Bourdieu, P. (1987). *Distinction. A social critique of the judgement of taste.* Harvard University Press.

Bowlby, J. (1982). *Attachment and loss: Vol.1. Attachment.* New York: Basic Books.

Breeuwsma, G. (1993). *Alles over de ontwikkeling. De grondslagen van de ontwikkelingspsychologie*. Boom/Amsterdam: Open Universiteit.

Breeuwsma, G. (2001). *De constructie van de levensloop*. Boom/Amsterdam: Open Universiteit.

Bruner, J. (1986). *Actual minds, possible worlds*. Cambridge, Massachusetts: Harvard University Press.

Bruner, J. (1990). *Acts of meaning*. Harvard: Harvard University Press.

Burnham, J. (2009). Workshop: *Creativity and play in conversations with children, adolescents and their families*. 12 June 2009, Antwerp.

Burnham, J. (2012). Developments in social GGRRAAACCEEESSS: Visible-invisible, voiced-unvoiced. In I. Krause (Ed.), *Cultural reflexivity*. London: Karnac.

Byng-Hall, J. (1995). Creating a secure family base: Some implications of attachment theory for family therapy. *Family Process, 34*, 45–58.

Carr, A. (2012). *Family therapy. Concepts, process and practice* (3rd ed.). Oxford: Wiley-Blackwell.

Carter, B., & McGoldrick, M. (2004). *The expanded family life cycle. Individual, family, and social perspectives*. Boston: A Pearson Education Company.

Cecchin, G. (1987). Hypothesising, circularity and neutrality revisited: An invitation to curiosity. *Family Process, 26*, 405–413.

Cecchin, G., Lane, G., & Ray, W. (1992). *Irreverance: A strategy for therapist's survival*. London: Karnac.

Cooklin, A. (2001). Eliciting children's thinking in families and family therapy. *Family Process, 40*(3), 293–312.

Cornfeld, E. (2018). *Quantum leaps from the safe space: A week long 'Intensive' narrative family gathering in response to childhood sexual abuse*. Adelaide: Dulwich Centre.

Crittenden, Claussen P., & Claussen, A. (2003). *The organization of attachment relationships. Maturation, culture and context*. Cambridge: University Press.

Dallos, R. (2005). Narratives of young offenders. In A. Vetere & E. Dowling. *Narrative therapies with children and their families*, 219–238. London: Routledge.

Dallos, R. (2006). *Attachment narrative therapy*. Maidenhead: Open University Press.

Daniel, G. (2018). *Family dramas: Intimacy power and systems in Shakespeare's tragedies*. London: Routledge.

Daniel, G., & Wren, B. (2005). Narrative therapy with children in families where a parent has a mental health problem. In A. Vetere & E. Dowling. *Narrative therapies with children and their families*, 119–139. London: Routledge.

De Botton, A. (2000). *The consolations of philosophy*. Hamish Hamilton.

Decraemer, K. (2010). Vele wegen leiden naar trauma. *Systeemtheoretisch Bulletin, 28*(2), 115–139.

Decraemer, K. (2021). Trauma in Verbinding. Over individuele systemische trauma exposure. *Systemisch Bulletin, 38*(3), 197–227.

De Jaegher, H., & Di Paolo, E. (2007). Participatory sense-making. *Phenomenology and the Cognitive Sciences, 6*(4), 485–507.

De Mol, J., & Buysse, A. (2008a). The phenomenology of children's influence on parents. *Journal of Family Therapy, 30*, 163–193.

De Mol, J., & Buysse, A. (2008b). Understandings of children's influence in parental-child relationships: A Q-methodological study. *Journal of Social and Personal Relationships, 25*, 359–379.

De Mol, J., & Rimé, B. (2017). Depressie bij jongeren: Het gezin als bron van verandering en een plaats voor het delen van emoties met anderen. Of hoe mijn depressie ook mijn vriend kan worden. In S. Vermeire & J. Sermijn (Eds.), *Wegen naar her-binding – Narratieve, collaboratieve en dialogische praktijken* (pp. 219–228). Antwerpen: Interactie-Academie.

De Mol, J., Reijmers, E., Verhofstadt, L., & Kuczynski, L. (2018). Reconstructing a sense of relational agency in family therapy. *Australian & New Zealand Journal of Family Therapy, 39*, 54–66.

De Saint-Exupéry, A. (1995). *The little prince*. Hertfordshire: Wordsworth.

Deleuze, G., & Guattari, F. (2013). *A thousand plateaus*. London: Bloomsbury Academic.

Dell, P. (1989). Violence and the systemic view. The problem of power. *Family Process, 28*(1), 1–14.

Denborough, D. (2005). A framework for receiving and documenting testimonies of trauma. *International Journal of Narrative Therapy & Community Work, 3/4*, 34–42.

Denborough, D. (2008). *Collective narrative practice. Responding to individuals, groups, and communities who have experienced trauma.* Adelaide: Dulwich Centre Publications.

Denborough, D. (2012). A storyline of collective narrative practice: A history of ideas, social projects and partnerships. *The International Journal of Narrative Therapy and Community Work, 1*, 40–56.

Denborough, D. (2018). *Do you want to hear a story? Adventures in collective narrative practice*. Adelaide: Dulwich Centre Publications.

Denborough, D. (2019). Travelling down the neuro-pathway: Narrative practice, neuroscience, bodies, emotions and the affective turn. *Journal of Narrative Therapy and Community Work, 3*, 13–53.

Duncan, B.L., Miller, S.D., Wampold, B.E., & Hubble, M.A. (2010). *The heart and soul of change. Delivering what works in therapy*. Washington: American Psychological Association.

Duvall, J., & Béres, L. (2011). *Innovations in narrative therapy. Connecting practice, training, and research*. New York: W.W. Norton & Company.

Epston, D. (2017). Narrative therapy in Wonderland. In Personal Workshop Conversations and Notes, 9–10 October 2017. Rotterdam, The Netherlands.

Epston, D., & White, M. (1992). *Experience, contradiction, narrative & imagination. Selected papers of David Epston & Michael White 1989–1991*. Adelaide: Dulwich Centre Publications.

Ericksson, M., & Lindstrom, B. (2007). Antonovsky's sense of coherence scale and its relation with quality of life. A systematic review. *Journal of Epidemiology and Community Health, 61*, 938–944.

Faes, M. (2005). Bespiegelingen. De zelfbeleving van kinderen. In E. Reijmers, L. Cottyn, M. Faes (Eds.), *Spelen met werkelijkheden. Systeemtheoretische psychotherapie met kinderen en jongeren* (pp. 88–101). Houten: Bohn Stafleu Van Loghum.

Fisher, A. (2005). Power and the promise of innocent places. *Narrative Network News, 34*, 12–14.

Flaskas, C. (2007). Holding hope and hopelessness: Therapeutic engagements with the balance of hope. *Journal of Family Therapy, 29*, 186–202.

Focht-Birkerts, L., & Beardslee, W.R. (2000). A child's experience of parental depression: Encouraging relational resilience in families with affective illness. *Family Process, 39*, 417–434.

Fonagy, P., & Target, M. (1997). Attachment and reflective function: Their role in selforganization. *Development & Psychopathology, 9*(4), 679–700.

Foucault, M. (1980). *Power/Knowledge. Selected interviews and other writings. 1972–77.* New York: Harvester Wheatsheaf.

Foucault, M. (2007). *Discipline, toezicht en straf. De geboorte van de gevangenis.* Groningen: Historische uitgeverij.

Fox, H. (2003). Using therapeutic documents: A review. *The International Journal of Narrative Therapy and Community Work, 4,* 26–36.

Fredman, G. (2004). *Transforming emotions. Conversations in counselling and psychotherapy.* London: Whurr.

Fredman, G. (2014). Weaving networks of hope with families, practitioners and communities. Inspirations from systemic and narrative approaches. *Australian and New Zealand Journal of Family Therapy, 35,* 54–17.

Fredman, G., & Fruggle, (2000). Parents with mental health problems: Involving the children. In P. Reder, M. McClure, & A. Jolley (Eds.), *Family matters: Interfaces between child and adult mental health.* London: Routledge.

Freedman, J. (2014). Witnessing and positioning: Structuring narrative therapy with families and couples. *The International Journal of Narrative Therapy and Community Work, 1,* 11–17.

Freedman, J., & Combs, G. (1993). Invitations to new stories: Using questions to explore alternative possibilities. In S. Gilligan & R. Price (Eds.), *Therapeutic conversations* (pp. 291–303). New York: Norton.

Freedman, L., & Combs, G. (1996). *Narrative therapy: The social construction of preferred realities.* New York: W. W. Norton & Company.

Freedman, J., & Combs, G. (2002). *Narrative therapy with couples... and a lot more!* Adelaide: Dulwich Centre Publications.

Freeman, J., Epston, D., & Lobovits, D. (1997). *Playful approaches to serious problems: Narrative therapy with children and their families.* New York: W. W. Norton.

Fruggeri, (1992). Therapeutic process as the social construction of change. In Mc Namee & K. Gergen (Eds.), *Therapy as social construction* (pp. 40–53). London: Sage Publications.

Geertz, C. (1973). *The interpretation of culture.* New York: Basic Books.

Gergen, K. (1999). *An invitation into social constructionism.* Thousand Oaks: Sage Publications.

Gergen, K. (2009). *Relational being: Beyond self and community.* New York: Oxford University Press.

Gergen, K.J., Hoffman, L., & Anderson, H. (1996). Is diagnosis a disaster? A constructionist trialogue. In F.W. Kaslow (Ed.), *Handbook of relational diagnosis and dysfunctional family patterns* (pp. 102–118). New York: Wiley.

Golding, K.S., & Hughes, D.A. (2012). *Creating loving attachments. Parenting with PACE to nurture confidence and security in the troubled child.* London: Jessica Kingsley Publishers.

Goldner, V. (1998). The treatment of violence and victimization in intimate relationships. *Family Process, 37*(3), 263–286.

Guishard-Pine, J., McCall, S., & Hamilton, L. (2007). *Understanding looked after children: An introduction to psychology for foster care.* London: Kingsley Publishers.

Hedtke, L. (2014). Creating stories of hope: A narrative approach to illness, death and grief. *The International Journal of Narrative Therapy and Community Work, 1,* 1–10.

Herring, N. (2021). Young people, living in care and adopted, talk about their experiences of receiving an NHS therapeutic intervention. Qualitative research analysed using Interpretative Phenomenological Analysis. *Journal of Family Therapy*, *43*, 426–444.

Higgins, G. (1994). *Resilient adults: Overcoming a cruel past*. San Francisco: Jossey-Bass.

Holzman, L. (2009). *Vygotsky at work and play*. London: Routledge.

Hoogsteder, M., & de Vriese, S. (Eds.) (2012). *Hechting & loyaliteit. Derde druk*. Amsterdam: SWP.

Hughes, D.A. (2007). *Attachment-focused family therapy*. New York, London: W.W. Norton & Company.

Hughes, D.A., & Baylin, J. (2012). *Brain-based parenting: The neuroscience of caregiving for healthy attachment*. New York, London: W.W. Norton.

Jakob, P. (2011). Re-connecting parents and young people with serious behaviour problems. Child-focused practice and reconciliation work in non-violent resistance therapy. New Authority Network International. http://www.newauthority.net/data/cntfiles/146_.pdf.

Jakob, P. (2013). Nonviolence and families in distress: Cocreating positive family narratives against the backdrop of trauma, deprivation, substance misuse and challenging social environments. *Systeemtheoretisch Bulletin*, *31*, 5–27.

Jenkins, A. (2009). *Becoming ethical. A parallel, political journey with men who have abused*. Lyme Regis: Russell House Publishing.

Jenkins, A., Hall, R., & Joy, M. (2003). Forgiveness and child sexual abuse. A matrix of meanings. In Dulwich Centre Publications (Ed.), *Responding to violence*. Adelaide: Dulwich Centre Publications.

Jørring, N.T. (2022). *Narrative psychiatry and family collaborations*. London, New York: Routledge.

Kaseke, S. (2010). 'Standing together on a riverbank': Group conversations about sexual abuse in Zimbabwe. *The International Journal of Narrative Therapy and Community Work*, *2010*(4), 42–44.

Keefer, L.A., Landau, M.J., & Sullivan, D. (2014). Non-human support: Broadening the scope of attachment theory. *Social and Personality Psychology Compass*, *8*(9), 524–535. https://doi.org/10.1111/spc3.12129

Koestler, A. (1964). *The act of creation*. London: Hutchinson & Co. (Publishers) Ltd.

Konijn, C. (2021). *Fostering traumatized children*. Unpublished doctoral dissertation. Research Institute of Child Development and Education (RICDE). University of Amsterdam.

Kristensen, R. (2007). Invitations and integrity. In *A two hours interview with Peter Lang and Jesper Juul interviewed by René Kristensen*. DVD Denmark. https://www.youtube.com/watch?v=ONpkWUgLXnA

Kuczynski, L., & De Mol, J. (2015). Dialectical models of socialization. In W.F. Overton & P.C.M. Molenaar (Eds.), *Theory and method. Handbook of child psychology and developmental science* (7th ed., Vol. 1, pp. 323–368). Hoboken: Wiley. doi: 10.1002/9781118963418.childpsy109

Laing, R., Phillipson, H. and Lee, A.R. (1966). *Interpersonal perception: A theory and a method of research*. London: Tavistock Publications.

Lakoff, G., & Johnson, M. (1999). *Philosophy in the flesh: The embodied mind and its challenge to Western thought*. New York: Basic Books.

Lang, P., & Mc Adam, E., (2001). *Meetings for the first time: Making connections, openings to the best ways forward. Family and network consultations*. Unpublished manuscript, London: Kensington Consultation Centre.

Lobatto, W. (2002). Talking to children about family therapy: A qualitative research study. *Journal of family Therapy*, *24*, 330–343.

Lobatto, W. (2021). Using systemic principles in the design of mental health and wellbeing services for looked after children and young people – Bringing together research, theory and practice. *Journal of Family Therapy*, *43*, 469–488.

Luthar, Cicchetti, & Becker, (2000). The construct of resilience: A critical evaluation and Guidelines for future work. *Child Development*, *71*, 543–562.

Mackesy, C. (2019). *The boy, the mole, the fox and the horse*. London: Ebury Publishing.

MacLeod, J. (1997). *Narrative & psychotherapy*. London: SAGE Publications.

Madigan, S. (2011). *Narrative therapy*. Washington, DC: American Psychological Association.

Madigan, S., & Epston, D. (1998). From'Spy-chiatric Gaze' to communities of concern. From professional monologue to dialogue. In D. Epson (Ed.), *Catching up with David Epston: A collection of narrative practice-based papers published between 1991 & 1996* (chapter 11, pp. 127–148). Adelaide: Dulwich Centre Publications.

Madsen, W.C. (2007). *Collaborative therapy with multi-stressed families*. New York, London: The Guilford Press.

Madsen, W.C. (2009). Collaborative helping: A practice framework for family-centered services. *Family Process, 48,* 103–116.

Madsen, W.C., & Gillespie, K. (2014). *Collaborative helping. A strengths framework for home-based services*. Hoboken: John Wiley & Sons.

Madsen, W.C., Root, B., & Jørring, N.T. (2021). Mattering as the heart of health and human services. *Journal of Contemporary Narrative Therapy, 1,* 19–32.

Malinowski, (1923). The problem of meaning in primitive languages. In C. Ogden, & I. Richard (Eds.), *The meaning of meaning* (pp. 315–336). London: Routledge and Paul Kegan.

Marsten, D., Epston, D., & Markham, L. (2017). *Narrative therapy in Wonderland. Connecting with children's imaginative know-how*. New York: W.W. Norton.

Mattheeuws, A. (1977). Basisconcepten uit de communicatietheorieën en de algemene systementheorie: Toepassing in echtpaartherapie. In: H. Janssens, A. Mattheeuws, M. Nevejan, & J. Verhulst (Eds.), *Benadering van gezinsproblemen: een oriëntatie voor hulpverleners*. Antwerpen/Amsterdam: De Nederlandse Boekhandel.

McAdam, E., & Lang, P. (2003). Appreciërend en toekomstgericht werken binnen een residentiële setting voor jongeren. In Workshop Notes. 16 May 2003, Antwerp, Belgium.

McCarthy, I., & Simon, G. (Eds.) (2016). *Systemic therapy as transformative practice*. Farnhill: Everything is Connected Press.

McNamee, S., & Gergen, K.J. (Eds.) (1992). *Therapy as social construction*. Lonodon: Sage Publications, Inc.

Minuchin, S. (1974). *Families & family therapy*. Cambridge, MA: Harvard University Press.

Minuchin, S., Montalvo, B., Guerney, B., Rosman, B., & Schumer, F. (1967). *Families of the slums: An exploration of their structure and treatment*. New York: Basic Books.

Minuchin, P., Colapinto, J., & Minuchin, S. (1998). *Working with families of the poor* (2nd ed.). New York: Guildford Press.

Moore, L., & Bruna Seu, I. (2011). Giving children a voice: Children's positioning in family therapy. *Journal of Family Therapy*, *33*, 279–301.

Moscovici, S. (1984). The phenomenon of social representations. In R.M. Farr, & S. Moscovici (Eds.), *Social representations* (pp. 18–76). Cambridge: Cambridge University Press.

Mukamana, A. (2020). Survivors supporting survivors: Recalling the history of the Ibuka counseling team. An interview with Adelite Mukamana. *International Journal of Narrative Therapy and Community Work, 2,* 1–7.

Mukamana, A. (2021). Ways of living and survival by children born out of rape during genocide. *International Journal of Narrative Therapy and Community Work, 4,* 1–9.

Mullender, A., Hague, G., Imam, U., Kelly, L., Malos, E., & Regan, L. (2002). *Children's perspectives on domestic violence.* London: SAGE Publications Ltd.

Myerhoff, B. (1982). Life history among the elderly: Performance, visibility, and remembering. IN J. Ruby (Ed.), *A crack in the mirror: Reflexive perspective in anthropology* (99–117). Philadelphia: University of Pennsylvania Press.

Myerhoff, B. (2007). Stories as equipment for living. In M. Kaminsky & M. Weiss (Eds.), *Stories as equipment for living. Last talks and tales of Barbara Myerhoff* (pp. 17–27). Ann Arbor: University of Michigan Press.

Ncube, N. (2006). The tree of life project: Using narrative ideas in work with vulnerable children in Southern Africa. *International Journal of Narrative Therapy and Community Work, 1,* 3–16.

Newman, D. (2021). *Dictionary of obscured experiences.* Sydney Narrative Therapy & Dulwich Center. https://dulwichcentre.com.au/wp-content/uploads/2021/04/Dictionary-of-Obscure-Experiences-compiled-by-David-Newman.pdf

Nyirinkwaya, S. (2020). Games, activities and narrative practice: Enabling sparks to emerge in conversations with children and young people who have experienced hard times. *International Journal of Narrative Therapy and Community Work, 3,* 34–45.

Omer, H. (2004). *Non-violent resistance. A new approach to violent and self-destructive children.* Cambridge: Cambridge University Press.

Parker, P. (2019). *The art of gathering: How we meet and why it matters.* London: Penguin Books Ltd.

Pearce, W. (1989). *Communication and the human condition.* Carbondale, IL: Southern Illinois University Press.

Pearce, W., & Cronen, V. (1980). *Communication, action and meaning. The creation of social realities.* Westport, CT: Praeger.

Pederson, L. (2015). Sharing sadness and finding small pieces of justice: Acts of resistance and acts of reclaiming in working with women who've been subjected to abuse. *International Journal of Narrative Therapy and Community Work, 3,* 1–12.

Perry, B. (2006). Applying principles of neurodevelopment to clinical work with maltreated and traumatized children: The neurosequential model of therapeutics. In N.B. Webb (Ed.), *Working with traumatized youth in child welfare* (pp. 27–52). New York: The Guilford Press.

Perry, B., & Szalavitz, M. (2017). *The boy who was raised as a dog, 3rd Edition: And other stories from a child psychiatrist's notebook: What traumatized children can teach us about loss, love, and healing.* New York: Basic Books.

Portnoy, S., Girling, I., & Fredman, G. (2015). Supporting young people living with cancer to tell stories in ways that make them stronger: The Beads of Life approach. *Clinical Child Psychology and Psychiatry, 21,* 255–267.

Prilleltensky, I., & Prilleltensky, O. (2021). *How people matter: Why it affects health, happiness, love, work, and society.* New York: Cambridge University Press.

Ramaekers, S., & Suissa, J. (2012). *The claims of parenting: Reasons, responsibility and society.* London, New York, Dordrecht, Heidelberg: Springer.

Redstone, A. (2004). Researching people's experience of narrative therapy: Acknowledging the contribution of the 'Client' to what works in counselling conversations. *The International Journal of Narrative Therapy and Community Work*, *2*, 57–62.

Reynolds, V. (2011). Resisting burnout with justice-doing. *The International Journal of Narrative Therapy and Community Work*, *4*, 27–45.

Reynolds, V. (2012). An ethical stance for justice-doing in community work and therapy. *Journal of Systemic Therapies*, *31*, 18–33.

Reynolds, V. (2020). Trauma and resistance: 'Hang time' and other innovative responses to oppression, violence and suffering. *Journal of Family Therapy*, *42*(3), 347–364.

Richardson, C., & Wade, A. (2008). 'Taking Resistance Seriously: A Response-Based Approach to Social Work in Cases of Violence Against Indiginous Woman. In S. Strega & J.Carrière (Eds.), *Walking this talk together: Anti-racist and anti-oppressive child welfare practice*. Winnipeg: Fernwood Publishing.

Richardson, M., Peacock, F. Brown, G., Fuller, T., Smart, T., & Williams, J. (2016). *Fostering good relationships: Partnership work in therapy with looked after and adopted children*. London: Karnac.

Rimé, B. (2009). Emotion elicits the social sharing of emotion: Theory and empirical review. *Emotion Review*, *1*, 60–85. doi: 10.1177/1754073908097189

Rimé, B., Finkenauer, C., Luminet, O; Zech, E. and Philippot, P. (1998). Social sharing of emotion: New evidence and new questions. *European Review of Social Psychology*, *9*, 145–189.

Rimé, B., Herbette, G., & Corsini, S. (2004). The social sharing of emotion: Illusory and real benefits of talking about emotional experiences. In I. Nyklicek, L.R. Temoshok, & A.J.J.M. Vingerhoets, (Eds.), *Emotional Expression and Health: Advances in theory, assessment and clinical applications*. Hove and New York: Brunner-Routledge.

Rober, P. (1999). Reflections on ways to create a safe therapeutic culture for children in family therapy. *Family Process*, *37*, 201–213.

Rober, P. (2002). Some hypotheses about hesitations and their nonverbal expressions in family therapy session. *Journal of Family Therapy*, *24*, 187–204.

Rober, P. (2014). Het kind betrekken in de gezinstherapeutische sessie. In A. Savenije, M.J. van Lawick, & E. Reijmers (Red.), *Handboek systeemtherapie* (pp. 523–534). Utrecht: De Tijdstroom.

Rober, P. (2017). *In therapy together: Family therapy as a dialogue*. London: Palgrave Macmillan.

Rober, P., Van Esbeek, D., & Elliot, R. (2006). Talking about violence: A micro-analysis of narrative processes in a family therapy session. *Journal of Marital and Family Therapy*, *32*(3), 313–180.

Rober, P., Van Tricht, K., & Sundet, R. (2021). 'One step up, but not there yet': Using client feedback to optimise the therapeutic alliance in family therapy. *Journal of Family Therapy*, *43*, 46–63.

Rucinska, Z., & Reijmers, E. (2014). Between philosophy and therapy: Understanding systemic play through embodied and enactive cognition. *Interaction*, *6*, 37–52.

Rucińska, Z., Gallagher, S., & Fondelli, T. (2021). Embodied imagination & metaphor use in autism spectrum disorder. *Healthcare*, *9*(9), 200. https://doi.org/10.3390/healthcare9020200

Ruesch, J., & Bateson, G. (1951). *Communication, the social matrix of psychiatry*. New York: W. W. Norton & Company.

Rutter, M. (1999). Resilience concepts and findings: Implications for family therapy. *Journal of Family Therapy*, *21*, 119–144.

Sarawak Museum (2010). *Journal of Borneo international beads conference 2010*. Kuching: Crafthub Sdn. BhD.

Semin, G., & Gergen, K. (1990). *Everyday understanding: Social and scientific implications*. London: Sage.

Sen, S. (2018). *Reclaim your life*. Chennai: Westland.

Sermijn, J. (2020). How symbolic witnesses can help counter dominant Stories and enrich communities of concern. In S.Mc. Namee, M. Gergen, C. Camargo-Borges, & Rasera (Eds.), *The sage handbook of social constructionist* (p. 151–159). SAGE Publishing Ltd.

Sermijn, J., & Loots, G. (2015). The cocreation of crazy patchworks: Becoming rhizomatic in systemic therapy. *Family Process*, *54*, 533–544.

Sheinberg, M. (2014). Thinking and working relationally: Interviewing and constructing hypotheses to create compassionate understanding. *Family Process, 53*(4), 618–639.

Sheinberg, M., & Fraenkel, P. (2001). *The relational trauma of incest: A family based approach to treatment*. New York: Guilford Press.

Sheinberg, M., & True, F. (2008). Treating family relational trauma: A recursive process using a decision dialogue. *Family Process*, *47*(2), 173–195.

Shotter, J. (2010). *Social construction on the edge. 'With-ness'-thinking and embodiment*. Ohio: Taos Publications.

Smith, C., & Nylund, D. (1997). *Narrative therapies with children and adolescents*. New York, London: The Guilford Press.

Splingaer, G. (2020). Solvej en de draak. Gezinstherapeutisch werken met complex trauma. *Systeemtherapie*, *32*, 9–24.

Stead, H. (2021). Rites the passage for carelevers. *Journal of Family Therapy*, *43*(3), 445–457.

Stern,S., Doolan,M., Staples,E., Szmukler, L., & Eisler, I. (1999). Disruption and reconstruction: Narrative insights into the experience of family members caring for a relative diagnosed with serious mental illness. *Family Process*, *38*(3), 353–369.

Sykes, J. (2011). Negotiating stigma: Understanding mothers' response to accusations of child neglect. *Children and Youth Services Review*, *33*, 448–456.

Syrstad, E., & Ness, O. (2021). "It is not just about doing or saying the right things": Working systemically with parents whose children are placed in public care. *Journal of Family Therapy*, *43*, 458–468.

Tarren-Sweeney, M. (2021). A narrative review of mental and relational health interventions for children in family-based out-of-home care. *Journal of Family Therapy*, *43*(3), 376–391.

Tarren-Sweeney, M., & Vetere, A. (2014). *Mental health services for vulnerable children and young people: Supporting children who are, or have been, in foster care*. Oxford: Routledge.

Todes, S. (2001). *Body and world*. Cambridge, MA: The MIT Press.

Tomm, K. (1987). Interventive interviewing: Part II. Reflexive questioning as a means to enable self-healing. *Family Process*, *26*(1), 3–13.

Tomm, K. (1988). Interventive interviewing: Part III. Intending to ask lineal, circular, strategic, or reflexive questions? *Family Process*, *27*(1), 1–15.

Thys, K., & Huybrechts, A. (2021). Non-violent resistance-based interventions in residential care with teenage: Finding new ways. *Context*, *175*, 9–11.

Ungar, M. (2005). A thicker description for resilience. *The International Journal of Narrative Thrapy and Community Work, 3*, 89–96.

Valsiner, J. (2000). *Culture and human development.* London: Sage.

Van Daele, M. (2014). Settingwisseling. In A. Savenije, M.J. van Lawick, & E.T.M. Reijmers (Red.), *Handboek Systeemtherapie* (pp. 605–615, hoofdstuk 44). Utrecht: De Tijdstroom.

Van den Berge, L. (2013). Parenting support and the role of society in parental self-understanding: Furedi's paranoid parenting revisited. *Journal of Philosophy of Education, 47*(3), 391–406.

Van den Berge, L. (2017). Schrijven is luisteren, een gesprek met David Van Reybrouck. In S. Vermeire & J. Sermijn (Eds.), *Wegen naar her-binding. Narratieve, collaboratieve en dialogische praktijken*, 278–286. Antwerpen: Interactie-Academie.

Van der Kolk, B. (2014). *Body keeps the score. Brain, mind, and body in the healing of trauma.* London: Penguin Books Ltd.

Van der Pas, A. (2004). *A serious case of neglect: The parental experience of child rearing.* Delft: Eburon Academic Publishers.

van Gennep (1960). *The rites of passage.* Chicago: University of Chicago Press.

van Hennik, R. (2021). Practice based evidence based practice, part II: Navigating complexity and validity from within. *Journal of Family Therapy, 42*, 27–45.

Van Parys, H., Smith, J.A., & Rober, P. (2014). Growing up with a mother with depression: An interpretative phenomenological analysis. *The Qualitative Report, 19*(15), 1–18.

Van Riet, J. (2020). 'Ik ben zo blij dat ik naar het leven teruggekeerd ben'. [Interview David Grossman.] *De Standaard,* 24 oktober 2020.

Varela, F. (1999). *Ethical know-how, action, wisdom, and cognition.* Stanford: Stanford University Press.

Verhofstadt-Deneve, L., Van Geert, P., & Vyt, A. (2003). *Handboek voor ontwikkelingspsychologie. Grondslagen en theorieën.* Houten: Bohn Stafleu Van Loghum.

Vermeire, S. (2007). Verhalen brouwen bij 'ongelofelijke' problemen. Een speelse methode om het ondenkbare denkbaar en het ondoenbare doenbaar te maken. *Systeemtheoretisch Bulletin, 25*(2), 205–220.

Vermeire, S. (2011). Narratieve wegen tot herstel. Biografisch interviewen van jongeren met deviant of delinquent gedrag. *Systeemtheoretisch Bulletin, 29*, 123–142.

Vermeire, S.(2015). *Xander, Geplaatst!* Antwerpen: Interactie-Academie vzw.

Vermeire, S. (2017). What if... I were king? Playing with roles and positions in narrative conversations with children who experienced trauma. *The International Journal of Narrative Therapy and Community Work, 4*, 6–17.

Vermeire, S. (2019). Genograms at the kitchen table: Tea, teabags and sugar cubes: Playfully working with genograms and timelines with families in transition. *Context, 161*, 6–10.

Vermeire, S. (2020). No child is an island: From attachment narratives towards a sense of belonging. *Journal of Family Therapy, 42*, 1–17.

Vermeire, S., & Sermijn, J. (2017). *Wegen naar her-verbinding. Narratieve, collaboratieve en dialogische praktijken.* Antwerpen: Interactie-Academie vzw.

Vermeire, S., & Van den Berge, L. (2021). Widening the screen: Playful responses to the challenges in online therapy with children, families and their network. *Journal of Family Therapy, 43*, 329–345.

Vermeire, S., & van Hennik, R. (2017). Narratieve brieven en documenten: een rijkdom aan mogelijkheden. In S. Vermeire & J. Sermijn (Eds.), *Wegen naar her-binding. Narratieve, collaboratieve en dialogische praktijken* (pp. 26–39). Antwerpen: Interactie-Academie.

Vermeire, S., Beckers, W., Faes, M., & Decraemer, K. (2018). *What's the problem? Children/adults turn problems inside out.* Antwerpen: Interactie-Academie vzw.

Vermeire, S., Van den Berge, L., & Van Reybrouck, T. (2022). Parents in the grip of parental guilt. Narrative paths to rediscover a future. In R. Yilmaz & B. Koç (Eds.), *Narrative theory and therapy in the post-truth era.* IGI Global (in press).

Vetere, A., & Dowling, E. (eds.) (2005). *Narrative therapies with children and their families.* London/New York: Routledge.

Vygotsky, L.S. (1986). *Thought and language* (A. Kozulin, Trans.). Cambridge, MA: MIT Press.

Wade, A. (1997). Despair, resistance, hope: Response-based therapy with victims of violence. In C. Flaskas, I. McCarthy, & J. Sheenan (Eds.), *Hope and despair in narrative and family therapy* (pp. 62–74). New York: Routledge.

Walsh, F. (2003). Family resilience: A framework for clinical practice. *Family Process, 42,* 1–17.

Walsh, F. (2006). *Strenghtening family resilience.* New York: The Guilford Press.

Walsh, F. (2007). Traumatic loss and major disasters: Strenghtening family and community resilience. *Family Process, 46*(2), 207–227.

Wasserman, I., & Fisher-Yoshida, B. (2017). *Communicating possibilities: A brief introduction to the coordinated management of meaning (CMM).* Chagrin Falls Ohio, OH: TAOS Institute Publications.

Watzlawick, P., Beavin Bavelas, J., & Jackson, D. (1967). *Pragmatics of communication. Patterns, pathologies, and paradoxes.* New York: W.W. Norton & Co.

Weingarten, K. (1998). The small and the ordinary: The daily practice of a postmodern narrative therapy. *Family Process, 37,* 3–16.

Weingarten, K. (2003). *Common shock. Witnessing violence every day.* New York: Dutton, Penguin Group.

Weingarten, K. (2010). Reasonable hope: Construct, clinical applications, and supports. *Family Process, 49,* 5–25.

Werner, E.E. (2005). Resilience and recovery. Findings from the Kaiuai longitudinal study. *Focal Point: Research, Policy, and Practice in Children's Mental Health, 19*(1), 11–14.

Werner, E.E., & Smith, R.S. (2001). *Journeys from childhood to midlife: Risk, resilience and recovery.* Ithaca: Cornell University Press.

White, M. (1995). *Re-authoring lives: Interviews and essays.* Adelaide: Dulwich Centre Publications.

White, M. (2002). Addressing personal failure. *International Journal of Narrative Therapy and Community Work, 3,* 33–76.

White, M. (2004). *Narrative practice and exotic lives: Resurrecting diversity in everyday life.* Adelaide: Dulwich Centre Publications.

White, M. (2006a). Children, trauma and subordinate storyline development. In D. Denborough (Ed.), *Trauma: Narrative responses to traumatic experience* (pp. 143–165). Adelaide: Dulwich Centre Publications.

White, M. (2006b). Working with children who have experienced significant trauma. In M. White & A. Morgan (Eds.), *Narrative therapy with children and their families* (pp. 85–97). Adelaide: Dulwich Centre Publications.

White, M. (2006c). Working with people who are suffering the consequences of multiple trauma: A narrative perspective. In D. Denborough (Ed.), *Trauma: Narrative responses to traumatic experience* (pp. 25–85). Adelaide: Dulwich Centre Publications.

White, M. (2007). *Maps of narrative practice*. New York: W. W. Norton.

White, M. (2011). *Narrative practice: Continuing the conversations* (D. Denborough, Ed.). New York: W.W. Norton.

White, M., & Epston, D. (1990). *Narrative means to therapeutic ends*. New York: W.W. Norton.

Wilson, J. (1998). *Child-focused practice. A collaborative approach to children*. London: Karnac Books.

Wilson, J. (2005). Engaging children and young people. In A. Vetere & E. Dowling (Eds), *Narrative therapy with children and their families* (pp. 90–106). London: Routledge.

Wilson, J. (2007). *The performance of practice*. London: Karnac Books.

Wilson, J. (2021). Boxed in? Commentary on widening the screen: Playful responses to challenges in online therapy with children and families. *Journal of Family Therapy, 43*, 346–350.

Wittgenstein, L. (1953). *The philosophical investigations*. Oxford: Blackwell.

Young, K. (2011). When all the time you have is now: Re-visiting practices and narrative therapy in a walk-in clinic. In J. Duvall & L. Béres (Eds), *Innovations in narrative therapy. Connecting practice, training, and research*. New York: W.W. Norton & Company.

Yuen, A. (2007). Discovering children's responses to trauma: A response-based narrative practice. *International Journal of Narrative Therapy and Community Work, 4*, 3–18.

Yuen, A. (2009). Less pain, more gain: Explorations of responses versus effects when working with the consequences of trauma. *An E-Journal of Narrative Practice, 1*, 6–16.

Index

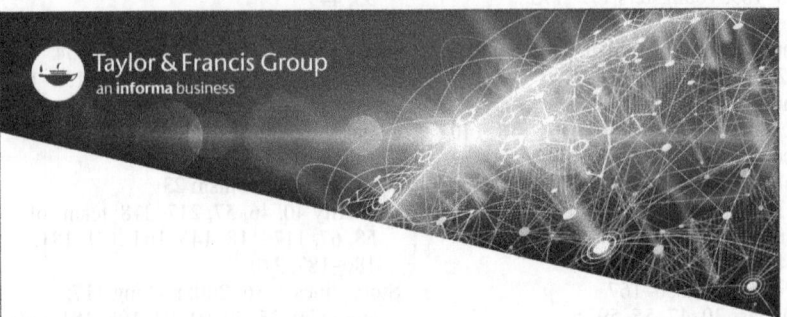
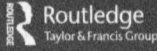
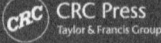